ESSENTIAL
MEDICAL TERMINOLOGY

FOURTH EDITION

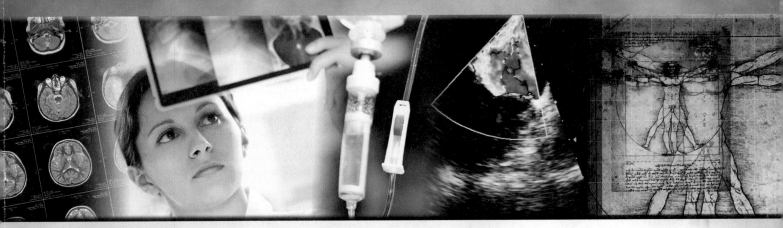

Peggy Stanfield, MS, RD/LD, CNS
Dietetic Resources
Twin Falls, Idaho

Y.H. Hui, PhD
Science Technology System
West Sacramento, California

Nanna Cross, PhD, RD/LD
Cross & Associates
Chicago, Illinois

JONES & BARTLETT
LEARNING

World Headquarters
Jones & Bartlett Learning
5 Wall Street
Burlington, MA 01803
978-443-5000
info@jblearning.com
www.jblearning.com

Jones & Bartlett Learning books and products are available through most bookstores and online booksellers. To contact Jones & Bartlett Learning directly, call 800-832-0034, fax 978-443-8000, or visit our website, www.jblearning.com.

Substantial discounts on bulk quantities of Jones & Bartlett Learning publications are available to corporations, professional associations, and other qualified organizations. For details and specific discount information, contact the special sales department at Jones & Bartlett Learning via the above contact information or send an email to specialsales@jblearning.com.

Production Credits

Chief Executive Officer: Ty Field
President: James Homer
Chief Product Officer: Eduardo Moura
Executive Publisher: William Brottmiller
Editorial Assistant: Sean Fabery
Production Editor: Jessica Steele Newfell
Marketing Manager: Grace Richards
VP, Manufacturing and Inventory Control: Therese Connell
Composition: Laserwords Private Limited, Chennai, India
Cover and Interior Design: Kristin E. Parker

Rights & Photo Research Coordinator: Amy Rathburn
Cover and Title Page Images: (MRI scan) © Kondor83/ShutterStock, Inc.; (female with x-ray) © Stokkete/ShutterStock, Inc.; (IV drip) © sfam_photo/ShutterStock, Inc.; (ultrasound machine) © sfam_photo/ShutterStock, Inc.; (Vitruvian Man) © juatasc/ShutterStock, Inc.; (EKG) © nulinukas/ShutterStock, Inc.; (light) sfam_photo/ShutterStock, Inc.
Printing and Binding: Courier Companies
Cover Printing: Courier Companies

To order this product, use ISBN: 978-1-284-03878-1

Library of Congress Cataloging-in-Publication Data
Stanfield, Peggy, author.
  Essential medical terminology / Peggy Stanfield, Y.H. Hui, Nanna Cross. — Fourth edition.
    p. ; cm.
  Includes bibliographical references and index.
  ISBN 978-1-284-02228-5 (pbk. : alk. paper)
  I. Hui, Y. H. (Yiu H.), author. II. Cross, Nanna, author. III. Title.
  [DNLM: 1. Terminology as Topic—Problems and Exercises. W 15]
  R123
  610.1'4—dc23
                    2013019527

6048

Printed in the United States of America
17 16 15 14 13   10 9 8 7 6 5 4 3 2 1

Brief Contents

UNIT I   Word Parts and Medical Terminology   1

CHAPTER 1   Word Pronunciations   3

CHAPTER 2   Word Parts and Word Building Rules   5

UNIT II   Root Words, Medical Terminology, and Patient Care   21

CHAPTER 3   Bacteria, Color, and Some Medical Terms   23

CHAPTER 4   Body Openings and Plural Endings   33

CHAPTER 5   Numbers, Positions, and Directions   41

CHAPTER 6   Medical and Health Professions   57

UNIT III   Abbreviations   69

CHAPTER 7   Medical Abbreviations   71

CHAPTER 8   Diagnostic and Laboratory Abbreviations   81

UNIT IV   Review   91

CHAPTER 9   Review of Word Parts from Units I, II, and III   93

UNIT V — Medical Terminology and Body Systems   109

CHAPTER 10 Body Organs and Parts   111

CHAPTER 11 Integumentary System   119

CHAPTER 12 Digestive System   137

CHAPTER 13 Respiratory System   159

CHAPTER 14 Cardiovascular System   177

CHAPTER 15 Nervous System   205

CHAPTER 16 Genitourinary System   225

CHAPTER 17 Musculoskeletal System   249

CHAPTER 18 Eyes and Ears   275

CHAPTER 19 Endocrine System   293

CHAPTER 20 Cancer Medicine   307

Contents

Preface to *Fourth Edition*   xi
Preface to *First Edition*   xiii
Acknowledgments   xv
How to Use This Book   xvii

UNIT I	Medical Terminology 1

CHAPTER 1   **Word Pronunciations**   3

CHAPTER 2   **Word Parts and Word Building Rules**   5
Objectives   5
Lesson One: Materials to Be Learned   5
Parts of a Medical Term   5
Listing of Word Parts   7
Prefixes, Word Roots with Combining Forms, and Suffixes   8
Lesson Two: Progress Check Part A   15
Lesson Two: Progress Check Part B   18

UNIT II	Root Words, Medical Terminology, and Patient Care 21

CHAPTER 3   **Bacteria, Color, and Some Medical Terms**   23
Objectives   23
Lesson One: Materials to Be Learned   24
Root Words for Bacteria   24
Prefixes for Color   24
Commonly Used Prefixes   25
Lesson Two: Progress Check   29

CHAPTER 4   **Body Openings and Plural Endings**   33
Objectives   33
Lesson One: Materials to Be Learned   34
Body Openings   34
Plural Endings   35
Lesson Two: Progress Check   37

CHAPTER 5   **Numbers, Positions, and Directions**   41
Objectives   41
Lesson One: Materials to Be Learned   41
Part 1: Prefixes for Numbers   41
Part 2: Prefixes for Positions and Directions   43
Part 3: Terms for Directions and Positions   45
Units of Weight and Measurement   47
  Weights and Measures   50
  Common Weights and Measures   51
Frequently Used Symbols   52
Lesson Two: Progress Check   53

CHAPTER 6   **Medical and Health Professions**   57
Objectives   57
Lesson One: Materials to Be Learned   58
Scientific Studies   58
Specialties and Specialists   59
  Physicians and Medical Specialties   59
  Other Health Professions   61
  Additional Professions   64
Lesson Two: Progress Check   65

UNIT III   **Abbreviations**   69

CHAPTER 7   **Medical Abbreviations**   71
Objectives   71
Lesson One: Materials to Be Learned   71
Abbreviations for Services or Units in a Healthcare Facility   72
Abbreviations for Frequencies   73
Abbreviations for Units of Measure   73
Abbreviations for Means of Adminstering Substances into the Body   74
Abbreviations for Diet Orders   75
Abbreviations for Activity and Toiletry   76
Abbreviations for Laboratory Tests, X-Ray Studies, and Pulmonary Function   76
Abbreviations for Miscellaneous Terms   77
Lesson Two: Progress Check   79

CHAPTER 8   **Diagnostic and Laboratory Abbreviations**   81
Objectives   81
Lesson One: Materials to Be Learned   82
Diagnostic Abbreviations   82
Laboratory Abbreviations   84
A List of Common Diagnostic and Laboratory Abbreviations   84
Lesson Two: Progress Check   87

UNIT IV — Review 91

CHAPTER 9 **Review of Word Parts from Units I, II, and III** 93
Objectives 93
Lesson One: Materials to Be Learned 94
Review A: Suffixes 94
Review B: Prefixes 95
Review C: Root Words for Body Parts 97
Review D: Descriptive Word Elements 99
Review E: Additional Medical Terms 100
Lesson Two: Progress Check 104

UNIT V — Medical Terminology and Body Systems 109

CHAPTER 10 **Body Organs and Parts** 111
Objectives 111
Lesson One: Materials to Be Learned 112
Structural Units of the Body 112
Body Cavities and Planes 114
Metabolism and Homeostasis 116
Lesson Two: Progress Check 117

CHAPTER 11 **Integumentary System** 119
Objectives 119
Lesson One: Materials to Be Learned 123
Parts of the Skin 123
Functions of the Skin 124
Surgical Processes and the Skin 125
Skin Growths 125
Biologic Agents and Skin Infection 126
Allergy and the Skin 128
Skin Disorders from Systemic Diseases 128
Skin Tests 129
Vocabulary Terms and the Skin 129
Lesson Two: Progress Check 132

CHAPTER 12 **Digestive System** 137
Objectives 137
Lesson One: Materials to Be Learned 141
Major and Accessory Organs 145
Clinical Disorders 146
Surgery 148
Medical Tests 149
Abdominal Reference Terms 151
Digestive Processes 151
Miscellaneous Terms 153
Lesson Two: Progress Check 154

CHAPTER 13 **Respiratory System** 159
Objectives 159
Lesson One: Materials to Be Learned 162

The Respiratory System   162
Respiratory Body Parts   164
Common Disorders of the Respiratory System   165
Diagnostic, Surgical, and Medical Procedures and General Terms   168
Lesson Two: Progress Check   172

CHAPTER 14   **Cardiovascular System**   177
Objectives   177
Lesson One: Materials to Be Learned   183
The Cardiovascular System   183
  Parts of the Heart   183
  The Circulatory System   186
  Types of Blood Vessels   189
  Blood Components   189
  Blood Pressure   190
  Clinical Disorders Affecting the Cardiovascular System   191
  Surgery, Lab, and Medical Tests   193
  Abbreviations   195
Lesson Two: Materials to Be Learned   196
The Lymphatic System   197
  Components of the System   197
  Parts and Functions of the System   197
  Pathologic Conditions of the Lymph System   198
Lesson Three: Progress Check   199

CHAPTER 15   **Nervous System**   205
Objectives   205
Lesson One: Materials to Be Learned   210
Central Nervous System   210
Autonomic Nervous System (Peripheral Nervous System)   210
Clinical Disorders   212
Terms Used in Diagnosis and Surgery   215
Psychiatric Terms   217
Special Terms   218
Lesson Two: Progress Check   220

CHAPTER 16   **Genitourinary System**   225
Objectives   225
Urinary System   226
Reproductive System   227
  Male Reproductive System   227
  Female Reproductive System   230
Lesson One: Materials to Be Learned   231
Urinary System   231
  Organs and Structures   231
  Clinical Conditions and Procedures   232
  Diagnostic Medical Terms   233
Reproductive System   235
  Male Organs   235
  Female Organs   237
  Male Clinical Conditions   238

Female Clinical Conditions 238
Male and Female Conditions 240
Pregnancy and Birth 241
Lesson Two: Progress Check 244

CHAPTER 17 **Musculoskeletal System** 249
Objectives 249
Lesson One: Materials to Be Learned 255
The Skeletal System 257
Division 257
Body Bones 258
Head Bones 259
Joints and Accessory Parts 259
Bone Processes, Depressions, and Holes 260
The Muscular System 261
Muscles of the Body 263
Motion 264
Physiologic Status of Muscles 264
Injuries 265
Clinical Disorders 265
Medical Management 268
Abbreviations (Musculoskeletal System) 269
Lesson Two: Progress Check 270

CHAPTER 18 **Eyes and Ears** 275
Objectives 275
Lesson One: Materials to Be Learned 279
Eyes 279
Structure of the Eye 279
Eye Disorders 280
Eye Diagnosis and Surgery 282
Common Medical Eye Terms 283
Ears 284
Structure of the Ear 284
Ear Disorders 285
Ear Surgery 286
Common Medical Ear Terms 286
Lesson Two: Progress Check 288

CHAPTER 19 **Endocrine System** 293
Objectives 293
Lesson One: Materials to Be Learned 296
Classification and Function of the Endocrine System 296
Disorders of the Endocrine System 298
Miscellaneous Terms 302
Lesson Two: Progress Check 303

CHAPTER 20 **Cancer Medicine** 307
Objectives 307
Lesson One: Materials to Be Learned 309
Medical Terms in Cancer Medicine 309

Cancer: Classification, Terminology, and Types   309
  Basic Classification   309
  Cancer with Specific Names   312
Screening and Early Detection   312
Medical Terms Related to the Diagnosis of Cancer   313
Special Cancer Diagnostic Tests   314
Methods of Cancer Treatment   315
  Cancer Treatment   315
Medical Terms Related to the Treatment of Cancer   316
Different Surgical Procedures Used to Treat Cancer   318
Breast Cancer and Medical Illustrations   318
Medical Terms Related to Types of Cancer   320
Lesson Two: Progress Check   322

APPENDIX A   **Answer Keys**   325
APPENDIX B   **Bibliography**   359
Index   361

Preface to the *Fourth Edition*

As we move forward into the advancing fields of medicine and health practices we find an ever increasing need to make changes and add new material. We asked our students for feedback, their instructors for suggestions, and our reviewers for contributions in expertise and experience. We received many valuable suggestions and comments and have included much constructive input wherever space permits. We hope that the resulting changes from us and from them will continue to improve the contents of *Essential Medical Terminology, Fourth Edition* and facilitate your effort in learning medical terminology. This revision is divided into two categories: changes in the contents of the *Third Edition* and the addition of new didactic tools, as explained here.

The original contents of the *Third Edition* have been revised extensively as follows:

- Objectives are added to the chapters.
- New terms are added throughout the text.
- Selected old terms in text are replaced with new ones.
- New test questions are added throughout the text.
- The bibliography in Appendix B is replaced with a new one.
- Special corrections or replacements are made in Chapters 15, 16, and 20.
- Standard minor changes are made throughout the whole text wherever the need arises.

We have added new didactic materials in specially designed enclosures to catch the attention of students and satisfy their curiosity. Your responsibility to learn such materials is at the discretion of your instructor and your own personal interest. They include the following:

- Alerts to commonly confusing medical terms
- The connection between drugs and medical terms
- Types of professions available in the allied health field
- New full-color photographs and illustrations showing common clinical disorders and associated medical terms appearing in the text

Several electronic aids are included. Access to a companion website featuring an audio glossary is included with each access code. Resources also have been prepared for instructors.

We hope you will notice that this is a full-color book to brighten your learning spirit and increase your attention.

Thank you so much for your continued support and use of the book. Please keep sending us your suggestions for improvement. We will strive to accommodate your wishes.

Preface to the *First Edition*

Essential Medical Terminology is a brief, user-friendly text designed to aid students in mastering the medical vocabulary and terms they will encounter in allied health, nursing, and medical careers. The terms have been selected on the basis of their utility, practical value, and application to the real world of the healthcare work environment.

The intended audience includes students in nursing, nursing assistants/aides, vocational/practical nurses, medical secretaries, medical technologists, medical librarians, medical assistants, physician's assistants, and other persons in the allied health and paramedical fields. This text is designed for use in one-semester or two-semester course, as it provides students with the basic principles of medical terminology and teaches vocabulary by applying terms in practice examples.

Although many instructors have expressed satisfaction with our 1989 text, *Medical Terminology: Principles and Practices,* others prefer a smaller text because their students need only a general knowledge of medical terminology. Therefore, we were ready when the publishers expressed an interest in a more compact text. To accomplish this goal, we made a careful selection of the most essential terms, exercises, illustrations, and other instructional materials that are of maximum benefit to those students required to take a general survey course of medical terminology.

After much hard work, we have succeeded in producing a text that has fewer than 400 pages. This condensed edition has many unique features that distinguish it from other medical terminology texts:

1. The selection of medical terms is unique, and, although some terms are found in other texts, many are not.
2. Half of the text is devoted to practice exercises or self-instructional modules.
3. The amount of descriptive text is minimal, allowing students to concentrate on learning the key terms.
4. Although the frame format is common in some texts, we have not adopted that didactic mode. Rather, we present medical terminology as it applies to the major body systems.
5. Students will find that learning by way of the major body systems is a meaningful and unifying method of mastering medical terminology and solidifying previously learned concepts of anatomy and physiology.

The text is organized into five units:

- Unit I   Word Parts and Medical Terminology (Chapters 1–2)
- Unit II   Root Words, Medical Terminology, and Patient Care (Chapters 3–6)
- Unit III   Abbreviations (Chapters 7–8)
- Unit IV   Review (Chapter 9)
- Unit V   Medical Terminology and Body Systems (Chapters 10–20)

With the exception of Chapter 1, all chapters contain two components: Lesson One: Materials to Be Learned and Lesson Two: Progress Check.

This unique text is accompanied by both traditional and modern supplementary teaching materials. The instructor's manual provides a spectrum of information: clinical case histories, practice tests, and student activities. It serves two important objectives: a wide selection of teaching materials and a reduction in class preparation time. For example, by using clinical case histories to supplement a complex topic in the classroom, the instructor can usually elicit enthusiastic participation and enliven classroom presentations. We also include full-color illustrations of human anatomy in this text, which detail the major body systems, special senses, and skin. These figures provide an anatomic reference for all of the medical terms in the text.

Our intention was to create a text that would serve the needs of both instructor and student. We strove to create a text that is both concise and thorough, thematically unified, easy to read, beautifully illustrated, and fully supplemented with supporting material to assure mastery of the material. We hope that both instructor and student will find *Essential Medical Terminology* a satisfactory and rewarding experience in teaching and learning medical terminology.

Acknowledgments

We acknowledge the invaluable assistance and advice provided by the editorial team at Jones & Bartlett Learning, who have helped move this edition from manuscript to publication. Thanks also to the production staff whose dedicated work and professionalism are evident in the quality of their work. You are the best judge.

We sincerely thank our reviewers who offered many valuable suggestions. Your comments were very helpful, and we incorporated as many of them into this edition as allocated page space would permit.

We do want to extend our appreciation to many students and their instructors for continued use of *Essential Medical Terminology* through the first three editions. We have tried to provide you with the updates and new information that you have asked for. We hope our mutual relationships continue with this *Fourth Edition* and beyond.

We also thank Mr. James Keating of Watsonville, Oregon. As the original acquisition editor of the *First Edition*, he gave us an unusual opportunity to educate many students for more than 25 years. We are indebted to him and his vision.

How to Use This Book

Essential Medical Terminology, Fourth Edition fits all types of medical terminology courses. It can be the primary text in either a one- or two-semester course.

One instructional mode other than formal classroom lecturing is as follows. The instructor serves as a supervisor and assigns materials in the text for self-study. The instructor may or may not enforce the following: class meetings between instructor and students, supervised or unsupervised tests, and preparation of tests with questions similar to those in this text.

Essential Medical Terminology offers a great deal of flexibility to instructors. Our recommendation is to progress through the table of contents as written. In any learning process, studying the information progressively provides sequence of thought and ensures that one does not overlook critical information.

The student, especially one studying independently of a formal class lecture, should read each chapter thoroughly and complete all exercises.

GENERAL GUIDELINES

We also offer the following guidelines to both instructors and students:

1. Read the table of contents to determine the syllabus or match up the contents to a prepared syllabus.
2. After studying the basis of pronunciation, students may start with any of the remaining chapters in Units I to IV. The chapters on body systems (10–19) can be taught in any order.
3. For each chapter after Chapter 1, the study procedure is simple. Read the materials to be learned a few times and proceed with the progress check. Students may want to repeat or review chapter materials before taking a test.
4. Once a chapter is started, finish it before proceeding to the next one.
5. Complete each chapter from beginning to end. Do not begin randomly within a chapter.
6. When students begin Unit V, they will find that each chapter contains an overview of a body system. Each body system can be studied in more depth with an anatomy and physiology text.

7. We encourage students to develop their own methods of memorizing unfamiliar words. Word associations are useful. Flashcards are a useful adjunct to study. Studying in pairs also is helpful for most students.

8. Students should review completed materials as often as possible to refresh their memories.

9. All of the answers to the Progress Checks are provided in Appendix A. Most instructors prefer that students do not look at the answers until they have completed the assigned exercise.

NEW DIDACTIC TOOLS

We have added a new category of didactic tools. These tools contain information related to but not included in this text. Each tool or tidbit of information is enclosed in a specially designed box within the outer margin. You may have to study them if they are included in class assignments by the teachers, or you may peruse them because they are of personal or general interest to you. No matter how these tools are used by you, they are supplementary to your text both in terms of unique information or a moment of escape from the more structured medical terms in the text. Each tool is explored in the following subsections.

Allied Health Professions

There was a time when the doctor, nurse, and an aide or two took care of a patient. Not very much interaction occurred unless the physician called for a conference with selected individuals. Today's medical facilities are run by teams of medical personnel including doctors, nurses, aides, pharmacists, laboratory personnel, technicians, dietary personnel, and social service workers. All have important roles in patient recovery. Are you interested in pursuing a career in this field? Chapter 1 shows a list of such professions in a special box. The boxes in Chapters 10–20 give a summary of each profession. You can contribute to patient care in each field if you select a career in the health professions.

Confusing Medical Terms

Many medical terms have derived from Latin and Greek, among other European languages. Sometimes, two terms with different medical meaning may differ only in one letter in their spellings. Sometimes, two terms with different medical meanings may sound alike though their spellings are completely different. Sometimes, two terms with the same medical meanings may be spelled entirely differently. Obviously, it is not possible to explain or list all such variations in a book of this size. Samples are provided in a special box, starting in Chapter 2.

Pharmacology and Medical Terminology

Most of us are familiar with such terms as *ulcer, chemotherapy*, and *antibiotic treatments*. This text does not have a chapter on pharmacology and medical terms. Instead, we have provided boxes in Chapters 11–20 relating medical terminology to drugs and their targeted medical treatments. Although they are examples only, they provide you with some perspectives about prescription and over-the-counter drugs. The ultimate objective is for you to learn some medical terms in pharmacology.

FULL-COLOR ILLUSTRATIONS AND PHOTOGRAPHS FOR CLINICAL DISORDERS

There is an old adage: A picture is worth a thousand words. We believe it is true, so we have included in this edition new full-color illustrations and photographs showing common clinical disorders and their assorted medical terms to enhance your understanding and identification of diseases and how they may be treated.

Medical Terminology

CHAPTER 1

Word Pronunciations

The pronunciation of each medical term is governed by the following rules. Pronunciation is indicated by a simple phonetic respelling of the term and these diacritical markings:

1. The primary accent is indicated by an underlining, e.g., cerebellum (ser-e-<u>bel</u>-um).
2. The secondary accent is indicated by (´), e.g., ser´-e-<u>bel</u>-um.
3. When an unmarked vowel ends a syllable, it is long, e.g., immune (i-mun´).
4. When a syllable ends with a consonant, its unmarked vowel is short, e.g., cranial (<u>kra</u>-ne-al).

   For ease of interpretation, the phonetic spellings used in this text have no other diacritical markings. However, the following basic rules apply to all pronunciation and are listed here for ease of interpretation of medical terms.

5. An unmarked vowel ending a syllable is *long*: It is indicated by a macron (¯), as in the examples below:

   a   urease (<u>u</u>-re-ās); abate (ah-bāt)
   e   electroscope (e-<u>lek</u>-tro-scōp); lead (lēd)
   i   askaracide (as-<u>kar</u>-i-sīd); bile (bīl)
   o   ohms (ōmz); ionophere (i-on-o-phēr); hormone (hor-mōn)
   u   union (ūn-ion); ampule (am-pūl)
   oo   oophoron (oo-fōr-on)

6. A short vowel that *is* the syllable or that *ends* the syllable is indicated by a breve (˘):

   a   apophysis (ă-<u>pof</u>-i-sis)
   e   edema (ĕ-<u>dēm</u>-ah); effusion (ĕ-<u>fūs</u>-ion)
   i   immunity (ĭ-<u>mūn</u>-ĭ-te´); oxidation (oks´-sĭ-<u>da</u>-shun)
   o   otic (ŏ-tic); official (ŏ-<u>fish</u>-al)
   u   avoirdupois (av-er-dŭ-poiz)
   oo   book (book)

ALLIED HEALTH PROFESSIONS

- *Dentistry:* dental hygienists, dental assistants
- *Dietetics:* dietitians, dietetic technicians, dietetic assistants
- *Emergency medical services:* emergency medical technicians and paramedics
- *Imaging modalities:* radiologic technologists and technicians, radiation therapists
- *Medicine:* cardiovascular technologists and technicians, nuclear medicine technologists, surgical technologists, medical assistants
- *Nursing:* registered nurses, licensed practical nurses, licensed vocational nurses
- *Optometry:* dispensing opticians
- *Pharmacy:* pharmacy technicians, pharmacy aides
- *Physical therapy:* physical therapists, physical therapist assistants and aides
- *Respiratory care practitioners:* respiratory therapists
- *Veterinary medicine:* veterinary technologists and technicians, animal care and service workers
- *Miscellaneous technologists and technicians:* clinical laboratory (medical) technologists and technicians; medical, dental, and ophthalmic laboratory technicians; nursing, psychiatric, and home health aides, medical assistants

Data from Stanfield, Peggy S., Cross, Nanna, and Hui, Y.H. *Introduction to the Health Professions*, 6th ed. Burlington, MA: Jones & Bartlett Learning; 2012.

Word Parts and Word Building Rules

LESSON ONE: MATERIALS TO BE LEARNED

Parts of a Medical Term
Listings of Word Parts
Prefixes, Word Roots with Combining Forms, and Suffixes

LESSON TWO: PROGRESS CHECK PART A

Matching
Spelling and Definition
Defining Medical Word Elements
Building Medical Words

LESSON TWO: PROGRESS CHECK PART B

Matching
Spelling and Definition
Building Medical Words
Defining Medical Terms

OBJECTIVES

After completion of this chapter and the exercises, the student should be able to:

1. List the basic parts of a medical term.
2. Define the terms *word root, combining vowel, combining form, prefix,* and *suffix.*
3. State the rules for building medical terms.
4. Divide medical words into their component parts.
5. Build medical words using combining forms, prefixes, and suffixes.
6. Use multiple word roots in a compound word.

LESSON ONE	Materials to Be Learned

PARTS OF A MEDICAL TERM

Words, including medical terms, are composed of three basic parts: word roots, prefixes, and suffixes. How the parts are combined determine their meaning. Changing any part of a word changes its meaning. Spelling and pronunciation also are very important because some medical terms sound similar, and some sound exactly alike but are spelled differently and therefore have different meanings. For example, the word *phagia* (fay-jee-ah) means eating or swallowing, and the word *phasia* (fay-zee-ah) means without speech.

Examples of words that are pronounced exactly alike but spelled differently are the terms *ileum* (ill-ee-um) and *ilium* (ill-ee-um). Ileum is part of the small intestine, but ilium is part of the hipbone.

1. *Prefix:* the word or element attached to the *beginning* of a word root to modify its meaning. Not all medical words have a prefix. A prefix keeps its same meaning in every

5

term in which it is used. *When defining a medical term that has both a prefix and a suffix, define the suffix first, the prefix second, and the word root last.*

Note in the following example how the meaning of the word changes: **peri-** = prefix for around, **cardi** = root word for heart, and **-itis** = suffix for inflammation.

Term: pericarditis
Definition: inflammation around the heart (muscle)

2. *Word root:* the *meaning* or *core* part of the word. Medical terms have one or more roots. By adding prefixes and suffixes to a word root, the meaning of a word is changed. Most medical words have at least one word root, and some have several. Word roots are joined by a combining vowel. A word root will have the same meaning in every word that contains it. When a word root is joined to a suffix, or to other root words to make a compound word, it requires the use of a combining vowel.

3. *Combining vowel:* usually an o and occasionally an i, used between compound word roots or between a word root and a suffix. Combining vowels make word pronunciation easier. When a vowel is added to a root word, it is called a *combining form.* It is usually marked with a diagonal, e.g., **arthr/o**.

    Combining vowels are kept between compound words even if the second word root does begin with a vowel, e.g., gastr/oentero/logy. Compound words are two or more root words joined with a combining vowel. Compound words also may have a suffix, which is joined to the word by a combining vowel. When the suffix begins with a vowel (usually an i), the combining vowel on the root word is dropped. When the suffix begins with a consonant, the combining vowel is kept. Examples are:

    - **mening/o** (root word and combining vowel) and **-itis** (suffix). The word is spelled *meningitis,* dropping the o. The term means inflammation of the meninges.
    - **hem/o** (root word and combining vowel) and **-rrhage** (suffix). The word is spelled *hemorrhage,* keeping the o. The term means escape of blood from the vessels. If the suffix and the combining vowel are the same vowel, the duplicate vowel is also dropped, e.g., **cardi/o** (root word for heart) and **-itis** (suffix). The word is spelled *carditis* (only one i is used). It means inflammation of the heart (muscle).

4. *Suffix:* the word part or element attached to the end of a root word to modify its meaning. Not all root words have a suffix, and some words have two suffixes, e.g., **psych/o/log/ic/al**. When a medical term has two suffixes (as *psychological* does), they are joined and considered one suffix, that is, **-ic/al** = **-ical**. Some suffixes are attached to a prefix only, e.g., **dia-** (prefix) and **-rrhea** (suffix), or *diarrhea.* When they form a complete word, as in this example (diarrhea), the resulting word may be considered a root word, depending on its use.

The literal meaning of a word may be shortened through usage, by common consent, or when understood without being expressed.

Please note the following two premises when studying:

1. Many columns carry the heading "word root." This is taken to mean that items under this column can be the word root itself or a word root with /o, that is, a combining form. This practice is to avoid excess repetition of the term "combining form" throughout the book.

CONFUSING MEDICAL TERMINOLOGY

-stasis Versus -stalsis

-stasis = control, stop, e.g., hemostasis (he-mo-<u>sta</u>-sis) refers to the interruption of blood flow or arrest of bleeding by the physiological properties of vasoconstriction and coagulation or by surgical means

-stalsis = contraction, e.g., peristalsis (per-uh-<u>stawl</u>-sis) refers to successive waves of involuntary contraction passing along the walls of a hollow muscular structure (as the esophagus or intestine) and forcing the contents onward

2. About 3–5% of the medical terms in this book that have not been presented in the lessons are included in the practice exercises. This is designed to:

- Encourage students to use the dictionary because the practice exercises are all open-book.
- Provide students an opportunity to practice dividing those words into their respective components according to the rules in the book.
- Give the instructor a choice whether to include these additional words.

Some textbooks on medical terminology use the same technique; others do not. Feedback from students and instructors will be noted. Word parts combine in various ways, as can be seen in the accompanying table.

Word Parts	Examples	Medical Terms
prefix + word root	**anti-** (prefix meaning against) + **thyroid** (root word for thyroid gland)	*antithyroid* • literal definition: against the thyroid • actual usage: (agent) suppressing thyroid activity
word root + suffix	**gastr** (word root for stomach) + **-ic** (suffix meaning pertaining to)	*gastric* • definition: pertaining to the stomach
combining form (word root + combining vowel) + suffix	**cardi** (root word for heart) + **/o** (a combining vowel) + **-logy** (suffix meaning study of)	*cardiology* • definition: study of the heart
prefix + suffix	**an-** (prefix meaning no, without) + **-emia** (suffix meaning blood)	*anemia* • literal definition: without (or no) blood • actual usage: decreased number of red blood cells or decreased hemoglobin in the cells
prefix + root word + suffix	**epi-** (prefix meaning above, over) + **gastr** (root word for stomach) + **-algia** (suffix meaning pain)	*epigastralgia* • literal definition: pain above the stomach • actual usage: pain in the upper region of the abdomen
compound word* + suffix	**ot/o** (root word for ear) + **rhin/o** (root word for nose) + **laryng/o** (root word for throat or larynx) + **-logy** (suffix meaning study of)	*otorhinolaryngology* • definition: the branch of medicine dealing with diseases of the ear, nose, and throat

* Two or more root words connected with a combining vowel.

LISTING OF WORD PARTS

You may or may not know most of the words presented in the table. Do not be concerned if you don't. There will be plenty of opportunity to learn more about them. In the next section, you are provided with listings of word parts. Many of the prefixes, combining forms, word roots, and suffixes are indicated. Eventually, you will have to be familiar with all of them. Here are some steps that will help you to learn:

1. Go through the lists of word parts once or twice.
2. Check your knowledge by covering all but the first column and see if you can provide meanings for some of the words.

CONFUSING MEDICAL TERMINOLOGY

ante- Versus anti-

ante- = before, forward, e.g., antepartum (an-te-<u>par</u>-tum) refers to occurring before childbirth

anti- = against, counter, e.g., anticoagulant (an-te-ko-<u>ag</u>-u-lant) is an agent that slows down the clotting process

PREFIXES, WORD ROOTS WITH COMBINING FORMS, AND SUFFIXES

TABLE 2-1	Prefixes Commonly Used in Medicine			
Prefix	**Definition**	**Word Example**	**Pronunciation**	**Definition**
a-, an-	no, not, without, lack of, apart	**an**oxia	an-ok´-se-ah	lack of sufficient oxygen in the blood
ad-	toward, near, to	**ad**hesion	ad-he´-zhun	union of two surfaces that are normally separate
bi-	two, double	**bi**cuspid	bi-kus´-pid	having two cusps
de-	down, away from	**de**generate	de-jen´-er-ate	to change from a higher to a lower form
di-	two, double	**di**plopia	di-plo-pe-ah	double vision
dia-	through, between	**dia**lysis	di-al´-i-sis	diffusion of solute molecules through a semipermeable membrane
dif-, dis-	apart, free from, separate	**dif**fusion	di-fu´-zhun	state or process of being widely spread
dys-	bad, difficult, painful	**dys**functional	dis-fungk´-zhun-al	disturbance, impairment, or abnormality of an organ
ec-, ecto-	out, outside, outer	**ecto**derm	ek-to-derm	outermost of the three primitive germ layers of the embryo
end-, endo-	within, inner	**endo**metrium	en-do-me´-tre-um	mucous membrane lining the uterus
ep-, epi-	upon, over, above	**epi**dural	ep-i-du-ral	situated upon or outside the dura mater
eu-	good, normal	**eu**phoria	u-fo´-re-ah	an exaggerated feeling of mental and physical well-being
ex-, exo-	out, away from	**ex**crete	ek-skreet´	to throw off or eliminate, as waste matter, by normal discharge
extra-	outside, beyond	**extra**uterine	ek-strah-u´-ter-in	situated or occurring outside the uterus
hyper-	above, beyond, excessive	**hyper**tension	hi-per-ten´-shun	persistently high blood pressure
hypo-	below, under, deficient	**hypo**dermic	hi-po-der´-mik	beneath the skin
in-	in, into, not	**in**fusion	in-fu´-zhun	steeping a substance in water to obtain its soluble principles
mega-	large, great	**mega**lgia	meg-al-je-ah	a severe pain
meta-	beyond, over, between, change	**meta**stasis	me-tas´-tah-sis	transfer of a disease from one organ to another not directly connected to it
para-	beside, alongside, abnormal	**para**colitis	par´-ah-ko-li´-tis	inflammation of the outer coat of the colon
poly-	many, much, excessive	**poly**cystic	pol´-e-sis´-tik	containing many cysts

TABLE	2-1	Prefixes Commonly Used in Medicine *(continued)*

Prefix	Definition	Word Example	Pronunciation	Definition
post-	after, behind	**post**natal	post-na´-tal	occurring after birth, with reference to the newborn
pre-	before, in front of	**pre**menstrual	pre-men´-stroo-al	preceding menstruation
pro-	before, in front of	**pro**otic	pro-ot´-ik	in front of the ear
super-	above, beyond	**super**nutrition	soo-per-nu-trish´-un	excessive nutrition
supra-	above, beyond	**supra**costal	soo-prah-kos´-tal	above or outside the ribs

TABLE	2-2	Word Roots and Combining Forms for Body Parts

Word Part	Definition	Word Example	Pronunciation	Definition
abdomin/o	abdomen	**abdomin**ocystic	ab-dom´-i-no-<u>sis</u>-tic	pertaining to the abdomen and gallbladder
aden/o	gland	**aden**itis	ad´-e-<u>ni</u>-tis	inflammation of a gland
an/o	anus	**an**oplasty	an´-oh-<u>plas</u>-te	plastic repair of the anus
andr/o	men	**andr**oid	<u>an</u>-droid	resembling a man
angi/o	vessel	**angi**ectomy	an´-je´-<u>ek</u>-to-me	excision of part of a blood vessel or lymph vessel
appendage	attached to or outgrowth	**append**ectomy	<u>ah</u>-pen-dek´-to-me	excision of the vermiform appendix
appendic/o	appendix	**appendic**olysis	ah-<u>pen</u>-di-kol´-i-sis	surgical separation of adhesions binding the appendix
arteri/o	artery	**arteri**ogram	ar-<u>te</u>-re-o-gram´	an x-ray picture of an artery
arthr/o	joint	**arthr**ocele	<u>ar</u>-thro-sel	a joint swelling
cardi/o	heart	**cardi**ology	<u>kar</u>-de-ol´-ogy	study of the heart
cephal/o	head	**cephal**ic	se´-phăl-ic	pertaining to the head
cerebr/o	cerebrum (part of the brain)	**cerebr**al	ser´-e-<u>bral</u>	pertaining to the brain
cyst/o	bladder	**cyst**ocele	<u>sis</u>-toh-seel	hernia of the bladder into the vagina
cyt/o	cell	**cyt**ology	si´-toh-lōgy	study of the body cells
encephal/o	brain	**encephal**oma	en-sef´-ah-<u>lo</u>-mah	a swelling or tumor of the brain

(continues)

TABLE	2-2	Word Roots and Combining Forms for Body Parts *(continued)*		

Word Part	Definition	Word Example	Pronunciation	Definition
enter/o	intestines	**enter**itis	en-<u>ter</u>-i´-tis	inflammation of the intestine (usually small intestine)
esophag/o	esophagus	**esophag**ism	e-<u>sof</u>-ah-jism	spasm of the esophagus
gastro/o	stomach	**gastro**pathy	gas-<u>trop</u>-ah-the	any disease of the stomach
gloss/o	tongue	**gloss**odynia	glos´-o-<u>din</u>-e-ah	pain in the tongue
gyne	woman	**gyne**phobia	jin´-e-<u>fo</u>-be-ah	morbid aversion to women
hem/o	blood	**hem**atoma	he-<u>ma</u>-toh´-mah	blood clot in an organ or under the skin
hepat/o	liver	**hepat**ocele	<u>hep</u>-ah-to-sel	hernia of the liver
hyster/o	uterus	**hyster**olith	<u>his</u>-ter-o-lith´	a uterine calculus (stone)
ile/o	ileum (small intestine)	**Ile**us	<u>il</u>-e-us	intestinal obstruction
irid/o	iris (eye)	**irid**omalacia	ir´-i-do-mah-<u>la</u>-she-ah	softening of the iris
kerat/o	cornea of eye; horny substance	**kerat**orrhexis	ker´-ah-to-<u>rek</u>-sis	rupture of the cornea
lamina, lamin/o	thin, flat part of vertebra	**lamin**otomy	lam´-i-<u>not</u>-o-me	transection of a vertebral lamina
lapar/o	abdominal wall	**lapar**orrhaphy	lap´-ah-<u>ror</u>-ah-fe	suture of the abdominal wall
lingua	tongue	nigra**lingua**	ni-gra-<u>ling</u>-gwah	black tongue
lob/o	lobe, as of lung or brain	**lob**otomy	lo-<u>bot</u>-o-me	cutting of nerve fibers connecting a lobe of the brain with the thalamus
mamm/o	breast	**mamm**ogram	<u>mam</u>-o-gram	x-ray recording of breast tissue
mast/o	breast	**mast**itis	mas-<u>ti</u>-tis	inflammation of the breast
my/o	muscle	**my**ocarditis	mi´-o-kar-<u>di</u>-tis	inflammation of the heart muscle
myel/o	bone marrow; spinal cord	**myel**ocyte	<u>mi</u>-e-lo-sit´	immature cell of bone marrow
myring/o	eardrum	**myring**oplasty	mi-<u>ring</u>-o-plas´-te	surgical reconstruction of the eardrum
nephr/o	kidney	**nephr**itis	ne-<u>fri</u>-tis	inflammation of the kidney
neur/o	nerve	**neur**algia	nu-<u>ral</u>-je-ah	pain in a nerve
oophor/o	ovary	**oophor**ocystosis	o-of´-o-ro-sis-<u>to</u>-sis	formation of an ovarian cyst
ophthalm/o	eye	**ophthalm**orrhagia	of-thal´-mo-<u>ra</u>-je-ah	hemorrhage from the eye
orchi/o	testicle	**orchi**opathy	or´-ke-<u>op</u>-ah-the	any disease of the testes

TABLE	2-2	Word Roots and Combining Forms for Body Parts (*continued*)

Word Part	Definition	Word Example	Pronunciation	Definition
orchid/o	testicle	**orchid**orrhaphy	or´-ki-<u>dor</u>-ah-fe	surgical fixation of an undescended testis into the scrotum by suturing
oste/o	bone	**oste**oporosis	os´-te-o-po-<u>ro</u>-sis	abnormal thinning of the skeleton
ot/o	ear	**ot**itis	o-<u>ti</u>-tis	inflammation of the ear
pancreat/o	pancreas	**pancreat**ogenous	pan´-kre-ah-<u>toj</u>-e-nus	arising in the pancreas
pharyng/o	pharynx	**pharyng**ismus	far´-in-<u>jis</u>-mus	muscular spasm of the pharynx
phleb/o	vein	**phleb**otomy	fle-<u>bot</u>-o-me	incision of a vein
pneum/o	lungs (air or gas)	**pneum**onectomy	nu´-mo-<u>nek</u>-to-me	excision of lung tissue
proct/o	rectum	**proct**odynia	prok´-to-<u>din</u>-e-ah	pain in the rectum
prostat/o	prostate gland	**prostat**itis	pros´-tah-<u>ti</u>-tis	inflammation of the prostate
pyel/o	pelvis of kidney	**pyel**ectasis	pi´-e-<u>lek</u>-tah-sis	dilation of the renal pelvis
rect/o	rectum and/or anus	**rect**ocele	<u>rek</u>-to-sel	hernial protrusion of part of the rectum into the vagina
ren/i	renal (kidney)	**ren**iform	<u>ren</u>-i-form	kidney-shaped
rhin/o	nose	**rhin**itis	ri-<u>ni</u>-tis	inflammation of the mucous membrane of the nose
sacr/o	sacrum	**sacr**olumbar	sa´-kro-<u>lum</u>-bar	pertaining to the sacrum and loins
salping/o	fallopian tube	**salping**ocyesis	sal-ping´-go-ci-<u>e</u>-sis	development of an embryo in the uterine tube; a tubal pregnancy
splen/o	spleen	**splen**optosis	sple-nop-<u>to</u>-sis	downward displacement of the spleen
spondyl/o	vertebra	**spondyl**odymus	spon´-di-<u>lod</u>-i-mus	twin fetuses united by the vertebrae
steth/o	chest	**steth**ospasm	<u>steth</u>-o-spasm	spasm of the chest muscles
stomat/o	mouth	**stomat**omalacia	sto-mah-to-ma-<u>la</u>-she-ah	softening of the structures of the mouth
ten/o	tendon	**ten**dolysis	ten-<u>dol</u>-i-sis	the freeing of tendon adhesions
thorac/a	thorax (chest)	**thorac**entesis	tho´-rah-sen-<u>te</u>-sis	surgical puncture and drainage of the thoracic cavity
thyr/o	thyroid gland	**thyr**oxine	thi-<u>rok</u>-sin	a hormone of the thyroid gland that contains iodine
trache/o	trachea	**trache**oscopy	tra´-ke-<u>os</u>-ko-pe	inspection of the interior of the trachea

(*continues*)

TABLE 2-2   Word Roots and Combining Forms for Body Parts (continued)

Word Part	Definition	Word Example	Pronunciation	Definition
tympan/o	eardrum	**tympan**um	tim-pah-num	part of the cavity of the middle ear, in the temporal bone
ureter/o	ureter	**ureter**opathy	u-re´-ter-op-ah-the	any disease of the ureter
vas/o	vessel	**vas**cular	vas-ku-lar	pertaining to blood vessels
ven/i	vein	**ven**ipuncture	ven´-i-punk-chur	surgical puncture of a vein

TABLE 2-3   Suffixes Used in Surgery

Suffix	Definition	Word Example	Pronunciation	Definition
-age	related to	tri/**age** (three)	tre-ahzh	sorting out and classification of casualties to determine priority of treatment
-centesis	surgical puncture	arthro/**centesis** (joint)	ar´-thro-sen-te-sis	puncture of a joint cavity for aspiration of fluid
-cid	kill	germi/**cid**al (germ)	jer-mi-si-dal	destructive to pathogenic microorganisms
-cis	cut, kill, excise	circum/**cis**ion (around)	ser-kum-sizh´-un	surgical removal of the foreskin of the penis
-clasis	to break down, refracture	oste/o**clasis** (bone)	os´-te-ok-lah-sis	surgical fracture or refracture of bones
-desis	binding, stabilization	arthr/o**desis** (joint)	ar´-thro-de-sis	surgical fusion of a joint
-ectomy	excision, removal	append/**ectomy**	ap´-en-dek-to-me	excision of the vermiform appendix
-iatry	healing (by a physician)	psych/**iatry** (mind)	si´-ki-ah-tre	healing of the mind
-ion	process	excerebrat**ion** (brain)	ek-ser-e-bra´-shun	process of removal of the brain
-lysis	loosen, free from adhesions, destruction	enter/o**lysis** (intestine)	en´-ter-ol-i-sis	surgical separation of intestinal adhesions
-osis	condition of	necr/**osis** (death)	ne-kro-sis	death of cells or tissues
-os/tomy	mouth, forming an opening	col/**ostomy** (colon)	ko-los-to-me	the surgical creation of an opening between the colon and the body surface
-pexy	fixation, suspension	gastro/**pexy** (stomach)	gas-tro-pek´-se	surgical fixation of the stomach
-plasty	formation, plastic repair	rhino/**plasty** (nose)	ri-no-plas´-te	plastic surgery of the nose

TABLE 2-3 Suffixes Used in Surgery *(continued)*

Suffix	Definition	Word Example	Pronunciation	Definition
-stasis	stop/control	hemo/**stasis** (blood)	he-mo-sta´-sis	stopping the escape of blood by either natural or artificial means
-therapy	treatment	chemo/**therapy** (drug)	ke-mo-ther´-ah-pe	treatment of illness by medication
-tomy	incision, to cut into	phlebo/**tomy** (vein)	fle-bot-o-me	incision of a vein
-tripsy	to crush	litho/**tripsy** (stone)	lith-o-trip´-se	the crushing of a stone in the bladder

TABLE 2-4 Suffixes for Diagnoses and Symptoms

Suffix	Definition	Word Example	Pronunciation	Definition
-algia	pain	cephal/**algia** (head)	sef´-a-lal-je-ah	headache
-cele	hernia, swelling	hepat/o**cele** (liver)	hep-ah-to-sel	hernia of the liver
-dynia	pain	cephal/o**dynia** (head)	sef´-ah-lo-din-e-ah	pain in the head
-ectasis	dilation, expansion	bronchi/**ectasis** (bronchus)	brong´-ke-ek-tah-sis	chronic dilation of one or more bronchi
-emia	blood	poly/cyth/**emia** (many)	pol-e-si-the´-me-ah	increase in total red cell mass of the blood
-gen	producing, beginning	carcin/o/**gen** (cancer)	car-sin-o-jen	any substance that causes cancer
-gram	record, picture	encephal/o/**gram** (brain)	en-sef-ah-lo-gram	the x-ray film obtained by encephalography
-graph	instrument for recording	cardi/o/**graph** (heart)	kar-de-o-graf´	an instrument used for recording electrical activity of the heartbeat
-graphy	process of recording	roentgen/o/**graphy**	rent´-gen-og-rah-fe	x-ray films (roentgenograms) of internal structures of the body
-iasis	abnormal condition, formation of, presence of	chole/lith/**iasis** (gallstone)	ko´-le-li-thi-ah-sis	the presence or formation of gallstones
-itis	inflammation	gastr/**itis** (stomach)	gas-tri-tis	inflammation of the stomach

(continues)

TABLE	2-4	Suffixes for Diagnoses and Symptoms (*continued*)		

Suffix	Definition	Word Example	Pronunciation	Definition
-logy	study of	bio/**logy** (life)	bi-<u>ol</u>-o-je	scientific study of living organisms
-malacia	softening	oste/o/**malacia** (bone)	os´-te-o-mah-<u>la</u>-she-ah	softening of the bones resulting from vitamin D deficiency
-megaly	enlargement	hepat/o/**megaly** (liver)	hep´-aht-o-<u>meg</u>-ah-le	enlargement of the liver
-meter	instrument for measuring	crani/o/**meter** (cranium)	kra´-ne-<u>om</u>-e-ter	an instrument for measuring skulls
-metry	process of measuring	pelvi/**metry** (pelvis)	pel-<u>vim</u>-e-tre	measurement of the capacity and diameter of the pelvis
-oid	resemble	lip/**oid** (fat)	<u>lip</u>-oid	fatlike; lipid (resembling a fat)
-oma	tumor	aden/**oma** (gland)	ad´-e-<u>no</u>-mah	a benign skin tumor in which the cells are derived from glandular epithelium
-osis	abnormal condition	dermat/**osis** (skin)	der´-mah-<u>to</u>-sis	any skin disease, especially one not characterized by inflammation
-pathy	disease	nephr/o/**pathy** (kidney)	ne-<u>frop</u>-ah-the	disease of the kidneys
-penia	decrease, deficiency	leuk/o/cyto/**penia** (white) (cell)	loo-ko-sit-o-<u>pe</u>-ne-ah	reduction of the number of leukocytes (white blood cells), the count being 5,000/mm³ or less
-phagia	eating, swallowing	dys/**phagia** (difficult)	dis-<u>fa</u>-je-ah	difficulty in swallowing or eating
-phasia	speech	a/**phasia** (without)	ah-<u>fa</u>-zhe-ah	defect or loss of the power of expression by speech, writing, or signs, or of comprehending spoken or written words
-phobia	fear	acr/o/**phobia** (extremities or top)	ak´-ro-<u>fo</u>-be-ah	morbid fear of heights
-plegia	paralysis	hemi/**plegia** (half)	hem´-e-<u>ple</u>-je-ah	paralysis of one side of the body
-ptosis	prolapse, falling, dropping	hyster/o/**ptosis** (uterus)	his´-ter-op-<u>to</u>-sis	metroptosis; downward displacement or prolapse of the uterus
-rrhage	burst forth	hem/o/**rrhage** (blood)	<u>hem</u>-o-rij	the escape of blood from the vessels; excessive bleeding
-rrhea	discharge, flow	men/o/**rrhea** (menses)	men´-o-<u>re</u>-ah	normal menstruation
-rrhexis	rupture	angi/o/**rrhexis** (blood vessel)	an´-je-or-<u>ek</u>-sis	rupture of a vessel, especially a blood vessel

Root Words, Medical Terminology, and Patient Care

Bacteria, Color, and Some Medical Terms

LESSON ONE: MATERIALS TO BE LEARNED

Root Words for Bacteria
Prefixes for Color
Commonly Used Medical Prefixes

LESSON TWO: PROGRESS CHECK

Multiple Choice
Matching
Write in the Prefix
Define the Prefix

OBJECTIVES

After completion of this chapter and the exercises, the student should be able to:

1. List and define the five major types of bacteria.
2. List and define prefixes that deal with color.
3. Change the meaning of a given word root by adding appropriate prefixes. Define, spell, and pronounce the new word.
4. Define, spell, and pronounce medical words used in this chapter.

CONFUSING MEDICAL TERMINOLOGY

-cele Versus celi/o

-cele = cyst, hernia, herniation, e.g., pharyngocele (fah-<u>rin</u>-jo-sel) refers to herniation of the throat

celi/o = abdomen, e.g., celioma (<u>se</u>-le-o-mah) an abdominal tumor

LESSON ONE	Materials to Be Learned

ROOT WORDS FOR BACTERIA

TABLE 3-1	Root Words for Bacteria			
Root Word	**Definition**	**Word Example**	**Pronunciation**	**Definition**
bacillus*	bacteria that are rod-shaped (plural is bacilli)	strepto**bacillus**	strep´-to-bah-<u>sil</u>-lis	rod-shaped bacteria that grow in twisted chains
coccus*	bacteria that are round in shape (plural is cocci, pronounced 'coc´-seye')	strepto**coccus**	strep´-to-<u>kok</u>-us	round bacteria that grow in twisted chains
dipl/o	pairs; bacteria that grow in pairs	**dipl**ococcus	dip´-lo-<u>kok</u>-us	round bacteria that grow in pairs
staphyl/o	bunches, like grapes; bacteria that grow in clusters	**staphyl**ococcus	staf´-i-lo-<u>kok</u>-us	round bacteria that grow in clusters
strept/o	twisted; bacteria that grow in twisted chains	**strepto**coccus	strep-to-<u>kok</u>-us	round bacteria that grow in twisted chains

* Both "bacillus" and "coccus" are Latin and considered regular scientific words. They are neither word roots nor combining forms. Although some consider them suffixes when written as "-bacillus," and "-coccus," others disagree. We place them under the heading "root word" because we do not want to start another column or invent another heading.

PREFIXES FOR COLOR

The prefixes used to denote color are very useful. The color of the cells, body fluids and reactions, skin, growths, and rashes are important indications used in diagnosing and treating conditions and diseases. Table 3-2 contains definitions and examples of some of the more commonly used prefixes for color.

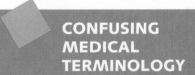

CONFUSING MEDICAL TERMINOLOGY

fasci/o Versus faci/o

fasci/o = fascia, fibrous band, e.g., fasciculation (fuh-sik-yuh-<u>ley</u>-shuh) refers to a brief spontaneous contraction affecting a small number of muscle fibers

faci/o = the face, form, e.g., facioplegia (fa-shi-o-<u>ple</u>-jia) refers to facial paralysis

TABLE 3-2	Prefixes for Color			
Prefix	**Definition**	**Word Example**	**Pronunciation**	**Definition**
alb-	white	**alb**ino	al-<u>bi</u>-no	a person with white hair, very pale skin, and nonpigmented irises
chlor/o-	green	**chlor**ophyll	<u>klo</u>-ro-fil	any of a group of green pigments that are involved in oxygen-producing photosynthesis
chrom/o-	color	**chrom**ocyte	<u>kro</u>-mo-sit	any colored cell or pigmented corpuscle
cirrh/o-	orange-yellow	**cirrh**osis	si-<u>ro</u>-sis	interstitial inflammation of an organ, particularly the liver (cirrhosis of the liver), showing orange-yellow discoloration in organ pigments
cyan/o-	blue	**cyan**osis	si´-ah-<u>no</u>-sis	a bluish discoloration of skin and mucous membranes
erythr/o-	red	**erythr**ocyte	e-<u>rith</u>-ro-sit	a red blood cell or corpuscle containing hemoglobin and transporting oxygen
leuk/o-	white	**leuk**ocyte	<u>loo</u>-ko-sit	white cell; a colorless blood corpuscle whose chief function is to protect the body against microorganisms causing disease
lutein/o-	saffron yellow	**lutein**	<u>loo</u>-te-in	a lipochrome from the corpus luteum, fat cells, and egg yolk
melan/o-	black	**melan**oma	mel´-ah-<u>no</u>-mah	malignant melanoma—"black tumor"
poli/o-	gray	**poli**omyelitis	po´-le-o-mi´-e-<u>li</u>-tis	an acute viral disease marked clinically by fever, sore throat, headache, vomiting, and often stiffness of the neck and back. It may attack the gray matter of the central nervous system (CNS) and brain, hence the common name "polio"
rhod/o-	red	**rhod**opsin	ro-<u>dop</u>-sin	visual purple; a photosensitive purple-red chromoprotein in the retinal rods
rubi/o-	reddish, redness	**rub**ella	roo-<u>bel</u>-ah	German measles; a mild viral infection marked by a pink macular rash, fever, and lymph node enlargement
xanth/o-	yellowish	**xanth**ochromia	zan´-tho-<u>kro</u>-me-ah	yellowish discoloration, as of the skin or spinal fluid

COMMONLY USED PREFIXES

The prefixes in Table 3-3 are commonly used in medical terminology. Many have been defined previously. They also appear throughout the text, especially as they relate to body systems. They are included in this chapter for easy reference.

TABLE	3-3	Commonly Used Prefixes		

Prefix	Definition	Word Example	Pronunciation	Definition
a-, an-	without, not	**a**febrile	a-<u>feb</u>-ril	without fever
		anoxia	an-<u>ok</u>-se-ah	absence of oxygen supply to tissues despite adequate perfusion of the tissue by blood; often used interchangeably with hypoxia to indicate a reduced oxygen supply
acro-	extremities; top or extreme point	**acro**dermatitis	ak-ro-der´-mah-<u>ti</u>-tis	inflammation of the skin of the hands or feet
aero-	air	**aero**bic	ar-<u>o</u>-bik	produced in the presence of oxygen
		an**aero**bic	an-ar-<u>o</u>-bik	produced without oxygen
aniso-	unequal	**aniso**cytosis	an-i´-so-si-<u>to</u>-sis	presence in the blood of erythrocytes showing excessive variations in size
brady-	slow	**brady**cardia	brad´-e-<u>kar</u>-de-ah	slowness of the heartbeat, as evidenced by slowing of the pulse rate to < 60
de-	take away, remove	**de**hydrate	de-<u>hi</u>-drat	remove water from, to dry; to lose water, become dry
dia-	through (as in running through)	**dia**rrhea	di´-ah-<u>re</u>-ah	abnormally frequent evacuation of watery stools
dif-, dis-	apart, free from, separate	**dif**fusion	di-fu´-zhun	state or process of being widely spread
dys-	bad, painful, difficult	**dys**tocia	dis-<u>to</u>-se-ah	abnormal labor or childbirth
		dysmenorrhea	dis´-men-or-<u>re</u>-ah	painful menstruation
ec-, ecto-	out, outside, outer	**ecto**derm	ek´-to-derm	outermost of the three primitive germ layers of the embryo
emia-	blood: condition of	an**emia**	an-<u>ne</u>-me-ah	reduction below normal of the number of erythrocytes, quantity of hemoglobin, or the volume of packed red cells in the blood; a symptom of various diseases and disorders
end-, endo-	within, inner	**endo**metrium	<u>en</u>-do-me´-tre-um	mucous membrane lining the uterus
eu-	good, easy	**eu**phoria	u-<u>fo</u>-re-ah	bodily comfort; well-being; absence of pain or distress
		euthanasia	u´-thah-<u>na</u>-zhe-ah	easy or painless death; mercy killing; deliberate ending of life of a person suffering from an incurable disease
extra-	outside, beyond	**extra**uterine	ek-strah-u´-ter-in	situated or occurring outside the uterus

TABLE 3-3	Commonly Used Prefixes *(continued)*

Prefix	Definition	Word Example	Pronunciation	Definition
hemi-	one side, half	**hemi**plegia	hem´-e-<u>ple</u>-je-ah	paralysis of one side of the body
hemo-	blood	**hemo**lysis	he-<u>mol</u>-i-sis	separation of the hemoglobin from the red cells and its appearance in the plasma
hetero-	different	**hetero**sexual	het´-er-o-<u>seks</u>-u-al	one who is sexually attracted to persons of the opposite sex
homo-	same	**homo**sexual	ho´-mo-<u>seks</u>-u-al	one who is sexually attracted to persons of the same sex
	resembling each other	**homo**geneous	ho´-mo-<u>je</u>-ne-us	of uniform quality, composition, or structure throughout
hydro-	water	**hydro**therapy	hi´-dro-<u>ther</u>-a-pe	the treatment of disease by the internal or external use of water
		hydrocephalus	hi´-dro-<u>sef</u>-ah-lus	a congenital or acquired condition marked by dilation of the cerebral ventricles and an accumulation of cerebrospinal fluid within the skull
hyper-	above normal, excessive, beyond	**hyper**tension	hi-per-<u>ten</u>-shun	persistently high arterial blood pressure; it may have no known cause or be associated with other diseases
hypo-	under, below normal	**hypo**glycemia	hi´-po-gli-<u>se</u>-me-ah	deficiency of glucose concentration in the blood, which may lead to nervousness, hypothermia, headache, confusion, and sometimes convulsions and coma
in-	in, into, not	**in**fusion	<u>in</u>-fu´-zhun	steeping a substance in water to obtain its soluble principles
iso-	equal, same	**iso**tonic	i´-so-<u>ton</u>-ik	of equal tension
		isothermal	i´-so-<u>ther</u>-mal	having the same temperature
lip-	fat	**lip**idemia	lip´-i-<u>de</u>-me-ah	hyperlipidemia: a general term for elevated concentrations of any or all of the lipids in the plasma
mal-	bad, poor	**mal**aise	mal-<u>az</u>	a vague feeling of bodily discomfort
		malocclusion	mal´-o-<u>kloo</u>-zhun	absence of proper relations of opposing teeth when the jaws are in contact
mega-	large, great	**mega**lgia	meg-al´-je-ah	a severe pain
		megavitamin	meg´-ah-<u>vi</u>-tah-min	a dose of vitamin(s) vastly exceeding the amount recommended for nutritional balance
megalo-	large (enlarged)	acro**megaly**	ak´-ro-<u>meg</u>-ah-le	abnormal enlargement of the extremities of the skeleton—nose, jaws, fingers, and toes

(continues)

TABLE 3-3 Commonly Used Prefixes (*continued*)

Prefix	Definition	Word Example	Pronunciation	Definition
meno-	menses (menstruation)	**meno**pause	<u>men</u>-o-pawz	cessation of menstruation
noct-	night	**noct**uria	nok-<u>tu</u>-re-ah	excessive urination at night
nyct-	night	**nyct**uria	nik-<u>tu</u>-re-ah	excessive urination at night
pan-	all, every	**pan**demic	pan-<u>dem</u>-ik	a widespread epidemic disease
para-	beside, beyond, accessory to	**para**cystic	par´-ah-<u>sis</u>-tik	situated near the bladder
per-	through	**per**forate	<u>pur</u>-fo-rat	to make a hole or holes through, as by punching or boring; to pierce, penetrate
peri-	around	**peri**toneum	per´-i-to-<u>ne</u>-um	the serous membrane lining the walls of the abdominal and pelvic cavities
poly-	many, much	**poly**uria	pol´-e-<u>u</u>-re-ah	excessive secretion of urine
post-	following, after	**post**partum	post-<u>par</u>-tum	occurring after childbirth, with reference to the mother
		postoperative	post-<u>op</u>-ra-tiv	following surgery
pre-	before	**pre**natal	pre-<u>na</u>-tal	preceding birth
pro-	preceding, coming before	**pro**gnosis	prog-<u>no</u>-sis	a forecast of the probable course and outcome of a disorder
pyo-	pus	**pyo**genic	pi´-o-<u>jen</u>-ik	producing pus
		pyorrhea	pi-o-<u>re</u>-ah	a copious discharge of pus
re-	put back	**re**hydrate	re-<u>hi</u>-drat	to restore water or fluid content to the body
super-	above, beyond	**super**nutrition	soo-per-nu-trish´-un	excessive nutrition
supra-	above, beyond	**supra**costal	soo-prah-kos´-tal	above or outside the ribs
syn-	going together, united	**syn**thesis	<u>sin</u>-the-sis	creation of a compound by union of elements composing it, done artificially or as a result of natural processes
		syndrome	<u>sin</u>-drome	a set of symptoms occurring together
tachy-	fast	**tachy**cardia	tak´-e-<u>kar</u>-de-ah	abnormally rapid heart rate

Body Openings and Plural Endings

LESSON ONE: MATERIALS TO BE LEARNED

Body Openings
Plural Endings

LESSON TWO: PROGRESS CHECK

Spelling and Definition
Word Construction
Building Medical Terms
Definitions

OBJECTIVES

After completion of this chapter and the exercises, the student should be able to:

1. Provide definitions for and use each term for the openings or orifices in the human body.
2. Identify singular and plural endings and provide word examples with pronunciations.

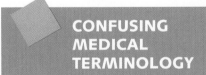

CONFUSING MEDICAL TERMINOLOGY

strata Versus striae

strata = plural of stratum, layers, e.g., strata (<u>strey</u>-tuh) of tissues refer to layers of tissues

striae = striae (<u>strahy</u>-ee) refers a slight or narrow furrow, ridge, stripe, or streak, especially one of a number in parallel arrangement, e.g., striae of muscle fiber, as in stretch marks

LESSON ONE	Materials to Be Learned

BODY OPENINGS

TABLE 4-1	Body Openings

Term	Pronunciation	Definition or Usage
aperture	ap-er-chur	an opening or orifice
canal (alimentary)	kah-nal	the musculomembranous digestive tube extending from the mouth to the anus
canal (vaginal)	kah-nal	the canal in the female from the vulva to the cervix uteri that receives the penis in copulation
cavity	kav-i-te	a hollow place or space, or a potential space, within the body or one of its organs
constriction	kon-strik-shun	making something narrow; to contract; to close (an opening)
dilatation, dilation	dil´-ah-ta-shun di-la-shun	stretched beyond normal dimensions; the widening of something; expansion, opening
foramen	for-ra-men	a natural opening or passage, especially one into or through a bone
hiatus	hi-a-tus	a gap, cleft, or opening
introitus	in-tro-itus	opening or entrance to a canal or cavity such as the vagina
lumen	loo-men	opening within a hollow tube or organ
meatus	me-a-tus	urinary passage or opening
orifice	or-i-fis	any orifice, such as the anal orifice
os	os	mouth opening; os uteri: mouth of the uterus, or cervix
patent	pa-tent	adjective, meaning open or not plugged, as in "the tube is patent"
perforation	per-fo-ra-shun	a hole in something, e.g., perforation of the stomach wall by a gastric ulcer
stoma	sto-mah	artificial opening established by colostomy, ileostomy, or tracheostomy
ventricle	ven-tri-kul	a small cavity or chamber, as in the brain or heart

PLURAL ENDINGS

Many medical terms have special plural forms. They are based on the ending of the word. Some of them are made plural in the same way you learned in English class. For example:

1. Adding an s to a singular noun. Example: singular, abrasion; plural, abrasions.
2. Singular nouns that end in s or ch form plurals by adding es. Example: singular, abscess; plural, abscesses.
3. Singular nouns that end in y preceded by a consonant form plurals by changing the y to i and adding es. Example: singular, artery; plural, arteries.

The following rules are commonly used for forming plurals for medical terms. If the word:

1. Ends in a, retain the a, and add e. Example: singular, bursa, vertebra; plural, bursae, vertebrae.
2. Ends in is, drop the is, and add es. Example: singular, crisis, diagnosis; plural, crises, diagnoses.
3. Ends in ix or ex, drop the ix or ex, and add ices. Example: singular, index, appendix; plural, indices, appendices.
4. Ends in on, drop the on, and add a. Example: singular, ganglion; plural, ganglia.
5. Ends in um, drop the um, and add a. Example: singular, ovum; plural, ova.
6. Ends in us, drop the us, and add i. Example: singular, nucleus, fungus; plural, nuclei, fungi.

There are exceptions to the rules. Some terms have more than one acceptable plural. If in doubt, consult your medical dictionary. Table 4-2 lists the plural endings to medical terms.

CONFUSING MEDICAL TERMINOLOGY

hidr/o Versus hydr/o

hidr/o = sweat, e.g., hidropoiesis (hid-roh-poi-ee-sis) refers to the production of sweat

hydr/o = water, relating to water, e.g., hydrencephalomeningocele (hi-dren-cef-al-o-men-in-jo-sel) refers to herniation of brain substance and meninges caused by a defect, with accumulation of cerebrospinal fluid along with brain substance in the sac

TABLE 4-2	Plural Endings				
Singular	**Word Example**	**Pronunciation**	**Plural**	**Word Example**	**Pronunciation**
a	bursa	ber-sah	ae	bursae	bur-sae
	vertebra	vur-ta-bra		vertebrae	vur-te-bre
ax	thorax	thor-aks	aces	thoraces	thor-a-sez
en	lumen	loo-men	ina	lumina	lu-mina
	foramen	for-ra-men	ina	foramina	for-ra-mina
is	crisis	kri-sis	es	crises	kri-ses
	diagnosis	di´-ag-no-sis		diagnoses	di´-ag-no-sez
	femoris	fe´-mo-ris	a	femora	fe´-mo-ra
ix	appendix	ah-pen-diks	ices	appendices	ah-pen-dises
inx	meninx	me-ninks	inges	meninges	me-nin-ges

(continues)

| TABLE 4-2 | Plural Endings | (continued) |

Singular	Word Example	Pronunciation	Plural	Word Example	Pronunciation
nx	phala*nx*	fa-lanks	ges	phalan*ges*	fa-lan-ges
on	spermatozo*on*	sper´-ma-to-zo-on	a	spermatozo*a*	sper´-ma-to-zo-a
um	diverticul*um*	di´-ver-tik-u-lum	a	diverticul*a*	di´-ver-tik-u-la
	ov*um*	o-vum		ov*a*	o-va
us	nucle*us*	nu-kli-us	i	nucle*i*	nu-clei
	thromb*us*	throm-bus		thromb*i*	throm-bi
ur	fem*ur*	fe-mur	ora	femor*a*	fem-ora
y	arter*y*	ar-ter-e	ies	arter*ies*	ar-ter-es
	ovar*y*	o-var-e		ovar*ies*	o-var-es

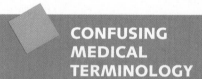

CONFUSING MEDICAL TERMINOLOGY

sarc/o Versus sacr/o

sarc/o = flesh (connective tissue), cancer of connective tissue, e.g., sarcocele (sar´-ko-sel) refers to a fleshy tumor or sarcoma of the testis

sacr/o = sacrum, e.g., sacrum (sak-ruhm) refers to a bone resulting from the fusion of two or more vertebrae between the lumbar and the coccygeal regions, in humans being composed usually of five fused vertebrae and forming the posterior wall of the pelvis; it means the area of the tailbone

Numbers, Positions, and Directions

LESSON ONE: MATERIALS TO BE LEARNED

Part 1: Prefixes for Numbers
Part 2: Prefixes for Positions and Directions
Part 3: Terms for Directions and Positions
Units of Weight and Measurement
  Weights and Measures
  Common Weights and Measures
Frequently Used Symbols

LESSON TWO: PROGRESS CHECK

Compare and Contrast
Identify the Location
Matching: Positions
Define the Term
Matching: Metric Units
Short Answer
Fill-in

OBJECTIVES

After completing this chapter and the exercises, the student should be able to:

1. Identify the location of any given body part.
2. Use appropriate prefixes to describe the direction of any movement and part of the body.
3. Give the meaning of prefixes that denote number and define given examples.
4. Identify commonly used prefixes that describe locations.
5. Describe body positions that indicate placement of a patient for a procedure or treatment.
6. Define the three major systems of weight and measurement used most often in medicine.
7. Convert Celsius to Fahrenheit or Fahrenheit to Celsius as needed.
8. Recognize commonly used symbols and abbreviations.
9. Define given word elements and transition to another system if required.

| LESSON ONE | Materials to Be Learned |

PART 1: PREFIXES FOR NUMBERS

Prefixes that denote number tell you whether something is one-half, one, two, three, or more; whether it is single or multiple; and whether it involves one side, two sides, or more. Table 5-1 contains definitions and examples of some of the commonly used prefixes for numbers.

TABLE 5-1		Prefixes for Numbers		

Prefix	Definition	Word Example	Pronunciation	Definition
uni- (mono-)	one	**uni**lateral	u´-ni-<u>lat</u>-er-al	affecting only one side
bi- (diplo-)	two (double), twice	**bi**lateral	bi-<u>lat</u>-er-al	having two sides; pertaining to both sides
		bicuspid	bi-<u>kus</u>-pid	having two points or cusps, e.g., bicuspid (mitral) valve; a bicuspid (premolar) tooth
gemin-	double, pair	**gemin**i	<u>jim</u>-in´-eh	twins
tri-	three	**tri**cuspid	tri-<u>kus</u>-pid	having three points or cusps, as a valve of the heart; the valve that guards the opening between the right atrium and right ventricle
		triceps	<u>tri</u>-seps	a muscle of the upper arm having three heads
quadri-	four	**quadri**plegic	kwod´-ri-<u>ple</u>-jic	paralysis of all four limbs
tetra-	four	**tetra**somic	tet-rah-some-ik	having four chromosomes where there should be only two
quint-	five	**quint**ipara	kwin-<u>tip</u>-ah-rah	a woman who has had five pregnancies that resulted in viable offspring (Para V)
sext-, sexti-	six	**sext**uplet	<u>sexs</u>-tu-plit	any one of six offspring produced at the same birth
sept-, septi-	seven	**sept**uplet	<u>sep</u>-tu-plit	one of seven offspring produced at the same birth
octa- (octo-)	eight	**octa**hedron	ok-ta-<u>he</u>-dron	an eight-sided solid figure
nona-	nine	**nona**n	<u>no</u>-nan	having symptoms that increase or reappear every ninth day; malarial symptoms are an example
deca-	ten	**deca**gram	<u>dek</u>-a-gram	a weight of 10 grams
multi-	many (more than one)	**multi**cellular	mul´-ti-<u>sel</u>-u-lar	composed of many cells
primi-	first	**primi**gravida	pri-mi-<u>grav</u>-i-dah	a woman pregnant for the first time
semi-	half (partially)	**semi**circular	sem´-i-<u>ser</u>-ku-lar	shaped like a half circle
hemi-	half, also one-sided	**hemi**anopsia	hem´-e-ah-<u>nop</u>-se-ah	defective vision or blindness in half of the visual field
ambi-	both or both sides	**ambi**dextrous	am´-bi-<u>deks</u>-trus	able to use either hand with equal dexterity
		ambivalence	am-<u>biv</u>-ah-lens	simultaneous existence of conflicting emotional attitudes toward a goal, object, or person
null-	none	**null**ipara	null-eh-<u>pair</u>-ah	a woman with no children
pan-	all	**pan**cytopenia	pan-site-<u>oh</u>-peen´-ee-ah	decreased number of all blood cells

PART 2: PREFIXES FOR POSITIONS AND DIRECTIONS

Prefixes that indicate directions describe a location. They tell you whether the location is above, below, inside, in the middle, around, near, between, or outside a body structure. Table 5-2 contains definitions and examples of commonly used prefixes that describe locations.

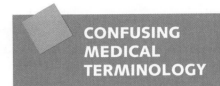

CONFUSING MEDICAL TERMINOLOGY

salping/o Versus salping/o

salping/o = uterine (fallopian) tube, e.g., salpingitis (sal-pin-gi-tis) refers to inflammation of the fallopian tube

salping/o = auditory (Eustachian) tube, e.g., salpingitis (sal-pin-ji-tis) refers to inflammation of the Eustachian tube

TABLE 5-2	Prefixes for Positions and Directions			
Prefix	**Definition**	**Word Example**	**Pronunciation**	**Definition**
ab-	away from	**ab**duction	ab-duk-shun	to draw away from; the state of being abducted
ad-	toward	**ad**duction	ah-duk-shun	to draw toward a center or median line
ante-	before, in front	**ante**cubital	an-tee-cu-bi-tol	"the space" in front of the elbow
circum-	around	**circum**cision	ser´-kum-sizh-un	surgical removal of all or part of the foreskin, or prepuce, of the penis
contra-	opposition, against	**contra**indicated	kon´-tra-in-di-ka-ted	any condition that renders a particular line of treatment improper or undesirable
de-	down, away from	**de**cay	deh-kay´	waste away (from normal)
dia-	through	**dia**gnosis	dahy-uh-g-noh-sis	knowledge through testing
ecto-, exo-	outside	**ecto**pic	ek-top-ik	located away from normal position; arising or produced at an abnormal site or in a tissue where it is not normally found
		exogenous	ek-soj-e-nus	originating outside or caused by factors outside the organism
		exocrine	ek-so-krin	secreting externally via a duct; denoting such a gland or its secretion
endo-	within	**endo**crine	en-do-krin	pertaining to internal secretions; hormonal
		endogenous	en-doj-e-nus	produced within or caused by factors within the organism
epi-	upon, over	**epi**gastric	ep´-i-gas-tric	the upper and middle region of the abdomen

(continues)

TABLE	5-2	Prefixes for Positions and Directions *(continued)*

Prefix	Definition	Word Example	Pronunciation	Definition
extra-	outside	**extra**uterine	ek´-strah-<u>u</u>-ter-in	situated or occurring outside the uterus
infra- (sub)	below, under	**infra**sternal	in´-frah-<u>ster</u>-nal	beneath the sternum
intra-	inside	**intra**cellular	in-tra-<u>sel</u>-u-lar	inside a cell
ipsi- (iso)	same (equal)	**ipsi**lateral	ip´-si-<u>lat</u>-er-al	situated on or affecting the same side
ir-	into, toward	**ir**rigate	ir´-reh-<u>gate</u>	wash into
meso-	middle, pertaining to mesentery	**meso**derm	<u>mez</u>-o-derm	the middle of the three primary germ layers of the embryo
meta- (supra)	after, beyond, over; change or transformation; following in a series	**meta**stasis	me-<u>tas</u>-tah-sis	the transfer of disease from one organ or part to another not directly connected with it
		metabolism	me-<u>tab</u>-o-lizm	the sum of the physical and chemical processes by which living organized substance is built up and maintained and by which large molecules are transformed into energy
		metamorphosis	met´-ah-<u>mor</u>-fo-sis	change of structure or shape; transition from one developmental stage to another
para-	near, beside	**para**medical	par´-ah-<u>med</u>-i-kal	having some connection with or relation to the science or practice of medicine
		paranormal	par´-ah-<u>nor</u>-mal	near-normal function
peri-	around, surrounding	**peri**odontal	per´-e-o-<u>don</u>-tal	around a tooth
		pericardium	per´-i-<u>kar</u>-de-um	pertaining to the fibrous sac enclosing the heart and the roots of the great vessels
retro-	behind, backward	**retro**peritoneal	ret´-ro-<u>per</u>-i-to-<u>ne</u>-al	behind the peritoneum
sub-	under, near	**sub**merged	sub-<u>mer</u>-j-ĕd	under the surface
trans-	across, through	**trans**verse	trans´-<u>verz</u>	positioned across
		transvaginal	trans´-<u>vaj</u>-i-nal	through the vagina

PART 3: TERMS FOR DIRECTIONS AND POSITIONS

Table 5-3 contains both prefixes and suffixes, many of which you learned in the preceding chapters and some of which are new. Both prefixes and suffixes are needed to describe body positions that indicate placement of a patient for procedures and/or treatments. Some words, such as Sims and Trendelenberg positions, are understood terms that denote the correct position without elaboration.

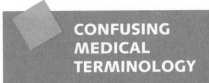

CONFUSING MEDICAL TERMINOLOGY

-tropia Versus -tropin

-tropia = turning, e.g., anatropia (an-ah-<u>tro</u>-pe-ah) refers to upward deviation of the visual axis of one eye when the other eye is fixing

-tropin = an affinity for, stimulating, e.g., thyrotropin (thi-<u>rot</u>-rah-pin), a thyroid-stimulating hormone; a hormone of the anterior pituitary gland having an affinity for and specifically stimulating the thyroid gland

---

TABLE 5-3   Terms for Directions and Positions

Term	Pronunciation	Definition
anterior	an-<u>ter</u>-e-or	situated at or directed toward the front; opposite of posterior
posterior	pos-<u>ter</u>-e-or	directed toward or situated at the back; opposite of anterior
cephalic	se-<u>fal</u>-ik	pertaining to the head, or the head end of the body
caudal	<u>kaw</u>-dal	situated toward the tail (coccygeal area)
decubitus	de-<u>ku</u>-bi-tus	the act of lying down; the position assumed in lying down
eversion	e-<u>ver</u>-zhun	a turning inside out; a turning outward
extension	ek-<u>sten</u>-zhun	the movement bringing the members of a limb into or toward a straight condition
flexion	<u>flek</u>-zhun	the act of bending or the condition of being bent
Fowler's	<u>fow</u>-lerz	the head of the patient's bed is raised 18–20 inches above level
internal	in-<u>ter</u>-nal	situated or occurring within or on the inside
external	eks-<u>ter</u>-nal	situated or occurring on the outside
knee-chest	<u>ne</u>-chest	the patient rests on his or her knees and chest; the head is turned to one side, and the arms are extended on the bed, the elbows flexed and resting so that they partially bear the weight of the patient
lateral	<u>lat</u>-er-al	situated away from the midline of the body; pertaining to the side
bilateral	bi-<u>lat</u>-er-al	having two sides; pertaining to both sides

(continues)

TABLE 5-3		Terms for Directions and Positions (*continued*)
Term	**Pronunciation**	**Definition**
lithotomy	li-<u>thot</u>-o-me	position in which the patient lies on his or her back, legs flexed on the thighs, thighs flexed on the abdomen and abducted
medial	<u>me</u>-de-al	situated toward the midline
oblique	o-<u>blēk</u>	slanting; incline
peripheral	pe-<u>rif</u>-er-al	an outward structure or surface; the portion of a system outside the central region
proximal	<u>prok</u>-si-mal	toward the center or median line; the point of attachment or origin
distal	<u>dis</u>-tal	remote; farther from any point of reference
quadrant	<u>kwod</u>-rant	one of four corresponding parts, or quarters, as of the surface of the abdomen or the field of vision
recumbent	re-<u>cum</u>-bent	lying down
rotation	ro-<u>ta</u>-shun	the process of turning around an axis
Sims'	simz	the patient lies on his or her left side and chest, the right knee and thigh drawn up, the left arm along the back
sinistro	<u>sin</u>-is-tro	left; left side
dextro	<u>dek</u>-stro	right; right side
superior	soo-<u>per</u>-e-or	situated above, or directed upward
inferior	in-<u>fer</u>-e-or	situated below, or directed downward
supine	<u>soo</u>-pīn	lying with the face upward or on the dorsal surface
supination	soo´-pi-<u>na</u>-shun	the act of placing or lying on the back
prone	prōn	lying face downward or on the ventral surface
pronation	prō-<u>nā</u>-shun	the act of assuming the prone position
trans	trans	through; across; beyond
Trendelenburg's	tren-<u>del</u>-en-bergz	the patient is supine on a surface inclined 45 degrees, the head lower than the legs
upright	<u>up</u>-rit	perpendicular; vertical; erect in carriage or posture

UNITS OF WEIGHT AND MEASUREMENT

This section contains weights and measures used most often in medicine. The transition between apothecary, avoirdupois, and metric is sometimes confusing to the beginning student. For the convenience of the learner, the units and equivalents are provided here, along with some symbols frequently encountered.*

TABLE 5-4	Units of Weight and Measurement	
Unit	**Abbreviation(s)**	**Definition**
Apothecaries' Weight (ah-poth-e-ka´-rez)		system used for measuring and weighing drugs and solutions, precious metals, and precious stones; fractions are used to designate portions of a unit and small Roman numerals are used to designate amounts, e.g., iss = one and one-half
grains	gr	
minims	m	
drams	dr	
ounces	oz	
pounds	lb (12 oz = 1 lb)	
Avoirdupois Weight (aver-du-poiz)		the system of measuring and weighing used in English-speaking countries for all commodities except drugs, precious stones, and precious metals
drops	gtt	
teaspoon	tsp	
tablespoon	T	
ounces	oz	
pound	lb (16 oz = 1 lb)	
Metric System (met-rik)		a system of weighing and measuring based on the meter and having all units based on the power of 10
Word Elements		
tera (10^{12})	T	monster: one trillion times the size of a unit
giga (10^{9})	G	one billion times the size of a unit
mega (10^{6})	M	one million times the size of a unit
kilo (10^{3})	k	one thousand times the size of a unit

(continues)

---

* Some textbooks in science and engineering use ML while others use both mL and ml. We use both of the latter abbreviations.

TABLE 5-4	Units of Weight and Measurement (continued)	

Unit	Abbreviation(s)	Definition
hecto (10^2)	h	one hundred times the size of a unit
deka (10)	dk	ten times the size of a unit
Unit Is One		
deci (10^{-1})	d	1/10 of a unit
centi (10^{-2})	c	1/100 of a unit
milli (10^{-3})	m	1/1000 of a unit
micro (10^{-6})	μ	1/1,000,000 of a unit
nano (10^{-9})	n	1/1,000,000,000 of a unit
pico (10^{-12})	p	1/1,000,000,000,000 of a unit
Metric Weight		
microgram	μg or mcg	1000 mcg = 1 milligram (mg)
milligram	mg	1000 mg = 1 gram (g or gm)
centigram	cg	100 cg = 1 g
decigram	dg	10 dg = 1 g
gram	g or gm	1 g = 1 g
dekagram	dkg	1 dkg = 10 g
hectogram	hg	1 hg = 100 g
kilogram	kg	1 kg = 1000 g
Metric Length		
millimeter	mm	1000 mm = 1 meter (m)
centimeter	cm	100 cm = 1 m
decimeter	dm	10 dm = 1 m
meter	m	1 m = 1 m
dekameter	dkm	10 m = 1 dkm
hectometer	hm	100 m = 1 hm
kilometer	km	1000 m = 1 km

TABLE 5-4	Units of Weight and Measurement *(continued)*

Unit	Abbreviation(s)	Definition
Metric Volume		
cubic centimeter	cc	1 cc = 1 ml (milliliter)
milliliter	ml or mL	1000 ml = 1 L (liter)
centiliter	cl	100 cl = 1 L
deciliter	dl	10 dl = 1 L
liter	l or L	1 L = 1 L
dekaliter	dkl	10 L = 1 dkl
hectoliter	hl	100 L = 1 hl
kiloliter	kl	1000 L = 1 kl
Equivalents (Equal to)		conversions from apothecary and avoirdupois to metric
weight	μg/mg	1000 μg = 1 mg
	mg/g	1000 mg = 1 g
	g/kg	1000 g = 1 kg
	kg/lb	1 kg = 2.2 lb
length	cm/in	2.5 cm = 1 in
volume	ml/cc/L	1000 ml = 1000 cc = 1 L
energy (joule)	J	1 J = 0.24 c
energy (calorie)	c	1 c = 4.18 J
Temperature (°T)		the degree (°) of sensible heat or cold expressed in terms of a specific scale
Celsius (or centigrade)	°C	scale at which the boiling point of water (H_2O) is 100° and the freezing point of H_2O is 0°
Fahrenheit	°F	scale at which the boiling point of H_2O is 212° and the freezing point of H_2O is 32°
conversion		to change from one scale or system to another
temperature		to convert Celsius to Fahrenheit, multiply by 9, divide by 5, and add 32: $°F = ([°C \times 9] \div 5) + 32$ to convert Fahrenheit to Celsius, subtract 32, multiply by 5, and divide by 9: $°C = ([°F - 32] \times 5) \div 9$

Weights and Measures

TABLE 5-5

U.S. System to Metric	
U.S. Measure	**Metric Measure**
Length	
1 in	25.0 mm
1 ft	0.3 m
Mass	
1 gr (grain)	64.8 mg
1 oz	28.35 g
1 lb	0.45 kg
Volume	
1 cu in	16.0 cm³
1 tsp	5.0 ml
1 T	15.0 ml
1 fl oz	30.0 ml
1 c	0.24 L
1 pt	0.47 L
1 qt (liq)	0.95 L
1 gal	0.004 m³
Energy	
1 cal (c)	4.18 J

Metric to U.S. System	
Metric Measure	**U.S. Measure**
Length	
1 mm	0.04 in
1 m	3.3 ft
Mass	
1 mg	0.015 g
1 gr (grain)	0.035 oz
1 kg	2.2 lb
Volume	
1 cm³	0.06 in³
1 ml	0.2 tsp
1 ml	0.07 T
1 ml	0.03 oz
1 L	4.2 c
1 L	2.1 pt
1 L	1.1 qt
1 m³	264.0 gal
Energy	
1 J	0.24 cal (c)

CONFUSING MEDICAL TERMINOLOGY

bi- Versus bi/o

bi- = two, twice, double, e.g., bicuspid (bi-<u>kus</u>-pid) refers to the valve that is situated between the left atrium and the left ventricle of the heart

bi/o or bio- = life, pertaining to life, e.g., biology (bahy-<u>ol</u>-uh-jee) refers to the study of life

Common Weights and Measures

TABLE 5-6

Measure	Equivalent
3 tsp	1 T
2 T	1 oz
4 T	1/4 c
8 T	1/2 c
16 T	1 c
2 c	1 pt
4 c	1 qt
4 qt	1 gal
1 tsp	5 g
1 T	15 g
1 oz	28.35 g
1 fl oz	30 g
1/2 c	120 g
1 c	240 g
1 lb	454 g
1 g	1 ml
1 tsp	5 ml
1 T	15 ml
1 fl oz	30 ml
1 c	240 ml
1 pt	480 ml
1 qt	960 ml
1 L	1000 ml

FREQUENTLY USED SYMBOLS

This section contains the symbols most frequently used in medical fields of practice.
A symbol is a graphic portrayal of words, phrases, or sentences.

TABLE 5-7

Symbol	Meaning
♂, □	male
♀, ○	female
*	birth
†	death
ā	before
p̄	after
℞	take (prescription)
°T	degree (temperature)
'	foot
"	inch
:	ratio (is to)
+	plus; positive; present
−	minus, negative; absent
ʒ	ounce
fʒ	fluid ounce
μg	microgram
c̄	with
s̄	without

Symbol	Meaning
↓	decreased, depressed
↑	increased, elevated
Θ	absent
∧	diastolic blood pressure
∨	systolic blood pressure
ʒ	dram
fʒ	fluidram
∞	infinity
±	indefinite (yes and no)
#	number; weight; gauge
/	per
Ⓛ	left
Ⓡ	right (also registered trademark)
≥	greater than or equal to
≤	less than or equal to
@	at
%	percent

Medical and Health Professions

LESSON ONE: MATERIALS TO BE LEARNED

Scientific Studies
Specialties and Specialists
Physicians and Medical Specialties
Other Health Professions
Additional Health Professions

LESSON TWO: PROGRESS CHECK

Multiple Choice: Scientific Studies
Matching
Short Answer
Completion
Multiple Choice: Professions
Abbreviations
Describe the Specialty

OBJECTIVES

After completion of this chapter and the exercises, the student should be able to:

1. Identify and define the medical terms and their word components for the major scientific health disciplines in medicine.
2. Identify and define the terms and their word components for physicians and professionals for each major medical specialty.

LESSON ONE	Materials to Be Learned

SCIENTIFIC STUDIES

TABLE 6-1

Root	Suffix	Word Example	Pronunciation	Definition
audi/o	-logy	**audi**ology	aw´-de-<u>ol</u>-o-je	the science concerned with the sense of hearing, especially the evaluation and measurement of impaired hearing and the rehabilitation of those with impaired hearing
bacteri/o		**bacteri**ology	bak-te´-re-<u>ol</u>-o-je	scientific study of bacteria
bi/o		**bi**ology	bi-<u>ol</u>-o-je	scientific study of living organisms
cardi/o		**cardi**ology	kar´-de-<u>ol</u>-o-je	study of the heart and its functions
dermat/o		**dermat**ology	der´-mah-<u>tol</u>-o-je	the medical specialty concerned with the diagnosis and treatment of skin diseases
endocrin/o		**endocrin**ology	en´-do-krin-<u>nol</u>-o-je	study of the endocrine system
gastr/oenter/o		**gastroenter**ology	gas´-tro-en´-ter-<u>ol</u>-o-je	study of the stomach and intestine and their diseases
gynec/o		**gynec**ology	gi´-ne-<u>kol</u>-o-je	the branch of medicine dealing with diseases of the genital tract in women
hemat/o		**hemat**ology	he´-mah-<u>tol</u>-o-je	the science dealing with the morphology of blood and blood-forming tissues and with their physiology and pathology
neur/o		**neur**ology	nu-<u>rol</u>-o-je	the branch of medical science that deals with the nervous system, both normal and diseased
onc/o		**onc**ology	ong-<u>kol</u>-o-je	the sum of knowledge regarding tumors; the study of tumors
ophthalm/o		**ophthalm**ology	of´-thal-<u>mol</u>-o-je	the branch of medicine dealing with the eye
path/o		**path**ology	pah-<u>thol</u>-o-je	the branch of medicine treating the essential nature of disease, especially changes in body tissues and organs that cause or are caused by disease
physi/o		**physi**ology	fiz´-e-<u>ol</u>-o-je	the science that treats the functions of the living organism and its parts, and the physical and chemical factors and processes involved
proct/o		**proct**ology	prok-<u>tol</u>-o-je	the branch of medicine concerned with disorders of the rectum and anus

TABLE 6-1 *(continued)*

Root	Suffix	Word Example	Pronunciation	Definition
psych/o	-logy	**psych**ology	si-<u>kol</u>-o-je	the science dealing with the mind and mental processes, especially in relation to human and animal behavior
radi/o		**radi**ology	ra´-de-<u>ol</u>-o-je	the branch of medical science dealing with the use of x-rays, radioactive substances, and other forms of radiant energy in the diagnosis and treatment of disease
ur/o		**ur**ology	u-<u>rol</u>-o-je	the branch of medicine dealing with the urinary system in the female and the genitourinary system in the male
phys	-iatry	**phys**iatry	<u>fiz</u>-e-ah-tree	the branch of medicine that deals with the physical restoration, rehabilitation, and maintenance of the body structures
psych		**psych**iatry	si-<u>ki</u>-ah-tree	the branch of medicine that deals with the study, treatment, and prevention of mental illness

SPECIALTIES AND SPECIALISTS

Physicians and Medical Specialties

TABLE 6-2

Root	Suffix	Word Example	Pronunciation	Definition
esthesia	-ologist	an**esthesi**ologist	an´-es-the´-ze-<u>ol</u>-o-jist	a physician who specializes in anesthesiology; an anesthesiologist administers anesthetics, of which there are two types: *general* anesthetics, which produce sleep, and *regional* anesthetics, which render a specific area insensible to pain
cardi/o		**cardi**ologist	kar´-de-<u>ol</u>-o-jist	a physician skilled in the diagnosis and treatment of heart disease
derm/o (dermat/o)		**derm**atologist	der´-mah-<u>tol</u>-o-jist	a physician who specializes in the treatment of infections, growths, and injuries related to the skin
endocrin/o		**endocrin**ologist	en´-do-kri-<u>nol</u>-o-jist	a physician skilled in the diagnosis and treatment of disorders of the glands of internal secretion
gastr/ oenter/o		**gastroenter**ologist	gas-tro-en´-ter-<u>ol</u>-o-jist	a physician who specializes in the study of the stomach and intestines and their diseases

(continues)

TABLE 6-2 *(continued)*

Root	Suffix	Word Example	Pronunciation	Definition
geriatric	-ician	geriatrician	jer´-e-a-<u>trish</u>-an	a physician who specializes in the diagnosis and treatment of the diseases of the aging and elderly
gynec/o	-ologist	gynecologist	gi´-ne-<u>kol</u>-o-jist	a physician who specializes in the diseases of the genital tract in women
hemat/o		hematologist	he´-mah-<u>tol</u>-o-jist	a physician who specializes in the science of blood and blood-forming tissues
intern	-ist	internist	in-<u>ter</u>-nist	a physician who specializes in internal organs of the body and their function
neur/o	-ologist	neurologist	nu-<u>rol</u>-o-jist	a physician who specializes in the science of the central nervous system
obstetric	-ian	obstetrician	ob´-ste-<u>trish</u>-an	a physician who specializes in pregnancy, labor, and the puerperium
onc/o	-ologist	oncologist	ong-<u>kol</u>-o-jist	a physician who specializes in the study of tumors
ophthalm/o		ophthalmologist	of´-thal-<u>mol</u>-o-jist	a physician who specializes in diagnosing and prescribing treatment for defects, injuries, and diseases of the eye
orth/o	-ist	orthopedist	<u>or</u>-tho-pe´-dist	a surgeon who specializes in the preservation and restoration of the function of the skeletal system, its articulation, and associated structures
ot/orhin/ olaryng/o	-ologist	otorhinolaryngologist	o´-to-ri´-no-lar-ing-<u>gol</u>-o-jist	a physician who specializes in the diseases of the ear, nose, and throat
path/o		pathologist	pah-<u>thol</u>-o-jist	a physician who specializes in diagnosing changes in body tissues and organs that cause or are caused by disease
pediatric	-ian	pediatrician	pe´-de-ah-<u>trish</u>-an	a physician who specializes in the diagnosis and treatment of children´s diseases
phys	-ist	physiatrist	fiz´-i-<u>a</u>-trist	a physician who specializes in prescribing and providing physical therapy and rehabilitation for patients requiring it
phys	-ician	physician	fi-<u>zish</u>-an	one who studies body function; an authorized practitioner of medicine
practice	-itioner	practitioner (family practice [MD, Doctor of Medicine] or general practice [DO, Doctor of Osteopathy])	prak-<u>tish</u>-a-ner	a physician who is schooled in six basic areas: internal medicine, obstetrics and gynecology, surgery, psychiatry, pediatrics, and community medicine; the practitioner can treat the whole family and coordinate specialty care if necessary

TABLE 6-2 *(continued)*

Root	Suffix	Word Example	Pronunciation	Definition
proct/o	-ologist	**proct**ologist	prok-<u>tol</u>-o-jist	a physician who specializes in the diagnosis and treatment of diseases of the rectum and anus
psych	-iatrist	**psych**iatrist	si-<u>ki</u>-a-trist	a physician who specializes in the diagnosis and treatment of mental disorders
radi/o	-ologist	**radi**ologist	ra´-de-<u>ol</u>-o-jist	a physician who specializes in the interpretation of x-rays and other radioactive substances used for diagnostic purposes

Other Health Professions

TABLE 6-3

Specialty	Title	Pronunciation	Definition
chiropractic (ki´-ro-prak-tik)	chiropractor (DC)	ki´-ro-<u>prak</u>-tor	a person trained in the manipulation of the vertebral column
dentistry (den-tis-tre)	dentist (DDS, DMD)	<u>den</u>-tist	a physician who is concerned with the teeth and associated structures
subspecialties of dentistry	endodontist	en´-do-<u>don</u>-tist	a dentist who specializes in conditions of the tooth pulp and root and the periapical tissues
	oral surgeon		a dentist who specializes in surgery of the mouth
	orthodontist	or´-tho-<u>don</u>-tist	a dentist who specializes in the treatment of irregularities of the teeth, malocclusion, and associated facial problems
	pedodontist	pe´-do-<u>don</u>-tist	a dentist who treats children´s teeth
	periodontist	per´-e-o-<u>don</u>-tist	a dentist who treats diseases of the gums
	prosthodontist	pros´-tho-<u>don</u>-tist	a dentist who constructs artificial appliances designed to restore and maintain oral function
related fields of dentisty	dental hygienist	<u>den</u>-tal hi´-<u>je</u>-nist	a dental specialist (not an MD) whose primary concern is maintenance of dental health and prevention of oral disease
	dental assistant		a person who assists the dentist at chairside
	dental technician		a person specially trained to prepare prosthetics, such as dentures, crowns, bridges, and partials

(continues)

TABLE 6-3 *(continued)*

Specialty	Title	Pronunciation	Definition
dietetics	registered dietitian (RD, MS, PhD)	reg-is-ter-ed di´-e-tish-an	a specialist schooled in the use of proper diet for the promotion of health, prevention of disease, and therapy for the treatment of disease
	dietetic technician (DTR)		a person with an associate of science degree trained to work under the guidance of a dietitian; can plan menus and/or nutritional care for patients
foot care	podiatrist (DMP)	po-di-ah-trist	a specialist who deals with the study and care of the foot
medical assisting	medical assistant		a person trained to assist physicians in examining and treating patients, routine laboratory testing, and assigned clerical duties
medical library	medical librarian (MLA)		a professional person skilled in providing large volumes of current information to professional staff and personnel in medicine, dentistry, nursing, pharmacy, and other allied health professions
medical records	medical record administrator		a person skilled in managing an information system that meets medical, ethical, and legal requirements, compiling statistics and directing and controlling medical record staff
	accredited record technician (ART)		a person who organizes, handles, and evaluates patient medical records
medical technology	medical technologist or clinical laboratory scientist (ASCP)		a person skilled in performing tests in a laboratory to identify and track disease
nursing	registered nurse (RN) or advanced practice nurse (APN)		a specialist licensed to work directly with patients, administering treatments as ordered by the physician
	nurse–midwife (RN, APN)	mid-wif	a professional nurse with additional training who specializes in the care of women throughout pregnancy, delivery, and the postpartum period
	nurse practitioner (RN, APN)		a registered nurse who has completed required additional training and certification; a nurse practitioner, with physician referral, is able to offer patients personal attention and follow-up care
	public health nurse (PHN)		a registered nurse concerned with the prevention of illness and care of the sick in a community setting rather than a healthcare facility

TABLE 6-3 *(continued)*

Specialty	Title	Pronunciation	Definition
nursing, practical	licensed practical nurse/licensed vocational nurse (LPN, LVN)		a person who has completed a 1-year program in a state-recognized school and has taken and passed the state licensing test; works under the supervision of an RN
	nursing assistant (CNA)		a person trained to help the RN and LPN in a clinical situation
physician assistant	physician assistant (PA)		a professional person trained in some medical procedures (not a physician) who performs limited duties under physician guidance
occupational therapy	occupational therapist (OTR)		a professional person schooled in the rehabilitation of fine motor skills who coordinates patient activities
optometry	optometrist (OD)	op-<u>tom</u>-e-trist	a professional person trained to examine the eyes and prescribe corrective lenses when there are irregularities in vision
pharmacy	pharmacist (RPh, PharmD)	<u>far</u>-mah-sist	one who is licensed to prepare, sell, or dispense drugs, compounds, and prescriptions
physical therapy	physical therapist (RPT)		a professional person skilled in the techniques of physical therapy and qualified to administer treatment prescribed by a physician or referred by a physician
psychology	psychologist (PhD, MS)	si-<u>kol</u>-o-jist	a person with advanced degrees who specializes in the treatment of disturbed mental processes and abnormal behavior; does not prescribe drugs
radiology	radiology technologist (ARRT)		one who specializes in the use of x-rays and radioactive isotopes in the diagnosis and treatment of disease and who works under the supervision of a radiologist
respiratory therapy	respiratory therapist (RRT)		one who holds at least an associate's degree in respiratory therapy and who assists patients to improve impaired respiratory functions under a physician's direction
social work	healthcare social worker (MSW, PhD)		a professional person skilled in helping patients and their families handle personal problems that result from long-term illness or disability
	psychiatric social worker (MSW, PhD, ACSW)		a professional person skilled in maintaining contact among patients with mental illness, their psychiatrist, and families and facilitating patients' return to community life
veterinary medicine	veterinarian (DVM)	vet´-er-i-<u>na</u>-re-an	a doctor trained and authorized to practice veterinary medicine and perform surgery on animals; may also do research

Additional Professions

Space limitations prohibit a complete presentation of known health professionals recognized by state and federal health authorities. Instead, Table 6-4 lists other health professions not covered previously.

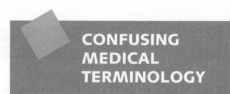

CONFUSING MEDICAL TERMINOLOGY

psychiatry Versus physiatry

psychiatry = treatment of mental disorders, e.g., psychiatry (si-<u>ki</u>-ah-tre) refers to the branch of medicine that deals with the treatment of mental disorders

physiatry = treatment of physical disorders, e.g., physiatry (fiz´-<u>i</u>-ah-tre) refers to the branch of medicine that deals with prescribing and providing physical therapy and rehabilitation for patients

---

TABLE 6-4   Additional Health Professions

• Animal Technicians	• Manual Arts Therapists
• Art Therapists	• Medical Illustrators
• Athletic Trainers	• Medical Secretaries
• Biological Photographers	• Medical Transcriptionists
• Community Health Educators	• Music Therapists
• Corrective Therapists	• Nuclear Medicine Technologists
• Dance Therapists	• Occupational Therapy Assistants
• Dietetic Assistants and Aides	• Opticians, Paraoptometrics
• Educational Therapists	• Orientation and Mobility Instructors for the Blind
• EEG Technologists and Technicians	• Paramedics
• EKG Technicians	• Pharmacy Assistants
• Emergency Medical Technicians (EMTs)	• Physical Therapy Assistants and Aides
• Healthcare Administrators	• Psychiatric/Mental Health Technicians
• Health Sciences Library Technicians	• Radiation Therapists
• Horticulture Therapists	• Radiology Technicians

Abbreviations

CHAPTER

7

Medical Abbreviations

LESSON ONE: MATERIALS TO BE LEARNED

Abbreviations for Services or Units in a Healthcare Facility
Abbreviations for Frequencies
Abbreviations for Units of Measure
Abbreviations for Means of Administering Substances into the Body
Abbreviations for Diet Orders
Abbreviations for Activity and Toiletry
Abbreviations for Laboratory Tests, X-Ray Studies, and Pulmonary Function
Abbreviations for Miscellaneous Terms

LESSON TWO: PROGRESS CHECK

Identify the Department
Identify the Prescription
Identify the Diet Order
Matching
Spell Out the Abbreviation

OBJECTIVES

After completion of this chapter and the exercises, the student should be able to:

1. Recognize medical abbreviations used by various services in a healthcare facility.
2. Identity abbreviations used when charting diet orders, activities, and medications for a patient.

LESSON ONE	Materials to Be Learned

The following information will help you in your study of medical abbreviations:

1. There are numerous medical abbreviations. Only samples are given in this chapter.
2. The necessity to learn certain medical abbreviations is directly related to a student's health career plan. For example, laboratory abbreviations and terms are essential for students planning to be Clinical Laboratory Technologists.
3. Physicians' handwriting, especially abbreviations, is difficult to read.
4. Purchase a medical abbreviations book recommended by your instructor.

ABBREVIATIONS FOR SERVICES OR UNITS IN A HEALTHCARE FACILITY

TABLE 7-1	
Abbreviation	**Definition**
A & D	admitting and discharge
CS	central service (or supply)
OR	operating room (surgery); MOR, minor surgery
RR	recovery room
PT & OT	physical therapy and occupational therapy (may be under PM & R, physical medicine and rehabilitation)
x-ray	radiology
lab	medical laboratory
MR	medical records
peds	pediatrics
Med-Surg	ward for medical and surgical patients (may be combined or separate)
OB	obstetrics (includes labor and delivery rooms, postpartum ward, and newborn nursery for healthy babies)
ICN or NICU	intensive care nursery, or newborn intensive care unit (for premature or unhealthy babies)
OPD	outpatient department
ER	emergency room; ED, emergency department
ENT	ear, nose, and throat
GU	genitourinary
NP	neuropsychiatric
SS	social service
CCU or ICU	coronary care unit or intensive care unit
DOU	definitive observation unit (less than intensive care, but more than "floor" care)
dietary (FS)	food service/dietary department
housekeeping	janitorial service
pharmacy	drugstore
morgue	unit for autopsies/holding the deceased
pathology (path)	laboratory for study of diseased tissues, including blood

ABBREVIATIONS FOR FREQUENCIES

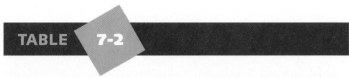

TABLE 7-2

Abbreviation	Definition
q	every
qd	once a day
qod	every other day
q ___ h	every ___ hours (insert hours)
bid	twice a day
tid	three times a day
qid	four times a day
hs	at bedtime (hour of sleep)
ac	before meals
pc	after meals
prn	when needed
ad lib	as desired
stat	immediately

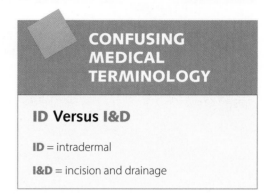

CONFUSING MEDICAL TERMINOLOGY

ID Versus I&D

ID = intradermal

I&D = incision and drainage

ABBREVIATIONS FOR UNITS OF MEASURE

TABLE 7-3

Abbreviation	Definition
tabs.	tablets, pills
g, gm	grams
gr.	grains
cc	cubic centimeters
mL, ml	milliliters

(continues)

TABLE 7-3 (continued)

Abbreviation	Definition
L	liter (1,000 cc or ml)
mEq	milliequivalent
U	units
gtts	drops
oz	ounces
dr.	drams

ABBREVIATIONS FOR MEANS OF ADMINSTERING SUBSTANCES INTO THE BODY

TABLE 7-4

Abbreviation	Definition
PO	by mouth (*per os*)
IV	intravenously (into a vein; usually a peripheral vein)
IM	intramuscularly (into a muscle)
H	hypodermically (with a needle)
subcu, subq	subcutaneously (through the skin, into the fatty tissue)
subling	sublingually (under the tongue)
R	rectally (by rectum)
parenteral	a solution given intravenously
enteral	tube feeding (into stomach or small intestine)
D_5W	5% glucose in distilled water; use IV
caps.	capsules
supp	suppository

TABLE 7-4	(continued)
Abbreviation	**Definition**
ss	one-half
mg	milligrams
N.S.	normal saline solution: isotonic solution
clysis	fluids given by needle, under skin (not in vein)
TKO	to keep open (vein)
KVO	keep vein open

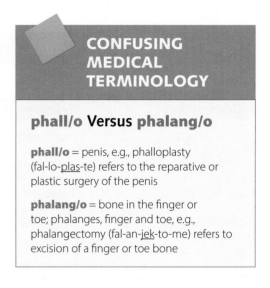

CONFUSING MEDICAL TERMINOLOGY

phall/o Versus phalang/o

phall/o = penis, e.g., phalloplasty (fal-lo-<u>plas</u>-te) refers to the reparative or plastic surgery of the penis

phalang/o = bone in the finger or toe; phalanges, finger and toe, e.g., phalangectomy (fal-an-<u>jek</u>-to-me) refers to excision of a finger or toe bone

ABBREVIATIONS FOR DIET ORDERS

TABLE 7-5	
Abbreviation	**Definition**
NPO	nothing *per os* (nothing to eat or drink orally)
I & O	intake and output (measured)
Cl Liq	clear liquids only: ginger ale, tea, broth, Jell-O, 7-Up, coffee
F Liq	full liquid: addition of milk and milk products; liquid at body temperature
Lo Salt, Low Na, Salt Free	restricted in sodium: ordered by mg or g of sodium desired, e.g., 2 g Na, 500 mg Na
NAS	no added salt packet; usually 4–6 g Na (mild restriction)
reg	regular diet ("house" or "normal" sometimes used); a balanced diet without restrictions as to the type of food texture, seasoning, or preparation method
mech soft	mechanical soft; a regular diet with alteration in texture only; sometimes called "edentulous"
med soft	medical soft; alterations in texture, preparation methods, and seasonings
bland	a medical soft diet further altered to omit acid-producing beverages and restrict seasonings; altered feeding intervals
Lo res	low residue; alteration in texture and a limited food selection to yield little intestinal residue
high fiber	a regular diet with increased amounts of foods containing dietary fiber
FF or PF	force or push fluids; increasing the liquid intake by addition of extra fluids

(continues)

TABLE 7-5   *(continued)*

Abbreviation	Definition
int fdg or int nour	interval feeding; supplemental nourishment served between meals
DAT	diet as tolerated
dysphagia pureed	regular diet pureed to a smooth, homogeneous, and cohesive consistency like pudding
consistent or controlled carbohydrate (CCHO)	consistent amounts of carbohydrate at meals and snacks to regulate blood glucose levels primarily for diabetes
Lo Fat, Lo Chol	low saturated fat, low cholesterol; a "Healthy Diet," based on *The Dietary Guidelines for Americans, 2010*, to reduce the risk of heart disease

ABBREVIATIONS FOR ACTIVITY AND TOILETRY

TABLE 7-6

Abbreviation	Definition
CBR	complete bed rest; ABR (absolute bed rest)
dangle	sit at edge of bed, legs over side
ambulate	walk
OOB	out of bed
BRP	bathroom privileges; may be up to bathroom only
commode	bedside toilet

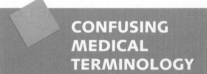

CONFUSING MEDICAL TERMINOLOGY

phren/o Versus phren/o

phren/o (phreno, phren, phreni, phrenic) = mind, e.g., phrenology (fri-<u>nol</u>-uh-jee) refers to a psychological theory or analytical method based on the belief that certain mental faculties and character traits (the mind) are indicated by the configurations of the skull

phren/o (phreno, phren, phreni, phrenic) = diaphragm, e.g., phrenogastric (fre-<u>no</u>-gas-trik) refers to the diaphragm and stomach

ABBREVIATIONS FOR LABORATORY TESTS, X-RAY STUDIES, AND PULMONARY FUNCTION

TABLE 7-7

Abbreviation	Definition
AP and Lat	routine x-ray picture of chest (front to back and side view)
up	upright x-ray picture
decub	decubitus (lying) position

TABLE 7-7 (continued)

Abbreviation	Definition
IVP	intravenous pyelogram (kidney)
BE	barium enema (colon)
2GI series	upper (barium swallow): x-ray of stomach/duodenum; lower (same as BE): x-ray of lower bowel/colon
GB series	gallbladder x-ray picture
MRI	magnetic resonance imaging; noninvasive procedure using a magnetic field that yields images for diagnosis
RAI, RAIU	radioactive iodine (uptake) for diagnosing thyroid function
SCAN	CT, CAT: computed tomography, computerized axial tomography
CBC	complete blood count
UA	urinalysis
VC	vital capacity (lungs)

ABBREVIATIONS FOR MISCELLANEOUS TERMS

TABLE 7-8

Abbreviation	Definition
qns	quantity not sufficient (lab requires a larger specimen); also refers to insufficient food/liquid intake
c̄	with (con)
s̄	without (sans)
dc	discontinue
TLC	tender loving care
stat	immediately
ASAP	as soon as possible
CPR	cardiopulmonary resuscitation

(continues)

TABLE 7-8 *(continued)*

Abbreviation	Definition
EUA	examination under anesthesia
DOA	dead on arrival
OD	overdose; also means right eye (refer to context where used)
prep	prepare
V/S	vital signs
ECG, EKG	electrocardiogram
EEG	electroencephalogram
Dx	diagnosis
Tx	treatment
Rx	prescription
Sx	symptoms
Na^+	natrium: sodium (chemical symbol for)
K^+	potassium (chemical symbol for)
Ca^{++}	calcium (chemical symbol for)
P^{+++}	phosphorus (chemical symbol for)
Cl^-	chloride (chemical symbol for)
I^-	iodine (chemical symbol for)
Fe^{++}	iron (chemical symbol for)
Hg^{++}	mercury (chemical symbol for)
DS	double strength
O.S.	left eye
PDR	*Physicians' Desk Reference*

CHAPTER

8

Diagnostic and Laboratory Abbreviations

LESSON ONE: MATERIALS TO BE LEARNED

Diagnostic Abbreviations
Laboratory Abbreviations
A List of Common Diagnostic and
    Laboratory Abbreviations

LESSON TWO: PROGRESS CHECK

Identify the Disease
Short Answer
Matching
Define the Abbreviation

OBJECTIVES

After completion of this chapter and the exercises, the student should be able to:

1. Use appropriate abbreviations for diagnostic, laboratory, and x-ray procedures.
2. Describe some abbreviations specific to a particular medical facility or specialty unit.

DIAGNOSTIC ABBREVIATIONS

TABLE 8-1

Abbreviation	Definition
A & P	auscultation and percussion
ASHD	arteriosclerotic heart disease
CA	carcinoma (cancer)
CBS	chronic brain syndrome
CC	chief complaint
CHD	coronary heart disease; congenital heart disease
CHF	congestive heart failure
c/o	complains of
COPD/COLD	chronic obstructive pulmonary (lung) disease
CP	cerebral palsy
CVA	cerebrovascular accident (stroke)
CVD	cardiovascular disease
DJD	degenerative joint disease (osteoarthritis)
Dx	diagnosis
FH	family history
FUO	fever of undetermined origin
GC	gonorrhea
HEENT	head, eyes, ears, nose, throat
Hx	history
(S)LE	(systemic) lupus erythematosus
m	murmur

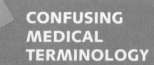

CONFUSING MEDICAL TERMINOLOGY

papill/o Versus papul/o

papill/o = nipple like, nipple, e.g., papillar (puh-<u>pil</u>-er) refers to resembling a nipple

papul/o = pimple, e.g., papule (<u>pap</u>-yool) refers to a small somewhat pointed elevation of the skin, usually inflammatory but nonsupportive

TABLE 8-1 (continued)

Abbreviation	Definition
MD	muscular dystrophy
MI	myocardial infarction
MS	multiple sclerosis
P & A	percussion and auscultation
PE	physical examination
PERRLA	pupils equal, round, react to light and accommodation (eyes)
PH	past history
PI	present illness
PID	pelvic inflammatory disease
RA	rheumatoid arthritis
R/O	rule out
Rx	recipe, take, prescription
SOB	short of breath
SR or ROS	systemic review or review of systems
Sx	symptoms
T & A	tonsillectomy and adenoidectomy
TIA	transient ischemic attack
TPR	temperature, pulse, respiration
URI	upper respiratory infection
UTI	urinary tract infection

LABORATORY ABBREVIATIONS

TABLE 8-2	
Abbreviation	**Definition**
AFB	acid-fast bacillus (tuberculosis organism)
C & S	culture and sensitivity
CATH	catheterize
CBC	complete blood count
Crit, Hct	hematocrit
diff	differential
ESR	erythrocyte sedimentation rate
FBS	fasting blood sugar
GTT	glucose tolerance test
Hb, Hgb	hemoglobin
RA	rheumatoid arthritis
RBC	red blood (cell) count (erythrocytes); red blood cells
STS	serologic test of syphilis
VDRL	venereal disease research laboratory
WBC	white blood (cell) count (leukocytes); white blood cells

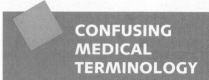

CONFUSING MEDICAL TERMINOLOGY

Hgb, HB, Hb Versus Hg

Hgb, HB, Hb = abbreviations for hemoglobin

Hg = abbreviation for mercury

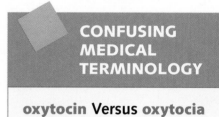

CONFUSING MEDICAL TERMINOLOGY

oxytocin Versus oxytocia

oxytocin = labor-inducing drug

oxytocia = rapid birth

A LIST OF COMMON DIAGNOSTIC AND LABORATORY ABBREVIATIONS*

TABLE 8-3	
Name of Test, Screening, Procedure, or Others	**Explanatory Notes**
cardio CRP™ (high-sensitivity C-reactive protein)	as stated in name
cervical biopsy	as stated in name
chlamydia tests	sexually transmitted diseases (STDs)
chloride (Cl)	blood/chemistry tests

TABLE 8-3	*(continued)*

Name of Test, Screening, Procedure, or Others	Explanatory Notes
cholesterol and triglycerides tests	blood/chemistry tests
chromosome analysis	as stated in name
CK (creatine kinase)	as stated in name
colon biopsy	as stated in name
colorectal cancer screen	as stated in name
complete blood count (CBC)	blood/chemistry tests
creatinine and creatinine clearance	blood/chemistry tests
C-reactive protein	as stated in name
cystic fibrosis test	screening
esophageal biopsy	as stated in name
fecal occult blood test	as stated in name
ferritin	blood/chemistry tests
folic acid	blood/chemistry tests
follicle-stimulating hormone (FSH)	as stated in name
glycohemoglobin (GHb)	as stated in name
gonorrhea test	sexually transmitted diseases (STDs)
Helicobacter pylori (H. pylori) tests	as stated in name
hemoglobin (part of CBC)	as stated in name
hepatitis B antigen and antibody tests	sexually transmitted diseases (STDs)
hepatitis C genotype	as stated in name
hepatitis C viral load	as stated in name
hepatitis C virus test	as stated in name
herpes test	sexually transmitted diseases (STDs)
HIV testing	sexually transmitted diseases (STDs)
HIV viral load	as stated in name
homocysteine	as stated in name

(continues)

TABLE 8-3 *(continued)*

Name of Test, Screening, Procedure, or Others	Explanatory Notes
HPV test (human papillomavirus)	sexually transmitted diseases (STDs)
human chorionic gonadotropin (hCG)	blood/chemistry tests
iron tests	blood/chemistry tests
lactic dehydrogenase (LDH)	blood/chemistry tests
lead	as stated in name
luteinizing hormone (LH)	as stated in name
magnesium (Mg)	blood/chemistry tests
maternal serum screening: alpha-fetoprotein (AFP) in blood estrogens, human chorionic gonadotropin (hCG), and maternal serum triple test	blood/chemistry tests
osteoporosis/bone mineral density testing	as stated in name
ovarian cancer	as stated in name
Pap test	as stated in name
parathyroid hormone (bio-intact PTH)	as stated in name
partial thromboplastin time (PTT)	as stated in name
phosphorus: phosphate in blood and phosphate in urine	blood/urine chemistry tests
potassium (K)	blood/chemistry tests
progesterone	as stated in name
prolactin	as stated in name
prostate biopsy	as stated in name
prostate-specific antigen (PSA)	as stated in name
prothrombin time (PT)	as stated in name
rheumatoid factor (RF)	as stated in name
rubella test	as stated in name
sedimentation rate	as stated in name
sickle cell testing	as stated in name
skin biopsy	as stated in name
sodium (Na)	blood/chemistry tests

Review

CHAPTER 9

Review of Word Parts from Units I, II, and III

LESSON ONE: MATERIALS TO BE LEARNED

Review A: Suffixes
Review B: Prefixes
Review C: Root Words for Body Parts
Review D: Descriptive Word Elements
Review E: Additional Medical Terms

LESSON TWO: PROGRESS CHECK

Compare and Contrast
Building Medical Terms
Fill-in
Define the Term
Matching
Short Answer: Root Words
Short Answer: Body Parts

OBJECTIVES

After completion of this chapter and the exercises, the student should be able to:

1. Define the meaning of given word elements.
2. Define whole medical terms by applying knowledge gained from previous study.
3. Recognize the meaning of new terms by dividing them into their respective elements.

This review chapter is designed to assist you by pulling together the terminology to reinforce your learning. These exercises are designed as learning tools. They give you the opportunity to write in your answers and test yourself. Check your answers carefully against the information contained in the previous three units. You also may use your medical dictionary. Check your spelling of the terms because spelling is very important to the meaning of medical words.

If you have audiotapes with your text, listen to each term for the correct pronunciation and repeat the word out loud several times so you will be comfortable using it in conversation.

LESSON ONE	Materials to Be Learned

REVIEW A: SUFFIXES

Write the meaning of each suffix in the space provided:

Suffix	Meaning
-algia	
-cele	
-dynia	
-ectasis	
-emia	
-gen	
-gram	
-graph	
-graphy	
-gravid	
-iasis	
-itis	
-logy	
-malacia	
-megaly	
-meter	
-metry	
-oid	
-oma	
-pathy	
-penia	
-phagia	
-phasia	
-phobia	

Suffix	Meaning
-plegia	
-ptosis	
-rrhage	
-rrhea	
-rrhexis	
-sclerosis	
-scopy	
-sis	
-spasm	
-stasis	

CONFUSING MEDICAL TERMINOLOGY

trop/o Versus troph/o

trop/o or tropo = turn, turning, change, e.g., tropocollagen (tro-po-<u>col</u>-la-gen) refers to the molecular component of a collagen fiber, consisting of three polypeptide chains coiled around each other; e.g., tropism (troh-piz-<u>uhm</u>) refers to an orientation (movement or bending) of an organism to an external stimulus (i.e., light, heat, gravity) especially by growth rather than by movement

troph/o = relation to nutrition, nourishment, development, growth, e.g., trophoplasm (<u>tra</u>-fo-plae-zem) refers to a type of protoplasm that provides nourishment to a cell

REVIEW B: PREFIXES

Write the meaning of each prefix in the space provided:

Prefix	Meaning
a-, an-	
ab-	
ad-	
aero-	
aniso-	
bi-	
brady-	
de-	
di-	
dia-	
dif-, dis-	
dys-	
ec-, ecto-	
end-, endo-	
ep-, epi-	

(continues)

Prefix	Meaning
eu-	
ex-, exo-	
extra-	
hemi-	
hemo-	
hetero-	
homo-	
hyper-	
hypo-	
in-	
iso-	
lip-	
mal-	
mega-	
megalo-	
meno-	
meta-	
noct-	
nyct-	
pan-	
para-	
per-	
peri-	
poly-	
post-	
pre-	
pro-	
pyo-	
pyro-	

CONFUSING MEDICAL TERMINOLOGY

per- Versus peri- Versus pre-

per- = excessive, through, e.g., pertussis (per-<u>tus</u>-is) refers to the medical form for whooping cough, a respiratory infection caused by the bacteria *Bordetella pertussis*, marked by a peculiar cough ending in a prolonged crowing or whooping respiration

peri- = around, surrounding, e.g., periatrial (per-re-<u>a</u>-tre-al) refers to around the area surrounding or around the atrium of the heart

pre- = before, in front of, e.g., premenstrual (pre-<u>men</u>-stroo-uh) refers to the one or two days before the menstrual period

CONFUSING MEDICAL TERMINOLOGY

peritone/o Versus perone/o Versus perine/o

peritone/o = membrane that lines the abdominal cavity, peritoneum, e.g., peritoneal (per-rih-<u>to</u>-ne-al) refers to pertaining to peritoneum

perone/o = fibula, e.g., perone (puh-<u>rohn</u>) refers to the small bone of the arm or leg, the fibula

perine/o = the space between the anus and external reproductive organs, perineum, e.g., episioperineoplasty (<u>ep</u>-iz-e-o-peh-rih-ne-o-plas-te) refers to plastic repair of the vulva and perineum

Prefix	Meaning
re-	
super-	
supra-	
syn-	
tachy-	

REVIEW C: ROOT WORDS FOR BODY PARTS

Many of the words in this section have been introduced to you in previous chapters. They should serve as a small review of root words.

Cover each definition in the right column and try to define the term before looking at the answer by using previous knowledge of word parts. A short definition is okay. The answer column contains a more detailed definition, but your answer may contain just the essential meaning of the word at this time.

TABLE 9-1

Root Word	Meaning	Word Example	Pronunciation	Definition
carp/o	wrist	meta**carp**al	met´-ah-<u>kar</u>-pal	the bones between the wrist and fingers
celi/o	abdomen			see *lapar/o*
cervic/o	neck	**cervic**al	<u>serv</u>-i-cal	pertaining to the neck or to the cervix
		cervix (of uterus)	<u>ser</u>-viks	the narrow lower end (neck) of the uterus
chondr/o	cartilage	**chondr**itis	kon-<u>dri</u>-tis	inflammation of a cartilage
colp/o	vagina	**colp**itis	kol-<u>pi</u>-tis	inflammation of the vagina; vaginitis
dent/o- odont	teeth	**dent**ist	<u>den</u>-tist	a person who has received a degree in dentistry and is authorized to practice dentistry
		orth**odont**ia	or-tho-<u>don</u>-ti-a	the branch of dentistry concerned with correcting and preventing irregularities of the teeth
esophag/o	esophagus	**esophag**itis	e-sof´-ah-<u>ji</u>-tis	inflammation of the esophagus
lapar/o	abdominal wall	**lapar**otomy	lap´-ah-<u>rot</u>-o-me	incision through the flank or, more generally, through any part of the abdominal wall
laryng/o	larynx	**laryng**itis	lar´-in-<u>ji</u>-tis	inflammation of the larynx

(continues)

TABLE **9-1** *(continued)*

Root Word	Meaning	Word Example	Pronunciation	Definition
myring/o	myringo (eardrum)	**myring**otomy	mir´-ing-<u>got</u>-o-me	incision of the tympanic membrane; tympanotomy
onych/o	nail	par**onych**ia	par´-o-<u>nik</u>-e-ah	inflammation in the folds of the tissue around the fingernail
oophor/o	ovary	**oophor**ectomy	o´-of-o-<u>rek</u>-to-me	excision of one or both ovaries
ophthalm/o	eye	**ophthalm**ologist	of´-thal-<u>mol</u>-o-jist	a physician who specializes in diseases of the eyes
pancreat/o	pancreas	**pancreat**itis	pan´-kre-ah-<u>ti</u>-tis	inflammation of the pancreas
pelv/i	pelvis	**pelv**imeter	pel-<u>vim</u>-e-ter	an instrument for measuring the pelvis
phleb/o	vein	**phleb**itis	fle-<u>bi</u>-tis	inflammation of a vein
pleur/o	pleura	**pleur**isy	<u>ploor</u>-i-se	inflammation of the pleura
pod/o	foot	**pod**iatry	po-<u>di</u>-ah-tre	specialized field dealing with the treatment and care of the foot
psych/o	mind	**psych**iatrist	si-<u>ki</u>-ah-trist	a physician who specializes in treatment of the mind
pub/o	pubes (pubic bones)	supra**pub**ic	soo´-prah-<u>pu</u>-bik	above the pubes
rhin/o	nose	**rhin**oplasty	<u>ri</u>-no-plas´-te	plastic surgery of the nose
salping/o	fallopian tube or Eustachian tube	**salping**itis	sal´-pin-<u>ji</u>-tis	inflammation of the uterine or auditory tube
soma	body	psycho**soma**tic	si´-ko-so-<u>mat</u>-ik	pertaining to the mind–body relationship; having bodily symptoms of psychic, emotional, or mental origin
splen/o	spleen	**splen**ectomy	sple-<u>nek</u>-to-me	excision of the spleen
spondyl/o	vertebra	**spondyl**itis	spon´-di-<u>li</u>-tis	inflammation of the vertebrae
stomat/o	mouth	**stomat**itis	sto´-mah-<u>ti</u>-tis	generalized inflammation of the oral mucosa
tars/o	ankle	meta**tars**al	met´-ah-<u>tar</u>-sal	bones between the ankle and toes
thorac/o	thorax (chest)	**thorac**entesis	tho´-rah-sen-<u>te</u>-sis	surgical puncture of the chest wall into the parietal cavity for aspiration of fluids
tympan/o	tympanum (eardrum or middle ear)	**tympan**otomy	tim´-pah-<u>not</u>-o-me	incision of the tympanic membrane
ureter/o	ureter	**ureter**itis	u-re´-ter-<u>i</u>-tis	inflammation of a ureter

Root Word	Meaning	Word Example	Pronunciation	Definition
urethr/o	urethra	**urethr**itis	u´-re-<u>thri</u>-tis	inflammation of the urethra
vas/o	vessel	cardio**vas**cular	kar´-de-o-<u>vas</u>-ku-lar	pertaining to the heart and blood vessels
ven/o	vein	intra**ven**ous	in´-trah-<u>ve</u>-nus	within a vein

TABLE 9-1 (continued)

REVIEW D: DESCRIPTIVE WORD ELEMENTS

TABLE 9-2

Root Word	Meaning	Word Example	Pronunciation	Definition
ankyl/o	stiffening or fusion	**ankyl**osis	ang´-ki-<u>lo</u>-sis	immobility and consolidation of a joint from disease, injury, or surgical procedure
carcin/o	cancer (malignancy)	**carcin**omo	kar´-si-<u>no</u>-mah	a malignant new growth made up of epithelial cells that may infiltrate surrounding tissues
cry/o	cold	**cry**osurgery	kri´-o-<u>ser</u>-jer-e	the destruction of tissue by application of extreme cold
crypt/o	hidden (small hidden sac)	**crypt**orchidism	krip-<u>tor</u>-ki-dism	failure of one or both testes to descend into the scrotum
esthesia	feeling	an**esthesia**	an´-es-<u>the</u>-ze-ah	loss of feeling or sensation, especially the loss of pain sensation induced to permit surgery
gravid/o	pregnant	primi**gravid**a	pri´-mi-<u>grav</u>-i-dah	a woman pregnant for the first time, gravida I
lip/o	fat	**lip**oma	li-<u>po</u>-mah	a benign fatty tumor
lith/o	stone	chole**lith**iasis	ko´-le-li-<u>thi</u>-ah-sis	the presence or formation of gallstones
necr/o	dead (decayed)	**necr**osis	ne-<u>kro</u>-sis	cell death: it may affect groups of cells or part of a structure or an organ
par-	to bear (children)	multi**para**	mul-<u>tip</u>-ah-rah	a woman who has had two or more pregnancies
path/o	disease state	osteo**path**y	os´-te-<u>op</u>-ah-the	any disease of a bone
phag/o-phagia	eating, swallowing	dys**phag**ia	dis-<u>fa</u>-je-ah	difficulty in swallowing

(continues)

TABLE 9-2 *(continued)*

Root Word	Meaning	Word Example	Pronunciation	Definition
-phasia	speech	a**phasia**	ah-<u>fa</u>-zhe-ah	defect or loss of the power of expression by speech, writing, or signs or of comprehending spoken or written language, caused by injury or disease of the brain centers
phon/o	voice	a**phon**ia	a-<u>fo</u>-ne-ah	loss of voice; inability to produce vocal sounds
schiz/o	split	**schiz**ophrenia	skit´-so-<u>fre</u>-ne-ah	any of a group of severe emotional disorders characterized by withdrawal from reality, delusions, hallucinations, and bizarre behavior
scler/o	hardening	arterio**scler**osis	ar-te´-re-o´-skle-<u>ro</u>-sis	hardening and thickening of the walls of arterioles
sta	slowed, halted, controlled	hemo**sta**sis	he´-mo-<u>sta</u>-sis	the arrest of bleeding, either by vasoconstriction and coagulation or by surgical means
therap	treatment	psycho**therapy**	si-ko-<u>ther</u>-ah-pe	treatment designed to produce a response by mental rather than physical effects
therm/o	heat	**therm**ometer	ther-<u>mom</u>-e-ter	an instrument for determining temperatures
thromb/o	clot, lump	**thromb**osis	throm-<u>bo</u>-sis	the formation or presence of a thrombus (clot)
traumat/o	injury, wound, damage from an external source	**traumat**openea	<u>traw</u>-ma-top-ne´-ah	passage of air through a wound in the chest wall

REVIEW E: ADDITIONAL MEDICAL TERMS

Review E on additional medical terms contains some words with which you will not be familiar. Test your ability to recognize the meaning of new medical terms by covering the definition column on the right side, dividing the word into its respective parts, and seeing if you can define it before you look at the answer.

TABLE 9-3

Word	Pronunciation	Definition
abdomen	<u>ab</u>-do´-men	that part of the body lying between the thorax and the pelvis and containing the abdominal cavity and viscera
abdominal	ab-<u>dom</u>-i-nal	pertaining to the abdomen
abortion	ah-<u>bor</u>-shun	expulsion from the uterus of the products of conception before the fetus is viable
abscess	<u>ab</u>-ses	a localized collection of pus in a cavity formed by disintegration of tissues

TABLE 9-3	*(continued)*	

Word	Pronunciation	Definition
acute	ah-<u>kut</u>	sharp; having severe symptoms and a short course
adhesion	ad-<u>he</u>-zhun	stuck together; abnormal joining of parts to one another
adnexa	ad-<u>nek</u>-sah	accessory structures of an organ: of the eye, including the eyelids and tear ducts; of the uterus, including the uterine tubes and ovaries
anomaly	ah-<u>nom</u>-ah-le	marked deviation from normal, especially as a result of congenital or hereditary defects
auscultation	aws´-kul-<u>ta</u>-shun	listening for sounds within the body, chiefly to detect conditions of the thorax, abdominal viscera, or a pregnancy
autoclave	<u>aw</u>-to-klav	a self-locking apparatus for the sterilization of materials by steam under pressure
axilla (axillary)	ak-<u>sil</u>-ah	the armpit
biopsy	<u>bi</u>-op-se	removal and examination, usually microscopic, of tissue from the living body, performed to establish precise diagnosis
catgut	<u>kat</u>-gut	an absorbable, sterile strand obtained from collagen derived from healthy mammals, used to suture
catheter	<u>kath</u>-e-ter	a tubular, flexible instrument passed through body cavities for withdrawal of fluids from (or introduction of fluids into) a body cavity
cervical	<u>ser</u>-vi-kal	pertaining to the neck or to the cervix
chronic	<u>kron</u>-ik	persisting for a long time
coccyx	<u>kok</u>-siks	triangular bone formed usually by fusion of last four vertebrae; the "tailbone"
congenital	kon-<u>jen</u>-i-tal	existing at the time of birth
defibrillator	de-fib´-ri-<u>la</u>-tor	an electronic apparatus used to produce defibrillation by application of brief electric shock to the heart directly or through electrodes placed on the chest wall
dilatation	dil´-ah-<u>ta</u>-shun	the condition of being stretched open beyond normal dimensions
dilation	di-<u>la</u>-shun	the act of dilating or stretching
edema	e-<u>de</u>-mah	an abnormal accumulation of fluid in intercellular spaces of the body (see **Figure 9–1**)
embolus	<u>em</u>-bo-lus	a clot or other plug brought by the blood from another vessel and forced into a smaller one, thus obstructing the circulation
emesis	<u>em</u>-e-sis	the act of vomiting; also used as a word termination, as in hematemesis
enema	<u>en</u>-e-mah	introduction of fluid into the rectum for evacuation of feces or as a means of introducing nutrient or medicinal substances, or the opaque material used in roentgenographic examination of the lower intestinal tract (BE)

(continues)

TABLE 9-3 (continued)

Word	Pronunciation	Definition
exacerbation	eg-zas´-er-<u>ba</u>-shun	increase in severity of a disease or any of its symptoms
excretion	eks-<u>kre</u>-shun	the act of eliminating waste
fascia	<u>fash</u>-e-ah	a sheet or band of fibrous tissue that lies deep to the skin or binds muscles and various body organs
febrile	<u>feb</u>-ril	pertaining to fever; feverish
fibrillation	fib´-ri-<u>la</u>-shun	a small, local, involuntary muscular contraction caused by activation of muscle cells or fibers
hemorrhage	<u>hem</u>-o-rij	the escape of blood from the vessels; bleeding
icterus	<u>ik</u>-ter-us	jaundice
immunization	im´-u-ni-<u>za</u>-shun	the process of providing immunity to disease processes
incontinence	in-<u>kon</u>-ti-nens	inability to control bowel and bladder functions
inflammation	in´-flah-<u>ma</u>-shun	a protective tissue response to injury or destruction of tissues
ischemia	is-<u>ke</u>-me-ah	deficiency of blood in a part, caused by functional constriction or actual obstruction of a blood vessel
jaundice	<u>jawn</u>-dis	icterus; yellowness of the skin, sclerae, mucous membranes, and excretions
metastasis	me-<u>tas</u>-tah-sis	transfer of disease from one organ or body part to another not directly connected with it
mucus	<u>mu</u>-kus	the free slime of the mucous membranes, composed of secretions of the glands, various salts, desquamated cells, and leukocytes
obese	o-<u>bes</u>	very fat; stout; corpulent
obesity	o-<u>bes</u>-i-te	an increase in body weight beyond the limitation of skeletal and physical requirements: the result of excessive accumulation of body fat
palpable	<u>pal</u>-pah-bul	felt by touching
paralysis	pah-<u>ral</u>-i-sis	loss or impairment of voluntary motor function
paralyzed	<u>par</u>-e-lizd	a condition of helplessness caused by inability to move; being ineffective or powerless
parietal	pah-<u>ri</u>-e-tal	pertaining to the walls of a cavity or located near the parietal bone
percussion	per-<u>kush</u>-un	the act of striking a part with short, sharp blows as an aid in diagnosing the condition of the underlying parts by the sound obtained
perineum	per´-i-<u>ne</u>-um	the pelvic floor and associated structures occupying the pelvic outlet
peritoneum	per´-i-to-<u>ne</u>-um	the serous membrane lining the walls of the abdominal and pelvic cavities and the contained viscera

Medical Terminology and Body Systems

CHAPTER 10

Body Organs and Parts

LESSON ONE: MATERIALS TO BE LEARNED

Structural Units of the Body
Body Cavities and Planes
Metabolism and Homeostasis

LESSON TWO: PROGRESS CHECK

Spelling and Definition
Fill-in
Definitions
Short Answer

OBJECTIVES

After completing this chapter and the exercises, the student should be able to:

1. Identify the parts of a cell and the specialized functions of tissues.
2. Identify the body systems.
3. Describe the functions of the body systems and how they work together.
4. Define the anatomic positions of the body and directional terms used to indicate them.
5. List the body cavities and the organs contained within them.
6. Identify nine body regions.
7. Use appropriate medical terms when describing locations of various parts of the body.

This chapter focuses on the way medical terms that you have previously learned relate to the body as a whole. To accurately understand and communicate data from medical reports, medical personnel use topographic anatomy. *Topographic* refers to the surface landmarks of the body. They are used as guides to the internal structures that lie beneath them, as well as the major regions of the body and their locations.

To describe the position of a structure or locate one structure in relation to another, medical professionals start with a position called the anatomical position. In this position, a person is standing erect, facing you, with hands at sides and palms forward, and feet and head pointed straight ahead. This is the position you will use to find the landmarks of the body. We begin with a discussion of cells, the structural and functional unit of all living matter.

ALLIED HEALTH PROFESSIONS

Dietitians and Dietetic Technicians

Dietitians are professionals trained in applying the principles of nutrition to food selection and meal preparation. They help prevent and treat illnesses by promoting healthy eating habits, scientifically evaluating clients' diets, and suggesting diet modifications. They counsel individuals and groups; set up and supervise food service systems for institutions such as schools, hospitals, and prisons; promote sound eating habits through education; and conduct research. Major areas of specialization include clinical, management, community, business and industry, and consultant dietetics. Dietitians also work as educators and researchers.

A dietetic technician, registered (DTR), works as a member of the food service, management, and healthcare team, independently or in consultation with a registered dietitian. The dietetic technician supervises support staff, monitors cost-control procedures, interprets and implements quality assurance procedures, counsels individuals or small groups, screens patients/clients for nutritional status, and develops nutrition care plans. The dietetic technician helps to supervise food production and service; plans menus; tests new products for use in the facility; and selects, schedules, and conducts orientation programs for personnel. The technician may also be involved in selecting personnel and providing on-the-job training. The dietetic technician obtains, evaluates, and uses dietary histories to plan nutritional care for patients. Using this information, the technician guides families and individuals in selecting food, preparing it, and planning menus based on nutritional needs. The dietetic technician has an active part in calculating nutrient intakes and dietary patterns.

INQUIRY

The Academy of Nutrition and Dietetics: www.eatright.org

Data from Stanfield, Peggy S., Cross, Nanna, and Hui, Y.H. *Introduction to the Health Professions*, 6th ed. Burlington, MA: Jones & Bartlett Learning; 2012.

LESSON ONE   **Materials to Be Learned**

STRUCTURAL UNITS OF THE BODY

TABLE 10-1

Unit	Pronunciation	Definition
Cells		
cell	sel	minute protoplasmic masses making up organized tissue, consisting of the nucleus surrounded by cytoplasm enclosed in a cell or plasma membrane. Fundamental, structural, and functional unit of living organisms. Each cell performs functions necessary for its own life. Cells multiply by dividing; this is called mitosis
nucleus	nu-kle-us	cell nucleus; a spheroid body within a cell, consisting of a thin nuclear membrane and genes or chromosomes
chromosomes	kroh´-moh-sohms	thread-like structures in the cell nucleus that control growth, repair, and reproduction of the body
cytoplasm	si-to-plasm	the protoplasm of a cell exclusive of that of the nucleus (nucleoplasm)
cell membrane	sel mem-bran	a thin layer of tissue, serving as the wall of a cell; selectively allows substances to pass in and out of the cell, and refuses passage to others

TABLE 10-1 (continued)		

Unit	Pronunciation	Definition
Tissues		
tissue	tish-u	a group of similarly specialized cells that together perform certain special functions
epithelial tissue	ep´-i-the-le-al tish-u	the skin and lining surfaces that protect, absorb, and excrete
connective tissue	ko-nek-tiv tish-u	the fibrous tissues of the body; that which binds together and is the ground substance of the various parts and organs of the body; examples are bones, tendons, and so on
muscle tissue	mus-el tish-u	tissue that contracts; consists of striated (striped), cardiac, and smooth muscle
nerve tissue	nerv tish-u	a collection of nerve fibers that conduct impulses that control and coordinate body activities
Organ		
organ	or-gan	tissues arranged together to perform a specific function; these internal structures are contained within the body cavities. Some examples include the heart, lungs, and organs of digestion, such as the liver and gallbladder, and the organs of reproduction
Systems		
system	sis-tem	a set of body organs that work together for a common purpose
integumentary system	in-teg´-u-men-ter-e sis-tem	skin serves as the external covering of the body; accessory organs of this system are nails, hair, and oil and sweat glands
musculoskeletal system	mus´-ku-lo-skel-e-tal sis-tem	skeleton and muscles: the 206 bones, the joints, cartilage, ligaments, and all of the muscles of the body
cardiovascular system	kar´-de-o-vas-ku-lar sis-tem	heart and blood vessels; blood pumped and circulated through the body
gastrointestinal system	gas´-tro-in-tes-ti-nal sis-tem	a long tube commonly called the GI tract: consists of mouth, esophagus, stomach, and intestines; accessory organs are pancreas, liver, gallbladder, and salivary glands
respiratory system	re-spi-rah-to´-re sis-tem	nose, pharynx, larynx, trachea, bronchi, and lungs; furnishes oxygen, removes carbon dioxide (respiration)
genitourinary system	jen´-i-to-u-re-ner´-e sis-tem	reproductive and urinary organs; also called urogenital system (GU or UG). The urinary organs are the kidneys, ureters, bladder, and urethra, and the reproductive organs are the gonads and various external genitalia and internal organs
endocrine system	en-do-krin sis-tem	glands and other structures that make hormones and release them directly into the circulatory system; ductless glands
nervous system	ner-vus sis-tem	brain and spinal cord make up the central nervous system (CNS); the autonomic nervous system (ANS), or peripheral nervous system, consists of 12 pairs of cranial nerves and 31 pairs of spinal nerves

BODY CAVITIES AND PLANES

Refer to **Figures 10–1, 10–2,** and **10–3** when studying body cavities and planes. The body has two main large cavities that contain the internal body organs—the *ventral* and *dorsal* cavities. Each of these cavities is further divided into smaller cavities that contain specific organs. *Ventral* refers to the front or belly portion of the body, and *dorsal* refers to the back portion of the body.

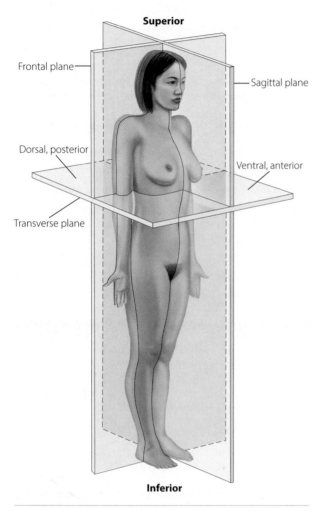

FIGURE 10–1 Body planes and directions

CONFUSING MEDICAL TERMINOLOGY

palpebrate Versus palpate Versus palpitate

palpebrate = blink or wink, e.g., palpebrate (pal-pee-<u>brit</u>) refers to winking

palpate = touch, e.g., palpate (<u>pal</u>-peyt) refers to the examination or exploring by touching (an organ or area of the body), usually as a diagnostic aid

palpitate = pulsate, quiver, throb, tremble, e.g., palpitate (<u>pal</u>-pi-teyt) as in "His heart palpitates wildly"

CONFUSING MEDICAL TERMINOLOGY

cyt/o Versus cyst/o

cyt/o = cell, e.g., cytoplasm (<u>sahy</u>-tuh-plaz-uhm) refers to gelatinous fluid outside the nucleus

cyst/o = bladder of a sac, urinary bladder, cyst, sac of fluid, e.g., cystoplasty (sis-to-<u>plas</u>-te) refers to plastic repair of the bladder

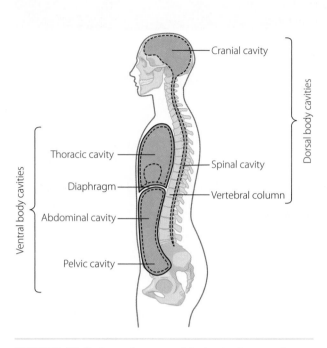

FIGURE 10–2 Sagittal section of the body, showing the dorsal and ventral body cavities

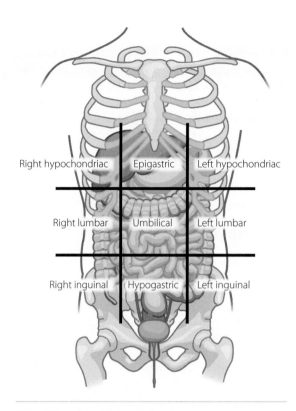

FIGURE 10–3 Abdominal regions

TABLE 10-2

Term	Pronunciation	Definition
Body Cavities		
body cavities		hollow spaces containing body organs
abdominal cavity	ab-<u>dom</u>-uh-nl <u>kav</u>-i-te	the cavity beneath the thoracic cavity that is separated from the thoracic cavity by the diaphragm; contains the liver, gallbladder, spleen, stomach, pancreas, intestines, and kidneys
pelvic cavity	<u>pel</u>-vik <u>kav</u>-i-te	the lower front cavity of the body located beneath the abdominal cavity; contains the urinary bladder and reproductive organs
pleural cavity	<u>pleu</u>´-ral <u>kav</u>-i-te	the thoracic cavity containing the lungs, trachea, esophagus, and thymus gland
thoracic cavity	tho-<u>rass</u>-ik <u>kav</u>-i-te	the chest cavity, which contains the lungs, heart, aorta, esophagus, and trachea
mediastinum	me´-de-ah-<u>sti</u>-num	the mass of tissues and organs separating the sternum in front and the vertebral column behind, containing the heart and its large vessels
peritoneal cavity	per´-i-to-<u>ne</u>-al <u>kav</u>-i-te	the space containing the stomach, intestines, liver, gallbladder, pancreas, spleen, reproductive organs, and urinary bladder

(continues)

TABLE 10-2 (continued)

Term	Pronunciation	Definition
cranial cavity	kra-ne-al kav-i-te	space enclosed by skull bones, containing the brain
spinal cavity	spi-nal kav-i-te	cavity containing the spinal cord
diaphragm	di-ah-fram	dome-shaped muscle separating the abdominal and thoracic cavities
Body Planes		
body planes		imaginary flat surfaces that divide (used in anatomic diagrams)
sagittal	saj-i-tal	a sagittal plane divides the body into right and left portions
midsagittal	mid-saj-i-tal	a plane that vertically divides the body, or some part of it, into equal right and left portions (medial)
coronal	ko-ro-nal	also called frontal; a plane that divides the body into anterior and posterior sections (front and back)
transverse	trans-vers	a plane that divides the body into superior and inferior sections (top and bottom)

METABOLISM AND HOMEOSTASIS

There are two important terms in medicine that have general application. They are described in Table 10-3.

TABLE 10-3

Term	Pronunciation	Definition
metabolism	me-tab-o-lizm	sum of the body's physical and chemical processes that convert food into elements for body growth, energy, building body parts (anabolism), and degrading body substances for recycling or excretion (catabolism)
homeostasis	ho´-me-o-sta-sis	a steady state: the tendency of stability in the normal physiologic systems of the organism to maintain a balance optimal for survival. Body temperature, osmotic pressure, normal cell division rate, and nutrient supply to cells are a few examples

CONFUSING MEDICAL TERMINOLOGY

perionychium Versus paronychia

perionychium = structure that surrounds the nail, e.g., perionychium (per-ee-oh-nik-ee-uhm) refers to the epidermis surrounding the base and sides of a fingernail or toenail

paronychia = infection of the nail e.g., paronychia (par-uh-nik-ee-uh) refers to inflammation of the epidermis (folds of skin) bordering a nail of a finger or toe, usually characterized by infection and pus formation

CHAPTER

11

Integumentary System

LESSON ONE: MATERIALS TO BE LEARNED

Parts of the Skin
Functions of the Skin
Surgical Processes and the Skin
Skin Growths
Biologic Agents and Skin Infection
Allergy and the Skin
Skin Disorders from Systemic
    Diseases
Skin Tests
Vocabulary Terms and the Skin

LESSON TWO: PROGRESS CHECK

Spelling and Definition
Write In
Matching: Skin Terms
Definitions
Matching: Skin Diseases
List the Functions
Word Puzzle on the Integumentary
    System

OBJECTIVES

After completion of this chapter and the exercises, the student should be able to:

1. Identify the structures of the skin and accessory organs.
2. List and describe the five functions of the skin.
3. Identify and describe the lesions and pathologic conditions that affect the integumentary system.
4. Describe laboratory tests and clinical procedures used in diagnosing and treating skin disorders.
5. Identify and define commonly used vocabulary terms that pertain to the skin.

ALLIED HEALTH PROFESSIONS

Dental Hygienists and Dental Assistants

Dental hygienists clean teeth and provide other preventive dental care; they also teach patients how to practice good oral hygiene. Hygienists examine patients' teeth and gums, recording the presence of diseases or abnormalities. They remove calculus, stains, and plaque from teeth; take and develop dental x-rays; and apply cavity preventive agents such as fluorides and pit and fissure sealants. In some states, hygienists administer local anesthetics and anesthetic gas; place and carve filling materials, temporary fillings, and periodontal dressings; remove sutures; and smooth and polish metal restorations.

Dental assistants perform a variety of patient care, office, and laboratory duties. They work at chairside as dentists examine and treat patients. They make patients as comfortable as possible in the dental chair, prepare them for treatment, and obtain dental records. Assistants hand instruments and materials to dentists and keep patients' mouths dry and clear by using suction or other devices. They also sterilize and disinfect instruments and equipment, prepare tray setups for dental procedures, and instruct patients on postoperative and general oral health care.

Some dental assistants prepare materials for making impressions and restorations, expose radiographs, and process dental x-ray film as directed by the dentist. State law determines which clinical tasks a dental assistant may perform, but in most states they may remove sutures, apply anesthetic and caries-preventive agents to the teeth and oral tissue, remove excess cement used in the filling process, and place rubber dams on the teeth to isolate them for individual treatment.

Those with laboratory duties make casts of the teeth and mouth from impressions taken by dentists, clean and polish removable appliances, and make temporary crowns. Dental assistants with office duties arrange and confirm appointments, receive patients, keep treatment records, send bills, receive payments, and order dental supplies and materials. Dental assistants should not be confused with dental hygienists, who are licensed to perform a wider variety of clinical tasks.

INQUIRY

Division of Education, American Dental Hygienists Association: www.adha.org
Dental Assisting National Board: www.danb.org
American Dental Assistants Association: www.dentalassistant.org
National Association of Dental Assistants: www.ndaonline.org

Data from Stanfield, Peggy S., Cross, Nanna, and Hui, Y.H. *Introduction to the Health Professions*, 6th ed. Burlington, MA: Jones & Bartlett Learning; 2012.

The skin and its accessory organs are called the *integumentary system*. The *integument* (skin) is a vital organ serving as a protective barrier that responds to internal and external stimuli and contributes to the maintenance of homeostasis. The integument forms the outer covering of the body. It consists of the skin and certain specialized tissues. Specialized tissues are hair, nails, *sebaceous* (oil) and *sudoriferous* (sweat) glands (see **Figure 11–1**), and mammary glands.

The skin is the largest organ of the body, weighing about 9 pounds and covering approximately 18 square feet in the adult. It consists of two layers of tissue, the *epidermis* and *dermis,* and a layer of *subcutaneous* tissue. Embedded in these layers are various accessory appendages. Skin components are defined in the section titled Parts of the Skin in Lesson One of this chapter. A brief discussion of the components and functions of the integument follows.

The epidermis is the skin's outer layer. It contains no blood vessels and receives its nourishment from the dermis. The cells are packed closely together, being thickest on the palms of the hands and soles of the feet. The epidermis is firmly attached to the dermis, the deeper layer of skin that lies below it. In turn, the dermis is attached through subcutaneous tissue to underlying structures such as muscle and bone. The appendages of fingernails and toenails are found only in humans and other primates, and hair is characteristic only of mammals.

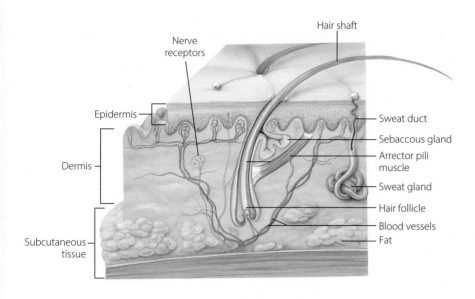

Hair shaft

Nerve
receptors

Epidermis

Sweat duct

Sebaccous gland

Arrector pili
muscle

Dermis

Sweat gland

Hair follicle

Blood vessels

Subcutaneous
tissue

Fat

FIGURE 11–1 Components of the epidermis, dermis, and subcutaneous tissue

A strand of hair is a tightly fused meshwork of horny cells filled with keratin. It has a root embedded in the hair follicle and a shaft, which is the visible part of hair. Each hair develops in the hair follicle as new growth forms from keratin located at the bottom of the follicle. Cutting the hair does not affect its rate of growth. Melanocytes located at the root of the hair follicle gives hair its color, and the color is dependent on the amount of melanin produced. As people age, melanocytes stop producing melanin and the hair turns gray or white.

Fingernails and toenails are composed of hard keratin plates that cover the dorsal surface of the tip of each toe and finger. The horny cells are tightly packed and cemented together and continue to grow indefinitely unless cut or broken off. Fingernails can be replaced in 3–5 months; toenails grow more slowly, requiring 12–18 months to be completely replaced.

The visible part of the nail is the nail body. At the base of the nail body and around the sides is a fold of skin called a *cuticle*. The *lunula* is a half-moon crescent at the base of the nail plate. Underneath the cuticle, the nail body extends into the root of the nail. It is nourished by the nail bed, an epithelial layer lying just beneath it, which contains a supply of blood vessels and gives the nails their pinkish coloring. Alterations in the growth and appearance can give an indication of systemic disease. For example, a flattened or spoon-shaped nail plate can result from iron-deficiency anemia.

Skin glands in humans include sebaceous glands, sudoriferous glands, and *mammary* glands, which are modified sweat glands. The glands of the ear canal that produce *cerumen* (ear wax) are also modified sweat glands, as are the specialized glands found in the *axilla* (armpit) and the *anogenital* area. A modified type of sweat gland, active only from puberty onward, is concentrated near the reproductive organs and in the armpits. These glands secrete an odorless sweat that contains substances that are quickly decomposed by bacteria on the skin. The end products of this breakdown are responsible for human body odor. Mammary glands are another type of modified sweat gland. They only secrete milk after a female has given birth. See **Figures 11–2** and **11–3** for a diagram of the skin and some injuries to the skin.

The skin performs five essential functions: protection, temperature regulation, communication, metabolism, and excretion.

1. *Protection:* the skin protects the body from microorganisms, fluid loss or gain, and other mechanical and chemical irritants. Melanin pigment provides some protection against the sun's ultraviolet rays.

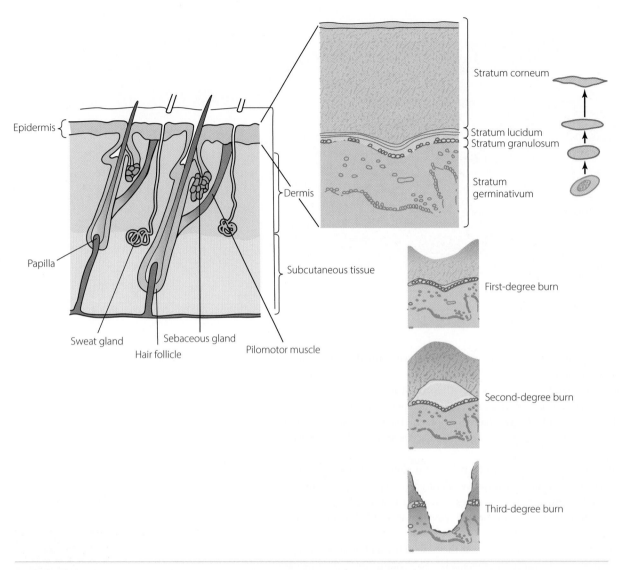

FIGURE 11–2 Diagram of the skin. The nucleated cell produced by the stratum germinativum dies (granulates) as it is forced outward to become the dead, scaly stratum corneum. The number of layers of the epidermis affected by the three types of skin burns is also shown. Only corneum cells are involved in first-degree burns. Damage to the upper three layers occurs in second-degree burns, forming a blister between layers 3 and 4. A third-degree burn involves all epidermal layers and, therefore, usually requires a skin graft to replace the stratum germinativum.

2. *Temperature regulation:* the blood supply to the skin nourishes the skin and helps regulate body temperature. Sweat glands also assist in the maintenance and regulation of body temperature.

3. *Communication:* all stimuli from the environment are received through the skin by receptors that detect temperature, touch, pressure, and pain. Skin is the medium of facial expression (e.g., smiles, frowns, grimaces).

4. *Metabolism:* in the presence of sunlight (ultraviolet radiation), the synthesis of vitamin D, essential for bone growth and development, is initiated from a precursor molecule (7-dehydrocholesterol) found in the skin.

5. *Excretion:* fatty substances, water, and salts (mainly the Na^+ ion) are eliminated from the skin.

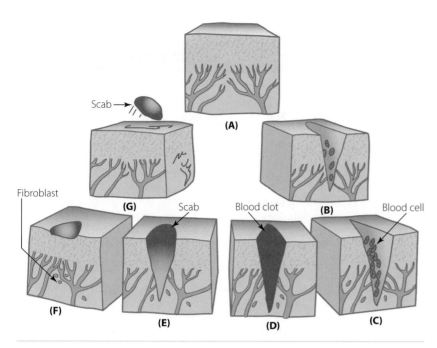

FIGURE 11–3 If normal skin (A) is injured deeply (B), blood escapes from dermal blood vessels (C), and a blood clot soon forms (D). The blood clot and dried tissue fluid form a scab (E), which protects the damaged region. Later, blood vessels send out branches, and fibroblasts migrate into the area (F). The fibroblasts produce new connective tissue fibers, and when the skin is largely repaired, the scab sloughs off (G).

The study of the skin is called *dermatology*, and the medical doctor who specializes in the study of the diseases and disorders of the skin is called a *dermatologist*. Details of the integumentary system are provided in succeeding sections of this chapter.

LESSON ONE	Materials to Be Learned

PARTS OF THE SKIN

TABLE 11-1

Part	Pronunciation	Definition
skin	skin	the outer covering of the body
epidermis (cuticle)	ep´-i-<u>der</u>-mis (<u>ku</u>-ti-kul)	the outermost, nonvascular layer of the skin; composed of, from within outward, five layers: basal layer, prickle-cell layer, granular layer, clear layer, and horny layer
dermis corium	<u>der</u>-mis <u>ko</u>-re-um	layer of the skin deep in the epidermis, consisting of a dense bed of vascular connective tissue and containing the nerves of terminal organs or sensation, the hair roots, and sebaceous and sweat glands

(continues)

| TABLE 11-1 (continued) | | |

Part	Pronunciation	Definition
hair, nails	hare, nales	appendages of the skin
subcutaneous	sub´-ku-ta-ne-us	beneath the skin, containing adipose tissue, connective tissue, vessels, and nerves
breasts	brests	mammary glands; the front of the chest. In female mammals, the breast contains milk-secreting elements for nourishing the young
squamous epithelium	skway-mus ep-ih-thee-lee-um	a layer of flattened platelike cells that cover internal and external body surfaces
stratum basale	strat-um bay-sil	in this layer of skin, new cells are formed and push older cells to the outermost surface of the skin
stratum corneum	strat-um cor-nee-um	outermost layer of skin where dead cells are converted to keratin, which flakes away

FUNCTIONS OF THE SKIN

| TABLE 11-2 | | |

Process or Part	Pronunciation	Definition
protection	pro-tek-shun	from microorganisms, injuries, and excessive exposure to the ultraviolet rays of the sun
sensory organ (receptor)	sen-so-re (re-cep-tor)	for the body to feel pain, cold, heat, touch, and pressure
temperature regulator	tem-per-ah-tur reg-u-la´tor	insulation against heat and cold, e.g., perspiration for cooling
metabolism	me-tab-o-lizm	in the presence of sunlight, synthesize vitamin D from a precursor molecule found in the skin
waste elimination	wast e-lim-i-na-shun	eliminate body wastes in the form of perspiration

CONFUSING MEDICAL TERMINOLOGY

-opia Versus -opsia

-opia = vision, e.g., presbyopia (prez-bee-oh-pee-uh) refers to "old eye" and is a vision condition involving the loss of the eye's ability to focus on close objects

-opsia = vision, e.g., hemianopsia (hem-ee-uh-nop-see-uh) refers to the loss of vision in one half of the visual field of one or both eyes

SURGICAL PROCESSES AND THE SKIN

TABLE 11-3

Process	Pronunciation	Definition
biopsy	<u>bi</u>-op-se	removal of tissue from body for examination
cautery	<u>kaw</u>-ter-e	tissue destruction by electricity
debridement	da-<u>bred</u>-ment	removal of contaminated or devitalized tissue from a traumatic or infected lesion
dermabrasion	der-mah-<u>bra</u>-shun	planing of the skin done by mechanical means, e.g., sandpaper or wire brushes
dermatome	<u>der</u>-mah-tom	an instrument for cutting thin skin slices for grafting
electrodesiccation	e-lek´-tro-des´-i-<u>ka</u>-shun	destruction of tissue by dehydration with high-frequency electric current
escharotomy	es-kah-<u>rot</u>-omy	removal of burn scar tissue
fulguration	ful´-gu-<u>ra</u>-shun	destruction of living tissue by electric sparks
graft	graft	a tissue or organ for implantation or transplantation; a piece of skin transplanted to replace a lost portion of the skin. Pigskin may be used as a temporary graft; a new type of synthetic collagen is now being used for permanent skin grafts
hyfracator	hi-fra-<u>cate</u>-or	a type of machine for destroying tissue (high-frequency eradicator)

SKIN GROWTHS

TABLE 11-4

Growth	Pronunciation	Definition
carcinoma	kahr-suh-<u>noh</u>-muh	a malignant new growth made up of epithelial cells tending to infiltrate surrounding tissues and give rise to metastases (see **Figure 11–4**)
keratosis	ker´-ah-<u>to</u>-sis	any horny growth, such as a wart or callosity
nevus (pl., nevi)	<u>ne</u>-vus	a mole or growth, e.g., birthmark; there are many types (see **Figure 11–5**)
steatoma	ste´-ah-<u>to</u>-mah	lipoma; a fatty mass retained within a sebaceous gland; sebaceous cyst
verruca(-ae)	ve-<u>roo</u>-kah	a wart, caused by viruses; a plantar wart is one on the sole or plantar surface of the foot

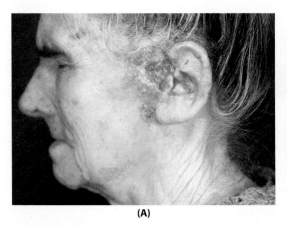

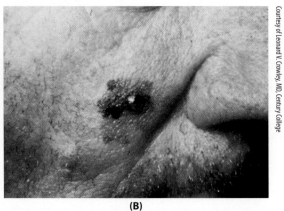

Courtesy of Leonard V. Crowley, MD, Century College

(A)   (B)

FIGURE 11–4 Common skin cancers caused by excessive sun exposure. (A) Cancer arising from keratinocytes (basal cell carcinoma). (B) Cancer arising from melanocytes (malignant melanoma).

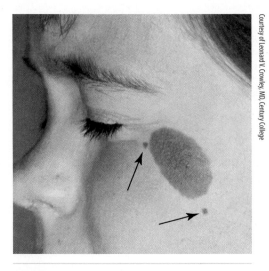

Courtesy of Leonard V. Crowley, MD, Century College

FIGURE 11–5 Benign nevi of skin; a large nevus is near the eye, and two smaller adjacent nevi are shown

BIOLOGIC AGENTS AND SKIN INFECTION

TABLE 11-5

Infection	Pronunciation	Definition
Bacteria		
acne vulgaris	<u>ak</u>-ne vul-<u>ga</u>-ris	an inflammatory disease of the skin with the formation of an eruption of papules or pustules; chronic acne, usually occurring in adolescence; may be caused by foods, stress, hereditary factors, hormones, drugs, and bacteria
carbuncle, furuncle	<u>kar</u>-bung-k´-l, <u>fu</u>-rung-k´-l	boils, abscesses, and pustular lesions

TABLE 11-5 *(continued)*

Infection	Pronunciation	Definition
cellulitis	sel´-u-<u>li</u>-tis	inflammation of the skin and subcutaneous tissue; may lead to ulceration and abscess
impetigo	im-pe-<u>ti</u>-go	a streptococcal or staphylococcal skin infection marked by vesicles or bullae that become pustular, rupture, and form yellow crusts, especially around the mouth and nose
Virus		
herpes genitalis	<u>her</u>-pez jen´-i-<u>tal</u>-is	blister-type inflammatory highly contagious skin disease of the genitals; a prevalent sexually transmitted disease; may harm an infant if the mother is infected at the time of delivery, causing damage to the child's nervous system
herpes ophthalmicus	<u>her</u>-pez oph-<u>thal</u>-mi-cus	severe herpes zoster involving the ophthalmic nerve (eye)
herpes simplex	<u>her</u>-pez <u>sim</u>-plex	an acute viral disease, often on the borders of the lips or nares (cold sores) or on the genitals
herpes zoster	<u>her</u>-pez <u>zos</u>-ter	shingles: an acute, unilateral, self-limited inflammatory disease of a nerve, e.g., on one side of the pelvis
verruca	ve-<u>ru</u>-kah	a wart
Fungus		
tinea	<u>tin</u>-e-ah	ringworm; a name applied to many different superficial fungal infections of different parts of the body
tinea barbae	<u>tin</u>-e-ah <u>bar</u>-bae	infection of the bearded parts of the face by ringworm
tinea capitis	<u>tin</u>-e-ah <u>kap</u>-i-tis	infection of the scalp by ringworm
tinea corporis	<u>tin</u>-e-ah <u>cor</u>-por-is	infection of the body by ringworm
tinea cruris	<u>tin</u>-e-ah <u>cru</u>-ris	infection of the groin by ringworm ("jock itch")
tinea pedis	<u>tin</u>-e-ah <u>pe</u>-dis	athlete's foot; a chronic superficial infection of the skin of the foot by ringworm
tinea unguium	<u>tin</u>-e-ah <u>un</u>-guium	infection of the fingernails by ringworm; the nails become opaque, white, thickened, and friable
Parasites		
pediculosis capitis	pe-dik´-u-<u>lo</u>-sis <u>kap</u>-i-tis	lice (head)
pediculosis corporis	pe-dik´-u-<u>lo</u>-sis cor-por-is	lice (body)
pediculosis pubis	pe-dik´-u-<u>lo</u>-sis <u>pu</u>-bis	pubic lice or crabs
scabies	<u>ska</u>-bez	a mite, a small parasite; can burrow under the skin

ALLERGY AND THE SKIN

TABLE 11-6		
Term	**Pronunciation**	**Definition**
eczema	<u>ek</u>-ze-ma	redness in skin, caused by some substance, e.g., food
neurodermatitis	nu´-ro-der´-mah-<u>ti</u>-tis	a dermatosis presumed to be caused by itching related to emotional causes or psychological factors
psoriasis	so-<u>ri</u>-ah-sis	a chronic, hereditary, recurrent dermatosis marked by discrete vivid red macules, papules, or plaques covered with silvery laminated scales

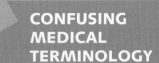

CONFUSING MEDICAL TERMINOLOGY

dermatome Versus dermatome Versus dermatome

dermatome (<u>dur</u>-muh-tohm) as in anatomy = an area of skin that is supplied with the nerve fibers of a single, posterior, spinal root

dermatome (<u>dur</u>-muh-tohm) as in surgery = an instrument that cuts thin slices of skin for grafting

dermatome (<u>dur</u>-muh-tohm) as in embryology = a mesodermal layer in early development, which becomes the dermal layers of the skin

SKIN DISORDERS FROM SYSTEMIC DISEASES

TABLE 11-7		
Disease	**Pronunciation**	**Definition**
diabetes mellitus	di´-ah-<u>be</u>-tez mel-<u>li</u>-tus	a disorder that can cause various skin lesions
erysipelas	er´-i-<u>sip</u>-e-las	a contagious disease of the skin and subcutaneous tissues caused by infection with streptococci organisms; redness and swelling of affected areas
histoplasmosis	his´-to-plaz-<u>mo</u>-sis	a systemic fungal disease caused by inhalation of dust contaminated by fungus
lupus erythematosus	<u>loo</u>´-pus er-i-<u>them</u>-a-to-sus	a chronic superficial inflammation of the skin; the lesions typically form a butterfly pattern over the bridge of the nose and cheeks
rubella	roo-<u>bel</u>-ah	German measles; a mild viral infection marked by a pink macular rash
rubeola	roo-<u>be</u>-o-lah	a synonym of measles in English and of German measles in French and Spanish
syphilis	<u>sif</u>-i-lis	a venereal disease; cutaneous lesions; caused by infection from direct sexual contact
varicella	var´-i-<u>sel</u>-ah	chickenpox; residues itch and later become scabs

SKIN TESTS

TABLE 11-8

Term	Pronunciation	Definition
coccidioidin	kok-sid´-e-<u>oi</u>-din	a sterile preparation injected intracutaneously as a test for valley fever (respiratory fungus disease)
Mantoux or PPD	man-<u>too</u>	a test for tuberculosis (TB), a bacterial disease
Dick test	dik test	an intracutaneous test for susceptibility to scarlet fever
Schick test	shik test	an intracutaneous test for diphtheria
sweat test	swet test	a test for presence of cystic fibrosis

VOCABULARY TERMS AND THE SKIN

TABLE 11-9

Term	Pronunciation	Definition
actinic	ak-<u>tin</u>-ik	referring to ultraviolet rays of the sun
albinism	<u>al</u>-bi-nizm	no body pigment; white skin and hair
alopecia	al´-o-<u>pe</u>-she-ah	baldness; hereditary or caused by chemotherapy
bulla(-ae)	<u>bul</u>-ah	large blisters, as in burns
burn	bern	thermal injury to tissues: first-degree burns show redness, second-degree burns produce blisters and are partial-thickness burns, and third-degree burns are full-thickness burns and involve subcutaneous tissue and muscle
callus	<u>kal</u>-us	localized hyperplasia of the horny layer of the epidermis (skin) caused by pressure or friction
cicatrix	<u>sik</u>-ah-triks	a scar
cyst	sist	a closed epithelium-lined cavity or sac, normal or abnormal, usually containing liquid or semisolid material
dermatology	der´-mah-<u>tol</u>-o-je	the medical specialty concerned with the diagnosis and treatment of skin diseases
ecchymosis	ek´-i-<u>mo</u>-sis	bruise, caused by bleeding under the skin
erosion	e-<u>ro</u>-shun	eating or gnawing away, e.g., an early ulcer

(continues)

TABLE 11-9		*(continued)*

Term	Pronunciation	Definition
eruption	e-<u>rup</u>-shun	breaking out; a rash
erythema	er´-i-<u>the</u>-mah	redness of the skin
eschar	<u>es</u>-kar	a slough (hard crust) produced by a thermal burn
exanthem	eg-<u>zan</u>-them	an eruptive (rose-colored) disease or fever
excoriation	eks-ko´-re-<u>a</u>-shun	a superficial loss of skin, e.g., by scratching
exfoliation	eks-fo´-le-<u>a</u>-shun	a falling off in scales or layers
fissure	<u>fish</u>-er	a narrow slit on the skin surface, e.g., anal fissure, athlete's foot lesion
gangrene	<u>gang</u>-gren	necrotic or dead tissue (see **Figure 11–6**)
hirsutism	<u>her</u>-soot-ism	abnormal hairiness, especially in women
keloid	<u>ke</u>-loid	a sharply elevated, progressively enlarging scar that does not fade with time
laceration	las´-e-<u>ra</u>-shun	cut; tearing; a torn wound
lesion	<u>le</u>-zhun	any pathologic or traumatic discontinuity of tissue, e.g., a sore
macule	<u>mak</u>-ul	a spot, or thickening, e.g., freckle, flat mole. Area is not raised above the surface
nodule	<u>nod</u>-ul	a small node that is solid and can be detected by touch; a rounded prominence, e.g., a boss
nummular	<u>num</u>-u-lar	coin-sized and coin-shaped
papulae	<u>pap</u>-u-le	a small, circumscribed, solid elevated lesion of the skin, e.g., wart, acne, mole
paronychia	par´-o-<u>nik</u>-e-ah	inflammation of the folds of tissue around the fingernail
petechia	pay-<u>tee</u>-kee-ee	small pinpoint hemorrhages of the skin
plaque	plak	any patch or flat area; used to describe the silvery scales of psoriasis
pruritus	proo-<u>ri</u>-tus	itching
pustule	<u>pus</u>-tul	a small, elevated, pus-containing lesion of the skin
scales, crusts	scalz, krusts	an outer layer formed by drying of a bodily exudate or secretion; flaking type of lesion, e.g., psoriasis, fungus
scar, cicatrix	sk-<u>ahr</u>, sik-<u>ah</u>-triks	a mark remaining after the healing of a wound or other morbid process
superfluous hair	soo-<u>pur</u>-floo-es har	excessive hair on the face of women
tumor	<u>too</u>-mor	swelling; may be benign or malignant; also called a neoplasm

TABLE 11-9 *(continued)*		
Term	**Pronunciation**	**Definition**
ulcer	<u>ul</u>-cer	a local destruction of tissue from sloughing of necrotic inflammatory tissue, e.g., varicose ulcer, decubitus ulcer
urticaria	er´-ti-<u>ka</u>-re-ah	hives; transient elevated patches (wheals)
vesicle	<u>ves</u>-i-k´-l	a small blister containing liquid
vitiligo	vit´-i-<u>li</u>-go	loss of pigment; white, patchy areas
wheal	hwel	a localized area of swelling on the body surface, e.g., produced by a skin test reaction
xanthoderma	zan-thoh-<u>der</u>-mah	yellow coloration of the skin
xeroderma	zee-roh-<u>der</u>-mah	rough and dry skin, a clinical and chronic condition

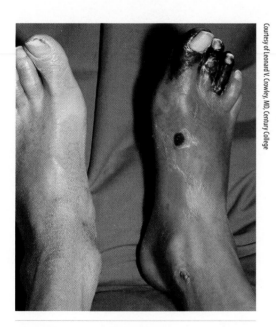

Courtesy of Leonard V. Crowley, MD, Century College

FIGURE 11–6 Gangrene of right foot as a result of arterial obstruction

PHARMACOLOGY MEDICAL TERMINOLOGY

Drug Classification	antihistamine (an-tih-_hiss_-tah-meen)	anti-inflammatory (an-tih-in-_flam_-ah-toh-ree)	anesthetic (an-ess-_thet_-ik)
Function	opposes the action of histamine, which is released in allergic reactions	counteracts inflammation in the body	partially or completely numbs or eliminates sensitivity with or without loss of consciousness
Word Parts	**anti-** = against; **histamine** = a chemical responsible for allergic reactions in human	**anti-** = against; **inflammatory** = pertaining to inflammation	**an-** = without; **esthesi/o** = feeling or sensation; **-tic** = pertaining to
Active Ingredients (samples)	diphenhydramine hydrochloride (Benadryl); brompheniramine maleate (Dimetane)	nabumetone (Relafen); naproxen sodium (Anaprox, Aleve)	lidocaine (Xylocaine)

LESSON TWO   Progress Check

🔷 SPELLING AND DEFINITION

Circle the correct spelling for the following terms and then define the term:

1. **(a)** epidermis   **(b)** epidermosis   **(c)** epedermis   **(d)** epodermasis
    Definition: _____

2. **(a)** subcutenous   **(b)** subcortenus   **(c)** subcuteneous   **(d)** subcutaneous
    Definition: _____

3. **(a)** biopse   **(b)** biopsy   **(c)** biospy   **(d)** bispoy
    Definition: _____

4. **(a)** debraidment   **(b)** debrisment   **(c)** debridement   **(d)** derbrement
    Definition: _____

5. **(a)** escharotomy   **(b)** scarotomy   **(c)** eschrotomy   **(d)** secharotomy
    Definition: _____

6. **(a)** keratinous   **(b)** keratosis   **(c)** karatosis   **(d)** karathosis
    Definition: _____

7. **(a)** steatanoma   **(b)** steteanoma   **(c)** steatoma   **(d)** stetusoma
    Definition: _____

8. **(a)** verracula   **(b)** verookah   **(c)** veracola   **(d)** verruca
    Definition: _____

9. **(a)** impitigo   **(b)** impetigo   **(c)** impecito   **(d)** imtipego
    Definition: _____

10. **(a)** pediculosis   **(b)** pedicleiosis   **(c)** pedicullosis   **(d)** pediculasis
    Definition: _____

11. (a) exema   (b) exczema   (c) eczema   (d) ekzema
Definition: _____

12. (a) posorasis   (b) psoriasis   (c) posorosis   (d) poriaahis
Definition: _____

13. (a) erisepilas   (b) erysipolus   (c) erisipilas   (d) erysipelas
Definition: _____

14. (a) varicella   (b) variccela   (c) variccella   (d) varecella
Definition: _____

15. (a) actomic   (b) actinic   (c) actinus   (d) actonus
Definition: _____

WRITE IN

Write in the medical terms for the following definitions:

1. _____ white skin and hair

2. _____ baldness

3. _____ medical specialty that deals with skin diseases

4. _____ redness of the skin

5. _____ a hard crust produced by a thermal burn

6. _____ coin-sized or coin-shaped

7. _____ small circumscribed solid elevated skin lesion

8. _____ transient elevated patches (wheals)

9. _____ small pus-containing lesion

10. _____ mark remaining after wound healing

11. _____ any horny growth, such as a wart or callosity

12. _____ highly contagious skin disease of the genitals

MATCHING: SKIN TERMS

Match the following terms to their definitions:

1. ecchymosis   a. scales or layers
2. erosion   b. scratching off (of the skin)
3. eruption   c. a rose-colored disease or fever
4. erythema   d. hard crust
5. eschar   e. redness
6. exanthema   f. breaking out
7. excoriation   g. eating or gnawing
8. exfoliation   h. a bruise

◆ DEFINITIONS

Describe the uses of the following tests:

1. mantoux _____

2. dick _____

3. schick _____

4. sweat _____

5. coccidioidin _____

6. histoplasmosis _____

◆ MATCHING: SKIN DISEASES

Match the terms on the left with their definitions on the right:

1. urticaria
2. vesicle
3. vitiligo
4. syphilis
5. gangrene
6. plaque
7. superfluous
8. callus
9. cyst

a. excessive
b. patch
c. venereal disease
d. hives
e. loss of pigment
f. dead tissue
g. small blister
h. a sac containing liquid
i. hyperplasia of the epidermis

◆ LIST THE FUNCTIONS

List the five major functions of the skin:

1. _____

2. _____

3. _____

4. _____

5. _____

WORD PUZZLE ON THE INTEGUMENTARY SYSTEM

Find the 46 words about the integumentary system by reading up, down, forward, backward, or diagonally. When the 46 words have been circled, the remaining letters will spell INTEGUMENTARY SYSTEM.

```
M  E  T  S  Y  S  Y  R  A  T  N  E  M  U  G  E  T  N  I  C
A  C  C  E  S  S  O  R  Y  O  R  G  A  N  S  R  A  C  S  O
E  I  N  B  A  S  A  L  C  E  L  L  T  F  A  H  S  U  E  N
L  M  U  I  L  E  H  T  I  P  E  S  W  E  A  T  B  T  B  N
C  K  E  R  A  T  I  N  I  Z  A  T  I  O  N  C  A  D  A  E
S  E  S  T  R  A  W  S  U  O  E  N  A  T  U  C  M  N  C  C
U  P  E  H  S  K  I  N  G  S  T  R  A  T  U  M  E  I  E  T
M  I  E  M  U  T  D  U  D  E  R  M  A  L  M  E  H  M  O  I
I  D  V  A  N  N  E  C  C  R  I  N  E  T  A  N  T  A  U  V
L  E  I  R  L  E  R  N  T  O  E  N  A  I  L  S  Y  T  S  E
I  R  T  K  I  M  M  A  L  O  P  E  C  I  A  T  R  I  A  T
P  M  C  E  G  G  I  R  U  P  A  P  I  L  L  A  E  V  Y  I
R  I  E  L  H  I  S  S  U  D  O  R  I  F  E  R  O  U  S  S
O  S  T  O  T  P  L  S  E  T  Y  C  O  N  A  L  E  M  Q  S
T  S  O  I  S  A  P  O  C  R  I  N  E  G  L  A  N  D  U  U
C  E  R  D  Y  Y  N  O  I  T  A  R  O  P  A  V  E  S  A  E
E  L  P  E  U  S  S  I  T  E  S  O  P  I  D  A  T  E  M  E
R  O  R  D  E  R  M  A  T  I  T  I  S  E  R  O  P  M  O  N
R  M  E  L  A  N  I  N  L  I  A  N  R  E  G  N  I  F  U  C
A  H  A  I  R  E  N  I  R  C  O  L  A  H  M  U  B  E  S  A
```

Words to Look for in the Word Puzzle

1. accessory organs	**13.** dermis	**25.** melanin	**37.** squamous
2. acne	**14.** eccrine	**26.** melanocytes	**38.** stratum
3. adipose tissue	**15.** epidermis	**27.** moles	**39.** subcutaneous layer
4. alopecia	**16.** epithelium	**28.** papilla	**40.** sudoriferous
5. apocrine gland	**17.** erythema	**29.** pigment	**41.** sunlight
6. arrector pili muscle	**18.** evaporation	**30.** pores	**42.** sweat
7. basal cell	**19.** fingernail	**31.** protective	**43.** tan
8. birthmark	**20.** hair	**32.** scars	**44.** toenails
9. connective tissue	**21.** halocrine	**33.** sebaceous	**45.** vitamin D
10. cutaneous	**22.** integumentary system	**34.** sebum	**46.** warts
11. dermal	**23.** keloid	**35.** shaft	
12. dermatitis	**24.** keratinization	**36.** skin	

WORD PUZZLE ON THE INTEGUMENT AND NERVOUS

CHAPTER

12

Digestive System

LESSON ONE: MATERIALS TO BE LEARNED

Major and Accessory Organs
Clinical Disorders
Surgery
Medical Tests
Abdominal Reference Terms
Digestive Processes
Miscellaneous Terms

LESSON TWO: PROGRESS CHECK

Write In
Matching: Digestive Tract
Definitions
Word Pool: Structure of the Digestive Tract
Matching: Surgical Procedures
Word Puzzle on the Digestive System

OBJECTIVES

After completion of this chapter and the exercises, the student should be able to:

1. Identify the organs of the digestive system.
2. Describe the location and label the structures of the digestive system.
3. List the function(s) of each organ and accessory organ in the digestive system.
4. Identify and define clinical disorders affecting the system.
5. Define and explain medical words pertaining to tests and procedures used in the diagnosis and treatment of digestive system disorders.

ALLIED HEALTH PROFESSIONS

Registered Nurses, Licensed Practical Nurses, Licensed Vocational Nurses and Nursing, Psychiatric, and Home Health Aides

Registered nurses (RNs), regardless of specialty or work setting, treat patients, educate patients and the public about various medical conditions, and provide advice and emotional support to patients' family members. RNs record patients' medical histories and symptoms, help perform diagnostic tests and analyze results, operate medical machinery, administer treatment and medications, and assist with patient follow-up and rehabilitation.

RNs teach patients and their families how to manage their illness or injury, explaining posttreatment home care needs; diet, nutrition, and exercise programs; and self-administration of medication and physical therapy. Some RNs work to promote general health by educating the public on warning signs and symptoms of disease. RNs also might run general health screening or immunization clinics, blood drives, and public seminars on various conditions.

Under the direction of physicians and registered nurses, licensed practical nurses (LPNs), or licensed vocational nurses (LVNs), care for people who are sick, injured, convalescent, or disabled. The nature of direction and supervision required varies by state and job setting.

LPNs care for patients in many ways. Often, they provide basic bedside care. Many LPNs measure and record patients' vital signs, such as height, weight, temperature, blood pressure, pulse, and respiration. They also prepare and give injections and enemas, monitor catheters, dress wounds, and give alcohol rubs and massages. To help keep patients comfortable, they assist with bathing, dressing, and personal hygiene, turning in bed, standing, and walking. They might also feed patients who need help eating. Experienced LPNs may supervise nursing assistants and aides.

Nursing and psychiatric aides help care for physically or mentally ill, injured, disabled, or infirm individuals in hospitals, nursing care facilities, and mental health settings. Home health aides have duties that are similar, but they work in patients' homes or residential care facilities. Nursing aides and home health aides are among the occupations commonly referred to as direct care workers because of their role in working with patients who need long-term care. The specific care they give depends on their specialty.

INQUIRY

National League for Nursing: www.nln.org
American Association of Colleges of Nursing: www.aacn.nche.edu
American Nurses Association: nursingworld.org
National Association for Practical Nurse Education and Service: www.napnes.org
National Federation of Licensed Practical Nurses: www.nflpn.org
National Association for Home Care and Hospice: www.nahc.org
Visiting Nurse Associations of America: www.vnaa.org
Center for the Health Professions: www.futurehealth.ucsf.edu

Data from Stanfield, Peggy S., Cross, Nanna, and Hui, Y.H. *Introduction to the Health Professions*, 6th ed. Burlington, MA: Jones & Bartlett Learning; 2012.

The digestive system, also called the gastrointestinal (GI) system or alimentary tract, contains the organs involved in the ingestion and processing of food. Its general description is that of a long muscular tube extending from mouth to anus and the accessory organs, which include the teeth, tongue, salivary glands, liver, gallbladder, and pancreas. The physician who specializes in diagnosis and treatment of disorders of the stomach and intestines is called a *gastroenterologist*.

The primary function of the GI system is to provide the body with food, water, and electrolytes by digesting nutrients to prepare them for absorption. The following processes are involved in this function:

1. *Ingestion:* taking food into the mouth
2. *Mechanical:* grinding or mincing food with the teeth and mixing with saliva from the salivary glands
3. *Peristalsis:* involuntary waves of smooth muscle contraction that move materials through the GI tract

4. *Digestion:* chemical breakdown of large molecules into small ones so that absorption can occur
5. *Absorption:* the movement of end products of digestion from the lumen of the digestive tract into the blood and lymph circulation so that they can be used by body cells
6. *Egestion (defecation):* elimination of undigested wastes and bacteria from the tract as feces

The major and accessory organs are defined in Lesson One; the structures are seen throughout this chapter. **Figures 12–1** and **12–2** illustrate the positions of the various organs. A brief discussion of the function of the major parts and accessory organs follows.

The upper digestive tract consists of the oral cavity, pharynx, esophagus, and stomach. The lower digestive tract is the small and large intestines. Accessory organs of the digestive system are the salivary glands, liver, pancreas, and gallbladder.

The digestive tract begins with the oral cavity (also known as *buccal cavity*). The major parts of the cavity are the lips, cheeks, hard palate, soft palate, and tongue.

The lips surround the opening of the cavity, and the cheeks, which are continuous with the lips and lined with mucous membrane, form the walls of the oval-shaped cavity (see **Figure 12–3**).

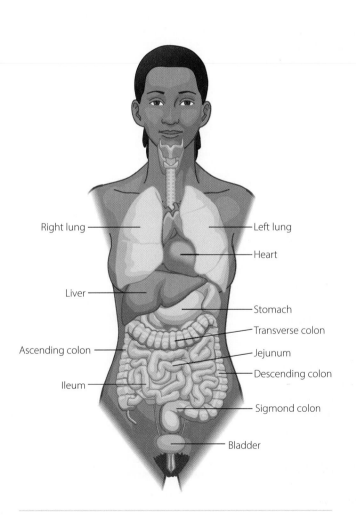

FIGURE 12–1 The viscera

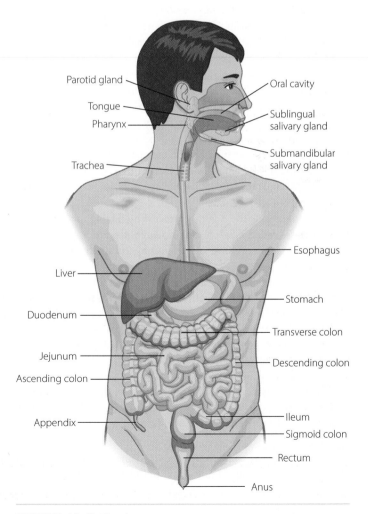

FIGURE 12–2 The digestive system

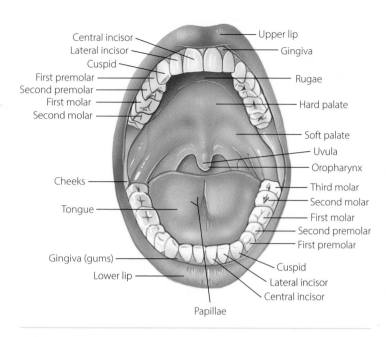

Central incisor
Lateral incisor
Cuspid
First premolar
Second premolar
First molar
Second molar

Upper lip
Gingiva

Rugae

Hard palate

Soft palate
Uvula
Oropharynx

Cheeks

Third molar
Second molar
First molar
Second premolar
First premolar

Tongue

Gingiva (gums)
Lower lip

Cuspid
Lateral incisor
Central incisor

Papillae

FIGURE 12–3 Oral cavity

The hard palate forms the anterior portion of the roof of the mouth, and the muscular soft palate lies posterior to it. The hard palate, or roof of the mouth, is supported by bone. It has irregular ridges in its mucous membrane lining called *rugae*. The soft palate is composed of skeletal muscle and connective tissue. Hanging from the soft palate is a small soft tissue called a *uvula*. This structure aids in producing sound and speech.

The tongue is a solid, strong, flexible structure covered with mucous membrane. It extends across the floor of the oral cavity and strong, flexible, skeletal muscles attach it to the lower joint bone (*mandible*). It is the principal organ of taste and also assists in chewing by moving the food around (*mastication*) and swallowing (*deglutition*).

Across the surface of the tongue are small, rough elevations known as *papillae*. They contain taste buds that detect sweet, sour, salty, and bitter tastes of food (or liquid) as they move across the tongue.

The tongue aids the digestive process by mixing food with saliva, shaping it into a small mass (called a *bolus*), and moving it toward the throat (*pharynx*) to be swallowed. The release of saliva is triggered by the smell, taste, and sometimes even the thought of food.

Salivary glands are exocrine glands, of which there are three pairs—the *parotids*, *submandibulars*, and *sublinguals*—and they secrete most of the saliva produced each day. Saliva is a watery secretion released by the salivary glands containing some mucus and digestive enzymes.

The gums are made of fleshy tissue and surround the sockets of the teeth. Every individual has two sets of teeth during his or her lifetime. The first set, known as "baby teeth," are primary or *deciduous* teeth. There are 20 teeth in this set, 10 in each jawbone, and the baby will begin to cut them at about 6 month of age. The second set of teeth, the permanent teeth, begin to appear around age 6 years and replace the deciduous teeth. There are 32 permanent teeth, 16 in each jawbone. The last of these teeth, the third molars, or wisdom teeth, usually start erupting at about age 17 years.

The shape of the tooth determines its name. The incisors have a chisel shape with sharp edges for biting, canine or cuspid teeth have a single cusp (point) used for grasping and tearing, and the bicuspids or premolars and the molars have flat surfaces with multiple cusps for crushing and grinding.

Beginning with the throat and ending at the anus is a long tube that has many parts and is connected to various other organs. Such parts and organs are listed here:

1. *Esophagus:* transports food from pharynx (throat) to *stomach* by peristalsis. Contains no digestive enzymes.
2. *Stomach:* primarily for food storage. Activity in the stomach results in formation of *chyme* and propels it into the *duodenum.* It secretes pepsin, hydrochloric acid, mucus, and intrinsic factor. The *gastric juices* initiate digestion of protein and fat.
3. *Small intestine:* completes digestion that started in the mouth and stomach by its intestinal enzymes, pancreatic enzymes, and bile from the liver. Also absorbs products of digestion. Peristalsis moves undigested residue to the large intestine.
4. *Pancreas:* the large, elongated gland located behind the greater curvature of the stomach. It contains both endocrine and exocrine glands. The endocrine cells, called islets of Langerhans, secrete the hormones insulin and glucagon. Exocrine glands secrete digestive enzymes, which allow them to digest protein, carbohydrate, and fat.
5. *Liver:* plays a major role in many body functions, as follows:

    a. Produces bile to emulsify fats
    b. Stores glycogen to maintain blood sugar levels
    c. Forms urea from excess amino acids and nitrogenous wastes
    d. Synthesizes fats from carbohydrate and protein
    e. Synthesizes cholesterol and lipoproteins from fats
    f. Synthesizes plasma proteins and blood clotting factors
    g. Stores minerals and fat-soluble vitamins
    h. Detoxifies drugs and toxins; inactivates hormones
    i. Produces heat
    j. Stores blood

6. *Gallbladder:* concentrates and stores bile.
7. *Large intestine:* performs the following functions:

    a. Absorbs 80–90% of water and electrolytes and reduces chyme to a semisolid mass
    b. Produces no digestive enzymes or hormones
    c. Bacteria present in the colon produce vitamin K, riboflavin, and thiamin
    d. Excretes waste and feces

The abdominal cavity and all its organs, including the organs of the GI system, are lined by a membrane called the *peritoneum.* The portion surrounding the abdominal organs is called the *visceral peritoneum* and that which lines the abdominal cavity is the *parietal peritoneum.*

LESSON ONE	Materials to Be Learned

The digestive system involves the processes of ingestion, digestion, absorption, and elimination of food and food products. The most essential medical terms related to

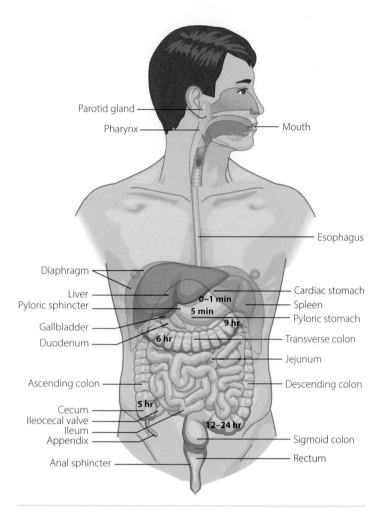

FIGURE 12–4 Human digestive tract; times indicated along the tract represent how long it takes food to pass through each area during the process of digestion

CONFUSING MEDICAL TERMINOLOGY

gastr/o Versus **abdomin/o, lapar/o,** and **celi/o**

gastr/o = stomach, e.g., gastroenterologist (gas-troh-en-tuh-rol-uh-jist) refers to a physician who specializes in the study of the stomach and intestine

abdomin/o, lapar/o, and **celi/o** = abdomen, belly; loin, flank, e.g., abdominocentesis (abdom-in-o-sen-te-sis) refers to surgical puncture of the abdomen; laparoscopy (lap-er-uh-skoh-pee) refers to use of a scope to penetrate the abdomen wall to study the abdominal cavity; celiotomy (se-li-ot-ah-me) refers to incision into the abdominal cavity

this system are described in this lesson. Study them in conjunction with **Figures 12–4** through **12–8**.

The digestive system is a large organ system, which includes the accessory organs. It has myriad functions. In such a complex system, there will be many clinical disorders and diseases, some of which will require surgery. To properly diagnose and treat these conditions, specific medical tests are used. Great accuracy in pinpointing the exact location of the problem is essential.

To provide a simple method of learning the major terms related to this system, this lesson is divided into six segments: the organ and accessory organs (and processes), selective clinical disorders, surgery terms, medical tests, identification of divisions and quadrants of the abdomen, and some general terminology related to the system.

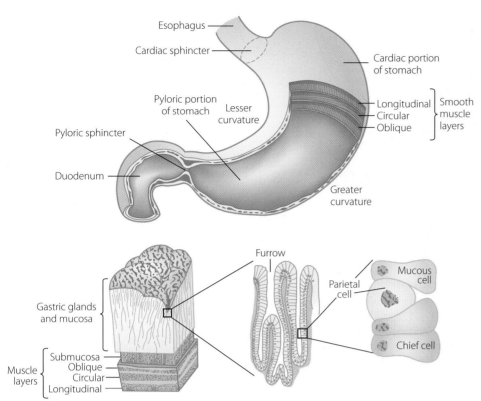

FIGURE 12–5 External and internal anatomy of the stomach

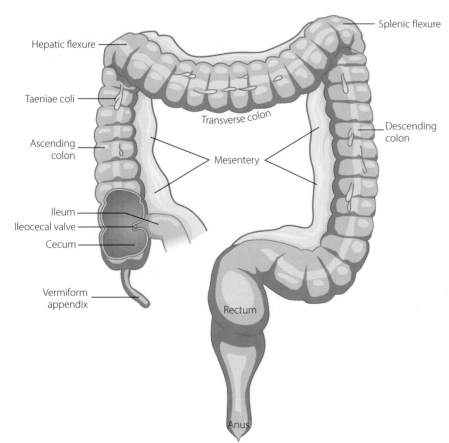

FIGURE 12–6 Large intestine; each segment is named according to the direction it travels or according to its shape

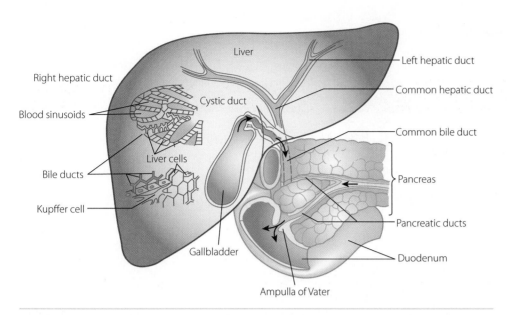

FIGURE 12–7 Liver and its interrelationship with the gallbladder, pancreas, and duodenum. A section has been removed from the liver and the area enlarged to show the arrangement of liver cells, bile ducts, Kupffer cells, and blood sinusoids to one another. Arrows indicate the direction of flow of bile from the gallbladder and liver and of digestive juices from the pancreas into the duodenum.

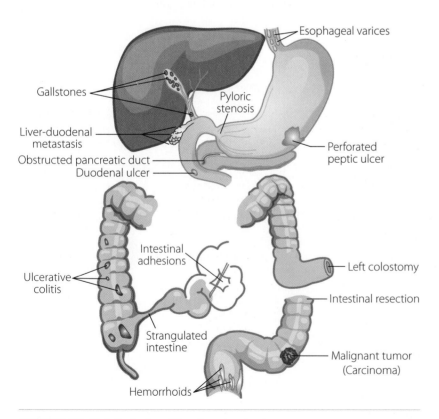

FIGURE 12–8 Pathologies of the alimentary tract

CONFUSING MEDICAL TERMINOLOGY

proct/o Versus prostat/o

proct/o = anus and rectum, e.g., proctology (prok-<u>tol</u>-o-je) refers to a branch of medicine concerned with disorders of the rectum and anus

prostat/o = prostate, prostate gland, e.g., prostatorrhea (pros-tat-or-<u>re</u>-ah) refers to a discharge from the prostate

MAJOR AND ACCESSORY ORGANS

TABLE 12-1

Major and Accessory Organ	Pronunciation	Definition
mouth	mowth	oral cavity forming the beginning of the digestive system
teeth	teeth	structures of the jaws for biting and masticating food
tongue	tung	chief organ of taste; aids in mastication, swallowing, and speech
salivary glands	<u>sal</u>-i-ver-e glands	pertaining to the saliva; glands in the mouth that secrete saliva
pharynx	<u>far</u>-ingks	the throat; the membranous cavity behind the nasal cavities and mouth and before the larynx
esophagus	e-<u>sof</u>-ah-gus	membranous passage extending from the pharynx to the stomach
stomach	<u>stum</u>-ak	the musculomembranous expansion of the digestive tract between the esophagus and duodenum, consisting of a cardiac part, a fundus, a body, and a pyloric part
duodenum	du-o-<u>de</u>-num	the first portion of the small intestine
jejunum	je-<u>joo</u>-num	part of the small intestine from the duodenum to the ileum
ileum	<u>il</u>-e-um	last portion of the small intestine, from jejunum to cecum
pancreas	<u>pan</u>-kre-as	a large, elongated gland situated transversely behind the stomach. Externally, it secretes digestive enzymes into the common duct; internally, its beta cells secrete insulin and glucagon. The alpha, beta, and delta cells of the pancreas form aggregates, called islets of Langerhans
liver	<u>liv</u>-er	the large, dark red gland in the upper part of the abdomen on the right side, just beneath the diaphragm; its functions include storage and filtration of blood, secretion of bile, conversion of sugars into glycogen, and many other metabolic activities (see overview)
gallbladder	<u>gall</u>-blader	the pear-shaped reservoir for bile, behind the liver; stores and concentrates bile
cecum	<u>se</u>-kum	the first part of the large intestine, a dilated pouch
ascending colon	a-<u>sen</u>-ding <u>ko</u>-lon	portion of the colon from the cecum to the hepatic flexure
transverse colon	trans-<u>vers</u> <u>ko</u>-lon	portion of the large intestine passing transversely across the upper part of the abdomen, between the hepatic and splenic flexure
descending colon	di-<u>send</u>-ing <u>ko</u>-lon	portion of the colon from the splenic flexure to the sigmoid colon
sigmoid colon	<u>sig</u>-moid <u>ko</u>-lon	portion of the large intestine between descending colon and rectum
rectum	<u>rek</u>-tum	the last portion of the large intestine
anus	<u>a</u>-nus	opening of the rectum on the body surface

CLINICAL DISORDERS

TABLE 12-2

Clinical Disorder	Pronunciation	Definition
adhesion	ad-<u>he</u>-zhun	union of two surfaces normally separate; also, any fibrous gland that connects them. Surgery within the abdomen may result in adhesions from scar tissue
alcoholism	<u>al</u>-ko-hol´-ism	excessive consumption of alcoholic beverages, interfering with personal health and economy; an addiction. Although this disease affects the entire body, the liver is the organ most involved
anorexia nervosa	an´-o-<u>rek</u>-se-ah ner-<u>vo</u>-sa	lack or loss of appetite for food; a psychophysiologic condition characterized by symptoms of undernutrition
appendicitis	ah-pen´-di-<u>si</u>-tis	inflammation of the appendix, which may rupture
borborygmus	bor-boh-<u>rig</u>-mus	audible abdominal sound produced by hyperactive intestinal peristalsis; they are rumbling, gurgling, and tinkling noises heard when listening with a stethoscope
botulism	<u>boch</u>-oo-lizm	an extremely severe type of food poisoning caused by a neurotoxin (botulinum) produced by *Clostridium botulinum* in improperly canned or preserved foods; can be fatal
carcinoma	kar´-si-<u>no</u>-ma	a malignant tumor
celiac disease	<u>ce</u>-li-ac <u>diz</u>-ez	damage to the lining of the small intestine caused by the inability to digest gluten found in wheat, resulting in malabsorption of nutrients and malnutrition, if untreated
cholelithiasis	ko´-le-li-<u>thi</u>-ah-sis	gallstones; hardened cholesterol stones formed from bile crystallization
cirrhosis	si-<u>ro</u>-sis	interstitial inflammation of an organ, particularly the liver; loss of normal architecture, with fibrosis and nodular regeneration
cleft lip/palate	cleft lip/<u>pal</u>-at	congenital fissure or split of the lip (cleft lip) or roof of the mouth (cleft palate)
colitis	ko-<u>li</u>-tis	inflammation of the colon, ulcerative or spastic
cryptitis	krip-<u>ti</u>-tis	inflammation of a crypt, especially the anal crypt
diverticulitis	di´-ver-tik´-u-<u>li</u>-tis	inflammation of the diverticula, the pouches that form in the walls of the large intestine
dysentery	<u>dis</u>-en-ter´-e	inflammation of the intestine, especially the colon, with abdominal pain, diarrhea, and blood and mucus in stools; most commonly associated with bacterial or parasitic infection
emaciation	ee-may-she-<u>ay</u>-shun	excessive leanness caused by disease or lack of nutrition
emesis	<u>em</u>-eh-sis	material expelled from the stomach during vomiting; vomitus
esophageal atresia	e-sof´-ah-<u>je</u>-al ah-<u>tre</u>-zhe-ah	congenital absence of the opening between esophagus and stomach

TABLE 12-2 *(continued)*

Clinical Disorder	Pronunciation	Definition
esophageal varices	e-sof´-ah-<u>je</u>-al <u>var</u>-i-sez	enlarged, incompetent veins in the distal esophagus, usually caused by portal hypertension in liver cirrhosis
esophagitis	e-sof´-ah-<u>ji</u>-tis	inflammation of the esophagus
femoral	<u>fem</u>-o-ral (pertaining to the groin)	hernia into the femoral canal
flexure	<u>flek</u>-sher	a bend or fold; as the hepatic flexure of the colon (near the liver)
gastric ulcers	<u>gas</u>-trik <u>ul</u>-serz	peptic or duodenal tissue inflammation of the stomach or intestinal linings, with pain and sometimes bleeding from perforation
gastritis	gas-<u>tri</u>-tis	inflammation of the stomach lining; a common stomach disorder
gastroenteritis	<u>gas</u>-tro-en´-ter-i-tis	inflammation of the stomach and intestine caused by ingested harmful bacterial toxin, with acute nausea and vomiting, cramps, and diarrhea
gastroesophageal reflux disease (GERD)	gas-tro-e-<u>soph</u>-a-<u>ge</u>-al re-<u>fluks</u> diz-<u>ez</u>	flow of gastric acid contents back up into the esophagus causing heartburn and, if chronic, esophagitis
glossitis	glo-<u>si</u>-tis	inflammation of the tongue
hepatitis	hep´-ah-<u>ti</u>-tis	inflammation of the liver; may be type A, type B, or type C; types D and E also have been identified
hernia	<u>her</u>-ne-ah	protrusion of a portion of an organ or tissue through an abnormal opening; there are many types
hiatal	hi-<u>a</u>-tal	protrusion of any structure through the esophageal hiatus of the diaphragm
Hirschsprung's disease	<u>hirsh</u>-sprungz diz-<u>ez</u>	congenital megacolon resulting from absence of autonomic ganglia in a segment of smooth muscle that normally stimulates peristalsis
impaction (fecal)	im-<u>pak</u>-shun (<u>fek</u>-al)	condition of being impacted; a collection of hardened feces in the rectum or sigmoid colon
inguinal	<u>ing</u>-gwi-nal (pertaining to the groin)	hernia into the inguinal canal; may be direct or indirect
intussusception	in´-tuh-suh-<u>sep</u>-shun	prolapse of a part of the intestine into the lumen of an immediately adjacent part
irritable bowel syndrome (IBS) or spastic colon	<u>eer</u>-uh-tuh-bul <u>bah</u>-wul <u>sin</u>-drohm <u>spas</u>-tic <u>coh</u>-lon	increased motility of the small or large intestine causing nausea, pain, anorexia, and trapping of gas throughout the intestinal tract

(continues)

TABLE 12-2   *(continued)*

Clinical Disorder	Pronunciation	Definition
melena	<u>mell</u>-eh-nah	abnormal black, tarry stool containing digested blood
nausea and vomiting (N & V)	<u>naw</u>-ze-ah and <u>vom</u>-it-ing	common symptoms in many GI disorders
obesity	o-<u>bes</u>-i-te	body mass index (BMI) of ≥ 30 using the formula: weight (kg) ÷ height squared (m^2)
oral leukoplakia	<u>or</u>-al loo-koh-<u>play</u>-kee-ah	precancerous lesion in the mouth
pancreatitis	pan´-kre-ah-<u>ti</u>-tis	inflammation of the pancreas
peritonitis	per´-i-to-<u>ni</u>-tis	inflammation of the peritoneal cavity; may be caused by chemical irritation or bacterial invasion
phenylketonuria (PKU)	fen-il-ke´-to-<u>nu</u>-re-ah	a congenital inability to metabolize phenylalanine, a component of protein; may lead to retardation
polyposis	pol´-i-<u>po</u>-sis	the formation of numerous polyps (growth hanging from a thin stalk)
pyloric stenosis	pi-<u>lor</u>-ik ste-<u>no</u>-sis	an obstruction of the pyloric orifice of the stomach, congenital or acquired
rectocele	<u>rek</u>-to-sel	hernia of the rectum through the vaginal floor
sialolith	si-<u>al</u>-o-lith	salivary duct stone
ulcers	<u>ul</u>-serz	a local defect of the surface of an organ or tissue
umbilical	um-<u>bil</u>-i-kal (pertaining to the umbilicus)	protrusion of the abdominal contents through the abdominal wall at the umbilicus

SURGERY

TABLE 12-3

Surgical Procedure	Pronunciation	Definition
anastomosis	ah-nas´-to-<u>mo</u>-sis	surgical formation of a connection between two parts; ileorectal anastomosis connects the ileum and rectum after removal of the colon
appendectomy	ap´-en-<u>dek</u>-to-me	excision of the appendix
biopsy	<u>bi</u>-op-se	removal of tissue for microscopic diagnosis

| TABLE | 12-3 | (continued) |

Surgical Procedure	Pronunciation	Definition
bypass	bi-pas	a shunt, e.g., a surgically created pathway
cheiloplasty	ki-lo-plas´-te	surgical repair of a lip defect
cholecystectomy	ko´-le-sis-tek-to-me	excision of the gallbladder
choledochoduodenostomy	ko-led´-o-ko-du´-o-de-nos-to-me	surgical formation of an opening into the duodenum that connects it with the common bile duct
colostomy	ko-los-to-me	surgical creation of an opening (stoma) between the colon and the body surface
gastrectomy	gas-trek-to-me	excision of the stomach, may be partial or subtotal
herniorrhaphy	her´-ne-or-ah-fe	surgical repair of a hernia
ileostomy	il´-e-os-to-me	surgical creation of an opening into the ileum with a stoma on the abdominal wall
laparotomy	lap´-ah-rot-o-me	incision through any part of the abdominal wall
portacaval shunt	por´-tah-ka-val shunt	connecting the portal vein and inferior vena cava to bypass a cirrhotic liver
stomach stapling (gastric bypass)	stum-ak sta-pling	part of the stomach stapled to permit passage of a small amount of food, used to treat gross obesity
vagotomy	va-got-o-me	cutting the vagus nerve to reduce stomach stimulation, used to treat an ulcer

MEDICAL TESTS

| TABLE | 12-4 |

Medical Test	Pronunciation	Definition
barium swallow	bah-ree-um swal-o	also called upper GI series; the oral administration of a radiopaque contrast medium to view the esophagus by x-ray, while swallowing, to detect abnormalities
biopsy	bi-op-se	removal and examination, usually microscopic, of tissue from the living body, performed for diagnosis
blood tests or laboratory tests	blud tests	chemical analyses of various substances in the blood to make diagnoses. Some tests evaluate electrolytes, albumin and bilirubin levels, blood urea nitrogen (BUN), cholesterol, total protein, and serum glutamic–oxaloacetic transaminase (SGOT)

(continues)

TABLE 12-4 *(continued)*

Medical Test	Pronunciation	Definition
cholangiography	ko-lan´-je-og-rah-fe	x-ray examination of the bile ducts, using a radiopaque dye as a contrast medium
colonoscopy	ko-lon-os-ko-pe	endoscopic examination of the colon, either transabdominally during laparotomy, or transanally by means of a colonoscope
digital examination	dig-i-tal eg-zam-i-na-shun	insertion of the gloved finger into the rectum or vagina
esophagogastroduodenoscopy (EGD)	e-sof´-ah-go-gas´-tro-du´-o-de-nos-ko-pe	using endoscopes to examine esophagus, stomach, and duodenum
extracorporeal shock wave lithotripsy (ESWL)	eks-trah-kor-por-ee-al shock wave lith-oh-trip-see	one treatment option for gallstones, using ultrasound to send shock waves to crush the gallstones, allowing contraction of the gallbladder to remove stone fragments
flat plate of abdomen	flat plate uv ab-do-men	an x-ray film of the abdomen
fluoroscopy	floo-or-oh-skop-ee	radiological technique to examine the function of an organ
gastrointestinal series (GIs)	gas´-tro-in-tes-ti-nal series	an examination of the upper gastrointestinal tract using barium as the contrast medium for a series of x-ray films; also called a barium meal
gastroscopy	gas-tros-ko-pe	inspection of the stomach's interior with a gastroscope
magnetic resonance imaging (MRI)	mag-neh-tic rez-oh-nans ima-ij-ing	noninvasive scanning to visualize fluid and soft and bone tissue; very precise and accurate
percutaneous transhepatic cholangiography (PTC)	per-kyoo-tay-nee-us trans-heh-pat-ik koh-lan-jee-og-rah-fee	a clinical method to examine the bile duct, using a needle to pass directly into the bile duct and inject a contrast medium that can be seen by specialized equipment
proctoscopy	prok-tos-ko-pe	inspection of the sigmoid and rectum with a proctoscope
scan	skan	an image produced using a moving detector or a sweeping beam of radiation, as in scintiscanning, B-mode ultrasonography, scanography, or CAT (computerized axial tomography)
serum glutamic oxalacetic transaminase (SGOT)	see-rum gloo-tam-ik oks-al-ah-see-tic trans-am-in-ays	an enzyme in high concentration in liver cells; high amounts in the blood indicate disease of liver cells
stool sample or specimen		a small stool sample for laboratory study, e.g., occult blood, parasites
ultrasonography	ul´-trah-son-og-rah-fe	using ultrasound to obtain a visual record of any organ

ABDOMINAL REFERENCE TERMS

TABLE 12-5

Area	Right	Left	Middle
quadrant (<u>kwod</u>-rant) (see **Figure 12–9**)	right upper quadrant (RUQ) and right lower quadrant (RLQ)	left upper quadrant (LUQ) and left lower quadrant (LLQ)	
divisions (nine)	right hypochondrium (hi´-po-<u>kon</u>-dre-um) (RH)	left hypochondrium (LH)	epigastric (ep´-i-<u>gas</u>-trik) (E)
	right lumbar (<u>lum</u>-bar) (RL)	left lumbar (LL)	umbilical (um-<u>bil</u>-i-kal) (U)
	right inguinal (<u>ing</u>-gwi-nal) or iliac (<u>il</u>-e-ak) (RI)	left inguinal or iliac (LI)	suprapubic (<u>soo</u>-prah-pu-bik) (S)

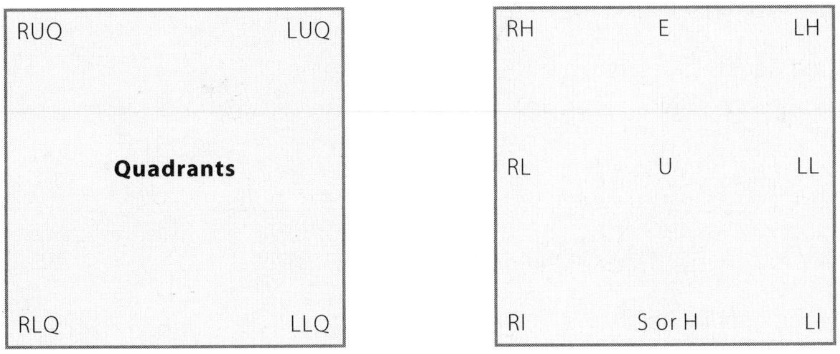

```
 RUQ           LUQ        RH        E        LH

                          RL        U        LL
      Quadrants

 RLQ           LLQ        RI      S or H     LI
```

FIGURE 12–9 Quadrants and divisions of the abdomen

CONFUSING MEDICAL TERMINOLOGY

hypo- Versus hyper-

hypo- = under, decreased, deficient, below, e.g., hypoglossal (hi-po-<u>glos</u>-al) refers to under the tongue

hyper- = above, over, excess, increased, beyond, e.g., hyperbilirubinemia (hi-per-bil-i-<u>ru</u>-bin-e-me-ah) refers to excessive bilirubin (a chemical made by the liver) in blood as a result of liver dysfunction or malfunction

DIGESTIVE PROCESSES

TABLE 12-6

Substance or Process	Pronunciation	Definition
absorption	ab-<u>sorp</u>-shun	the uptake from the intestine of fluids, solutes, proteins, fats, and other nutrients into the intestinal wall cells, blood, lymph, or body fluids
anabolism	a-<u>nab</u>-o-lizm	building up, using nutrients (proteins) for growth and development
catabolism	kah-<u>tab</u>-o-lizm	burning nutrients; breakdown in the presence of oxygen

(continues)

TABLE 12-6 (continued)

Substance or Process	Pronunciation	Definition
deciduous	de-<u>sid</u>-u-us	primary (baby) teeth replaced by permanent
deglutition	de´-glu-<u>ti</u>-shun	the act of swallowing
digestion	di-<u>jes</u>-chun	the act of converting food and fluids into chemical substances that can be absorbed and assimilated
elimination	e-lim-i-<u>na</u>-shun	excreting solid waste (feces)
epiglottis	epi-<u>glot</u>-is	thin leaf-shaped structure posterior to root of tongue
eructation	eh-ruk-<u>tay</u>-shun	a unique sound resulting from the body attempting to bring air from the stomach through the mouth
excretion	ek-<u>skre</u>-shun	excreting body solid and liquid waste (feces and urine)
incisors	in-<u>size</u>-orz	front teeth used for biting, tearing
ingestion	in-<u>jes</u>-chun	taking food, liquids, drugs, etc., by mouth
mandible	<u>man</u>-di-ble	lower jaw
mastication	mas-ti-<u>kay</u>-shun	chewing
maxilla	mak-<u>sil</u>-a	upper jaw
molars	<u>moh</u>-larz	crushing and grinding teeth
palate	<u>pal</u>-at	roof of the mouth
papillae	pah-<u>pill</u>-ay	small rough elevations on tongue and roof of mouth; contain taste buds
periodontal disease	pair-ee-oh-<u>don</u>-tal diz-<u>ez</u>	group of inflammatory gum disorders
peristalsis	peri-<u>stal</u>-sis	muscular movement of food and liquid through the GI tract
trachea	<u>tray</u>-kea	wide, short tube, commonly called the windpipe; starts below larynx and enters thoracic cavity
uvula	yoo-<u>vyoo</u>-lah	small cone-shaped tissue hanging from soft palate of the mouth

MISCELLANEOUS TERMS

TABLE	12-7	

Term	Pronunciation	Definition
achalasia	ak-al-<u>lay</u>-zee-ah	decreased mobility of the lower two-thirds of the esophagus, along with constriction of the muscle between the esophagus and stomach, the lower esophageal sphincter (LES)
anasarca	an´-ah-<u>sar</u>-kah	generalized massive edema
ascites	ah-<u>si</u>-tes	abnormal accumulation of (edematous) fluid within the peritoneal cavity
buccal	<u>buk</u>-al	pertaining to the cheek
cachexia	kah-<u>kek</u>-se-ah	severe malnutrition and wasting, emaciation
dental caries	<u>den</u>-tal <u>cair</u>-eez	tooth decay formed from microorganisms maintained in the mouth
enema	<u>en</u>-e-mah	introduction of fluid into the rectum to promote evacuation of feces or to administer nutrient or medicinal substances
enteropathy	en´-ter-<u>op</u>-ah-the	a disease of the intestine
enzyme	<u>en</u>-zim	a protein produced in a cell capable of facilitating a specific biologic or chemical reaction—enzymes perform this function without being destroyed or altered
fistula	<u>fis</u>-tu-lah	an abnormal passage between two internal organs, or leading to the body surface
gamma globulins	<u>gam</u>-ah <u>glob</u>-u-linz	substances containing antibodies; they provide passive immunity in some people against certain infectious diseases
gavage	gah-<u>vahzh</u>	forced feeding, especially through a tube passed into the stomach; common for premature infants, people who are unconscious, and those who are critically ill
glossal	<u>glos</u>-al	pertaining to the tongue
hyperalimentation	hi´-per-al´-i-men-<u>ta</u>-shun	an intravenous feeding program similar to total parenteral nutrition
lavage	lah-<u>vahzh</u>	washing out an organ, e.g., the stomach or bowel
lingual	<u>ling</u>-gwal	pertaining to the tongue; sublingual means "under the tongue"
nasogastric (ng)	na´-zo-<u>gas</u>-trik	a soft flexible tube introduced through the nose into the stomach for gavage, lavage, or suction
NPO (nothing per os)		no food or fluid by mouth or other body orifice (os means any body orifice)
parotid	pah-<u>rot</u>-id	near the ear
peritoneum	per´-i´-to-<u>ne</u>-um	membrane lining abdominal walls and pelvis, body cavities, and surrounding the contained viscera; the peritoneal cavity (see Figure 12–1)

(continues)

TABLE 12-7 *(continued)*

Term	Pronunciation	Definition
rugae	<u>roo</u>-gay	a ridge or fold, such as the rugae of the stomach that presents large folds in the mucous membrane of that organ
stoma	<u>sto</u>-mah	"mouth"; an artificially created opening (e.g., in colostomy) on the surface of the abdomen
thrush	thrush	fungal infection of the mouth caused by *Candida albicans* resulting in painful creamy white raised patches of the tongue and oral mucosa
total parenteral nutrition	pah-<u>ren</u>-ter-al nu-<u>trish</u>-un	intensive intravenous feeding most often introduced through a subclavian vein
viscera	<u>vis</u>-er-ah	a large interior organ in a body cavity, especially the abdomen
volvulus	<u>vol</u>-vyoo-lus	loop of bowel twisting on itself resulting in bowel obstruction

PHARMACOLOGY AND MEDICAL TERMINOLOGY

Drug Classification	antidiarrheal (an-tih-dye-ah-<u>ree</u>-ul)	antiemetic (an-tih-ee-<u>met</u>-ik)	antiulcer agent (an-tih-<u>ull</u>-ser)
Function	prevents or treats diarrhea	prevents or relieves nausea and vomiting	treats and prevents peptic ulcer and gastric hypersecretion
Word Parts	**anti-** = against; **diarrheal** = pertaining to diarrhea	**anti-** = against; **emetic** = pertaining to "vomiting"	**anti-** = against; **ulcer** = pertaining to an open sore with imflammation (e.g., stomach)
Active Ingredients (examples)	diphenoxylate-atropine sulfate (Lomotil); loperamide hydrochloride (Imodium)	chlorpromazine (Thorazine); meclizine hydrochloride (Bonine, Dramamine II, Antivert)	ranitidine hydrochloride (Zantac); nizatidine (Axid)

LESSON TWO　Progress Check

◆ WRITE IN

For each digestive disease or disorder described, write in the correct term.

1. abnormal fibers that bind one organ to another _____

2. a severe type of food poisoning caused by anaerobic bacteria _____

3. a malignant tumor anywhere in the body _____

4. the term for stones in the gallbladder _____

5. inflammation of the colon _____

6. pouches in the sigmoid colon _____

7. an inflamed area with tissue destruction in the gastric mucosa _____

8. inflammation of the stomach or intestines _____

9. inflammation of the tongue _____

10. protrusion of a part out of its natural place _____

11. telescoping of the intestine into itself _____

12. a hernia that causes a bowel obstruction _____

13. inflammation of the liver _____

14. the most common symptoms of GI disorders _____

15. having a body mass index (BMI) of 30 or greater _____

16. inflammation of the pancreas _____

17. inflammation of the peritoneal membrane _____

18. a disease of infancy in which the outlet of the stomach is too narrow for food to pass through _____

_____

19. foamy, bulky, foul-smelling stool high in fat content _____

20. replacement of liver cells by fibrous tissue _____

◥ MATCHING: DIGESTIVE TRACT

Match the parts of the digestive tract listed at the left with their respective functions listed on the right:

1. tongue
2. pharynx
3. parotid, submaxillary, sublingual
4. esophagus
5. gallbladder
6. liver
7. pancreas
8. ileum
9. gastric mucosa
10. gastric secretions

a. produces saliva
b. breaks up food for digestion
c. aids in swallowing
d. produces insulin and enzymes
e. stores bile
f. stores fat-soluble vitamins; manufactures bile
g. a tube that directs food to the next organ
h. carries food to the esophagus
i. digests and absorbs food
j. prevents acid from consuming the stomach

◥ DEFINITIONS

Give a definition for each of the following terms:

1. small intestine _____

2. gastroenterologist _____

3. digestion _____

4. absorption _____

5. alimentary canal _____

6. peristalsis _____

7. mucus _____

8. duodenum _____

9. pyloric sphincter _____

10. ampulla of Vater _____

11. mesentery _____

12. hemorrhoids _____

13. peritoneum _____

14. colon _____

15. cecum _____

16. caries _____

17. bicuspid _____

18. carcinoma _____

19. gavage _____

20. volvulus _____

◆ WORD POOL: STRUCTURE OF THE DIGESTIVE TRACT

Select appropriate terms from the word pool below to complete these sentences:

1. The first part of the digestive system is called the _____.

2. The chief organ of digestion is the _____.

3. The first part of the small intestine is called the _____.

4. The first part of the large intestine is called the _____.

5. Three accessory organs are _____.

6. Primary (baby) teeth replaced by permanent teeth are _____.

7. The lower part of the large intestine is called the _____.

8. The last part of the alimentary canal is the _____.

9. A structure whose common name is the apron is the _____.

10. The three divisions of the small intestine are the _____.

11. A term meaning roof of the mouth is the _____.

12. A group of inflammatory gum disorders is called _____.

Word Pool: anus, ascending, bicuspid, cecum descending, deciduous, duodenum, gallbladder, greater omentum, ileum, jejunum, liver, mouth or oral cavity, pancreas, periodontal disease, rectosigmoid, rectum, small intestine, transverse, palate

◆ MATCHING: SURGICAL PROCEDURES

Match the procedure on the left to its description on the right:

1. anastomosis
2. cholecystectomy
3. colostomy
4. gastrectomy
5. herniorrhaphy
6. ileostomy
7. laparotomy
8. stapling
9. shunt
10. vagotomy

a. creation of a new opening into the abdomen
b. exploratory incision into the abdomen
c. a bypass of an obstruction
d. closing off of part of the stomach to permit passage of only small amounts of food
e. surgical repair of a hernia
f. excision of the gallbladder
g. joining two parts together (intestine: ducts) when a portion has been removed
h. creating a stoma on the surface of the abdomen for excretion of waste
i. cutting the vagus nerve to reduce acid secretions
j. subtotal removal of the stomach

◆ WORD PUZZLE ON THE DIGESTIVE SYSTEM

There are 51 words about the digestive system contained in this puzzle. Find them by reading forward, backward, up, down, or diagonally. When you have located the 51 listed words, the remaining letters (from left to right) will spell DIGESTIVE SYSTEM.

```
A N U S L A N A C Y R A T N E M I L A F
I L E U M A E N H B D I S E P N D G A P
X A S D S M S A Y I E E V E T E D T Y A
I S R I T Y O L M L C L R R C E S L R N
D C E O O L C C E E A I I I S D O D A C
N E V M M A U A F V S N D C I R P I L R
E N S G A S L N L T S U E C I R A T L E
P D N I C E G A A I O N A C E Y L O I A
P I A S H O C L C U D C S D C R A R X T
A N R S R E S F S I I P D N E E T A A I
M G T A C I A U N R H A G I C T E P M C
R C L O S C G G O I L N A M U N U J E J
O O E T T A C L N B M C S A M E R P I U
F L V O H O H C L U G R T T U S E H E I
I O R P L C T L N S U E R I C E C A N C
M N O O O E A E V Y T A I V O M T R I E
R S N R R G D I L I P S C S S T U Y S D
E F D O S O L I V E R E T S A T M N P I
V Y H O U L A B S O R P T I O N M X E C
H C L D I G E S T I V E S Y S T E M P A
```

Words to Look for in the Word Puzzle

1. absorption
2. acid
3. alimentary canal
4. amylase
5. anal canal
6. anus
7. ascending colon
8. bile
9. cecum
10. CHO
11. chyme
12. deciduous
13. descending colon
14. digestive system
15. duodenum
16. esophagus
17. fats
18. feces
19. gallbladder
20. gastric
21. glucose
22. gut
23. HCl
24. hydrochloric acid
25. ileocecal valve
26. ileum
27. intrinsic factor
28. jejunum
29. lips
30. liver
31. maxillary
32. mesentery
33. mucosa
34. oral
35. os
36. palate
37. pancreas
38. pancreatic juice
39. parotid
40. pepsin
41. peristalsis
42. pharynx
43. pyloric sphincter
44. rectum
45. sigmoid
46. stomach
47. taste
48. transverse
49. vermiform appendix
50. villi
51. vitamin

CHAPTER 13

Respiratory System

LESSON ONE: MATERIALS TO BE LEARNED

The Respiratory System
Respiratory Body Parts
Common Disorders of the Respiratory System
Diagnostic, Surgical, and Medical Procedures and General Terms

LESSON TWO: PROGRESS CHECK

Matching
Multiple Choice
Definitions
Abbreviations
Naming
Matching: Breath Sounds
Word Puzzle on the Respiratory System

OBJECTIVES

After completion of this chapter and the exercises, the student should be able to:

1. Identify the organs of the respiratory system.
2. Describe the location and label the structures of the respiratory system.
3. List the functions of the respiratory system.
4. Identify and define clinical disorders affecting the respiratory system.
5. List and explain laboratory tests and medical procedures used to diagnose disorders of the respiratory system.

ALLIED HEALTH PROFESSIONS

Respiratory Therapists and Respiratory Therapy Technicians

The term *respiratory therapist* used here includes both respiratory therapists and respiratory therapy technicians. Respiratory care therapists work to evaluate, treat, and care for patients with breathing disorders. They work under the direction of a physician.

Most respiratory therapists work with hospital patients in three distinct phases of care: diagnosis, treatment, and patient management. In the area of diagnosis, therapists test the capacity of the lungs and analyze the oxygen and carbon dioxide concentrations and potential of hydrogen (blood pH), a measure of the acidity or alkalinity of the blood. To measure lung capacity, the therapist has the patient breathe into a tube connected to an instrument that measures the volume and flow of air during inhalation and exhalation. By comparing the reading with the norm for the patient's age, height, weight, and sex, the therapist can determine whether lung deficiencies exist.

To analyze oxygen, carbon dioxide, and pH levels, therapists need an arterial blood sample, for which they generally draw arterial blood. This procedure requires greater skill than is the case for routine tests, for which blood is drawn from a vein. Inserting a needle into a patient's artery and drawing blood must be done with great care; any slip can damage the artery and interrupt the flow of oxygen-rich blood to the tissues. Once the sample is drawn, it is placed in a gas analyzer, and the results are relayed to the physician.

INQUIRY

American Association for Respiratory Care: www.aarc.org
National Board for Respiratory Care: www.nbrc.org

Data from Stanfield, Peggy S., Cross, Nanna, and Hui, Y.H. *Introduction to the Health Professions*, 6th ed. Burlington, MA: Jones & Bartlett Learning; 2012.

The respiratory system consists of a series of tubes that transport air into and out of the lungs. Its function is to supply oxygen (O_2) to the body cells and to transport carbon dioxide (CO_2) produced by the body cells into the atmosphere. The respiratory organs also have important functions for normal speech, acid–base balance, hormonal regulation of blood pressure, and defense against foreign material. The respiratory system also allows humans to perceive odors and to filter and moisten air.

Respiration involves the following processes:

1. Pulmonary ventilation (breathing)
2. External respiration (diffusion of O_2 and CO_2 between air in the lungs and the capillaries)
3. Internal respiration (diffusion of CO_2 and O_2 between blood and tissue cells)
4. Cellular respiration (use of O_2 by the body cells in production of energy and release of CO_2 and H_2O)

The respiratory tract is divided into the upper respiratory tract, consisting of the *nose, pharynx,* and *larynx,* and the lower respiratory tract, the *trachea, bronchi,* and *lungs.* These structures are defined and illustrated in Lesson One (see **Figure 13–1**). A brief discussion of their respective functions follows:

1. *Nose* (nostrils or nares): the external portion of the respiratory tract filters small particles, warms and humidifies incoming air, and receives odors. It is the primary organ for the sense of smell.
2. *Pharynx* (throat): a 5-in. muscular tube that extends from the base of the skull to the esophagus. It is the airway that connects the mouth and nose to the larynx. Although it is a single organ, it is divided into three sections, the *nasopharynx, oropharynx,* and *laryngopharynx.* The nasopharynx is behind the nose and serves to equalize pressure on both sides of the tympanic membrane (eardrum). The oropharynx, behind the mouth, is a muscular soft palate containing the uvula and palatine tonsils. The laryngopharynx surrounds the opening of the

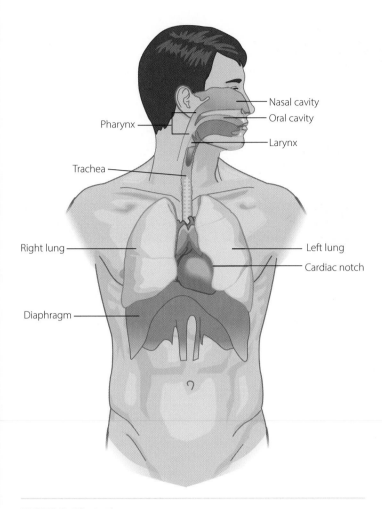

FIGURE 13–1 The respiratory system

esophagus, which is the gateway to the rest of the respiratory system. The pharynx is the common passageway for both air and food. To prevent food from entering the respiratory tract, a small flap called the *epiglottis* covers the opening of the larynx during the act of swallowing.

3. *Larynx* (voice box): connects the pharynx with the trachea. It is a short tube shaped like a triangular box and is supported by nine cartilages, three paired and three unpaired. It contains the vocal cords and supporting tissue that make vocal sounds possible.

4. *Trachea* (windpipe): a 10- to 12-cm-long tube, the trachea extends into the chest and serves as a passageway for air into the bronchi. It lies in front of the esophagus. It is kept permanently open by 16 to 20 C-shaped cartilaginous rings.

5. *Bronchi*: the trachea branches into two tubes called the bronchi (the bronchial tree). Each bronchus enters a lung. The right primary (main) bronchus is shorter than the left because the arch of the aorta displaces the lower trachea to the right. Foreign objects falling into the trachea are more likely to lodge in the right bronchus. Each bronchus subdivides into progressively smaller branches called *bronchioles*, which terminate in the *alveoli* (air space).

6. *Lungs*: pyramid-shaped, spongy, air-filled organs that are molded into the thoracic cavity that contains them. The right lung has three lobes, the left has two. In the lungs, alveoli are surrounded by a network of tiny blood vessels called capillaries: O_2 from the lungs passes into these capillaries for distribution

to the cells, and CO_2 from the blood cells passes into the lungs for removal (by exhalation). When O_2 is absorbed into the blood it attaches to *hemoglobin* and is released as needed.

The pleura are the serous membrane coverings that enclose each lung. The *parietal* pleura lines the *thoracic* (chest) cavity (rib cage, diaphragm, and mediastinum). The *visceral* pleura covers the lung and is continuous at the root of the lung, where it joins with the parietal pleura. The parietal and visceral pleura lie close together; between them is a thin film of lubricating fluid that prevents friction when the two slide against each other during respiration.

| LESSON ONE | Materials to Be Learned |

THE RESPIRATORY SYSTEM

The overview described the structure, function, and supporting systems of the respiratory system. The respiratory system involves the exchange of oxygen and carbon dioxide. We inhale oxygen (O_2) and exhale carbon dioxide (CO_2). This process is also known as *respiration (inspiration and expiration)*. To facilitate your learning of myriad medical terms within the respiratory system, the terms are divided into tables. Table 13-1 in Lesson One identifies the body parts, and Table 13-2 names and defines common respiratory diseases and disorders. Table 13-3 provides terms pertaining to the tests and diagnostic and/or surgical aspects of treatment, as well as terminology needed for an understanding of the respiratory system. Refer to **Figures 13–2** through **13–5** as needed.

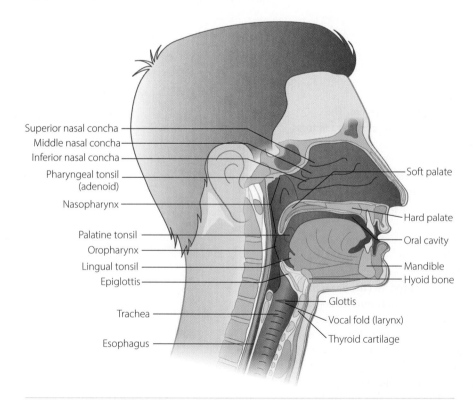

FIGURE 13–2 Sagittal section of the head and neck, showing the respiratory passage down to the bifurcation of the trachea

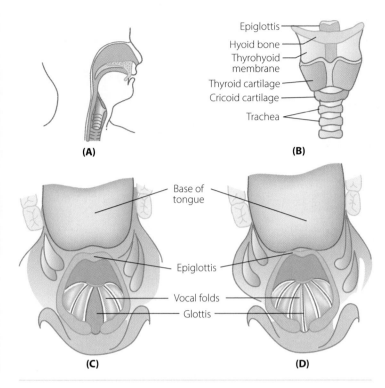

FIGURE 13–3 Larynx. (A) In relation to the head and neck. (B) Anterior aspect. (C) Superior aspect with vocal folds open. (D) Superior aspect with vocal folds closed.

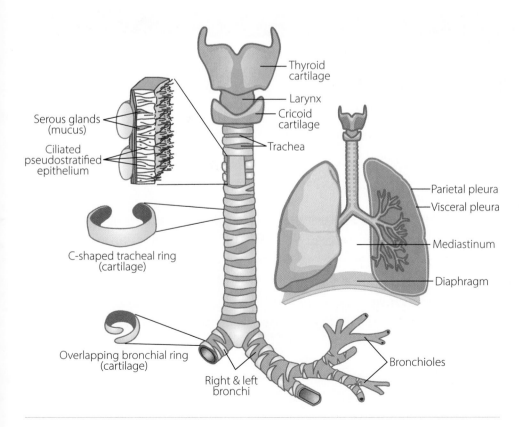

FIGURE 13–4 Anterior aspect of the human larynx, trachea, and bronchi

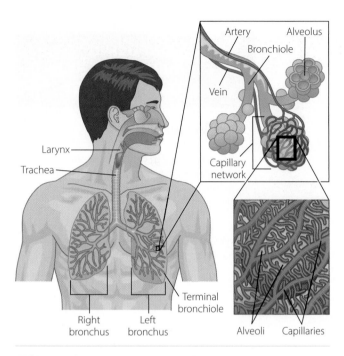

FIGURE 13–5 Internal structure of the lungs

RESPIRATORY BODY PARTS

TABLE 13-1

Body Part (Organ)	Pronunciation	Definition
nasal cavity	na-zal kav-i-te	nose, nares, cavity separated by septum
pharynx	far-ingks	throat, cavity behind the nasal cavities and mouth
larynx	lar-inks	voice organ, containing the vocal cords
trachea	tra-ke-ah	windpipe
lung	lung	two cone-shaped spongy organs consisting of alveoli, blood vessels, nerves, and elastic tissue; each is enveloped in a double-folded membrane called the pleura
parietal pleura	par-ry-e-tal ploo-rah	the serous membrane that lines the thoracic (chest) cavity
visceral pleura	viss-or-al ploo-rah	membrane that covers the lungs; this membrane and the parietal membrane are close together; between them is a thin film of lubricating fluid that prevents friction when they slide against each other

TABLE 13-1 (continued)		
Body Part (Organ)	**Pronunciation**	**Definition**
bronchus (pl., bronchi)	brong-kus (brong-ki)	one of the larger passages conveying air to (right or left principal lobe) and within the lungs
bronchioles	brong-ke-olz	one of the subdivisions of the branched bronchial tree
alveolus (pl., alveoli)	al-ve-o-lus (al-ve-ol-i)	a small saclike dilation (outpocketing) of the alveolar ducts
diaphragm	dye-ah-fram	muscular partition that separates the thoracic cavity from the abdominal cavity and aids in the process of breathing

COMMON DISORDERS OF THE RESPIRATORY SYSTEM

TABLE 13-2		
Condition	**Pronunciation**	**Definition**
abscess (lung)	ab-ses	a localized collection of pus in a cavity formed by the disintegration of tissues
anthracosis	an-thrah-koh-sis	accumulation of carbon deposits in the lung due to breathing smoke or coal dust, also known as black lung disease
ARDS		adult (acute) respiratory distress syndrome
asbestosis	as-beh-stoh-sis	lung disease caused by inhaling asbestos particles; associated with development of mesothelioma, a type of lung cancer
asphyxiation	as-fik-se-a-shun	suffocation
asthma	az-mah	spasm and narrowing of bronchi, leading to bronchial airway obstruction
atelectasis	at'-e-lek-tah-sis	incomplete expansion of the lungs at birth, or collapse of the adult lung
bradypnea	brad-ip-nee-ah	abnormally slow breathing
bronchiectasis	brong-ke-ek-tah-sis	chronic dilation of one or more bronchi
bronchitis	brong-ki-tis	inflammation of one or more bronchi
byssinosis	bis-ih-noh-sis	lung disease resulting from inhaling cotton, flax, or hemp, also know as brown lung disease
carcinoma	kar-si-no-mah	a malignant new growth made up of epithelial cells tending to infiltrate surrounding tissues and to give rise to metastases

(continues)

TABLE 13-2 *(continued)*

Condition	Pronunciation	Definition
coccidioidomycosis	kok-<u>sid</u>-e-oi-do-mi-<u>ko</u>-sis	a respiratory infection caused by spore inhalation of *Coccidioides immitis,* varying in severity from that of a common cold to symptoms resembling those of influenza; also called valley fever
COPD		chronic obstructive pulmonary (lung) disease, especially emphysema, chronic bronchitis, and asthma
cor pulmonale	kor <u>pul</u>-mo-nay-lee	heart failure from pulmonary disease
coryza	ko-ri-<u>zah</u>	profuse discharge from the mucous membrane of the nose; the common cold
cough	koff	a forceful expiration preceded by a preliminary inhalation and usually caused by irritation of the airways from dust, smoke, infection, or mucus; can be described as croupy, rasping, harsh, hollow, loose, dry, productive, brassy, bubbly, or wracking
croup	kroop	a childhood disease with symptoms including a barking cough, difficulty (suffocative) breathing, stridor, and spasm of the laryngx
cystic fibrosis	sis-<u>tik</u> fi-<u>bro</u>-sis	generalized hereditary disorder of infants, children, and young adults associated with malfunctioning of the pancreas and frequent respiratory infections
deviated septum	de-<u>vi</u>-ated <u>sep</u>-tum	defect in the wall between the nostrils that can cause partial or complete obstruction
diphtheria	<u>dif</u>-the-re-ah	an acute bacterial infection primarily affecting the membranes of the nose, throat, or larynx accompanied by fever and pain
effusion	e-fu-<u>zhun</u>	escape of a fluid; exudation or transudation
emphysema	em-fi-<u>se</u>-mah	a pathologic accumulation of air in tissues or organs
epistaxis	ep-ih-<u>staks</u>-is	hemorrhage from the nose; nosebleed
expectoration	ex-pek-toh-<u>ray</u>-shun	the act of spitting out saliva or coughing up material from the lungs
fibrosis	fi-<u>bro</u>-sis	formation of fibrous or scar tissue (in lungs) usually caused by previous infections
flail chest	flal chest	chest wall moves paradoxically with respiration as a result of multiple fractures of the ribs
"flu"	floo	popular name for influenza
hay fever	hay <u>fe</u>-ver	a hypersensitive state, e.g., allergy to pollen
hemothorax	he-mo-<u>tho</u>-raks	blood in the pleural thoracic cavity
hiatal hernia	hi-<u>a</u>-tal <u>her</u>-ne-ah	protrusion of part of the stomach into the chest through the esophageal hiatus defect of the diaphragm
hiccup	hik-<u>up</u>	sharp respiratory sound with spasm of the glottis and diaphragm
histoplasmosis	his-to-<u>plaz</u>-mo-sis	fungal infection of the lungs, may be symptomatic or asymptomatic, resembling tuberculosis

TABLE 13-2 *(continued)*

Condition	Pronunciation	Definition
hyaline	<u>hi</u>-ah-liln	glossy, translucent
hyaline membrane disease	<u>hi</u>-ah-lin mem-<u>bran</u> di-<u>zez</u>	lack of surfactant caused by a layer of hyaline material lining the alveoli, alveolar ducts, and bronchioles; leading cause of neonatal deaths
influenza	in-floo-en-zah	an acute viral infection of the respiratory tract; serious for the very young and old
laryngitis	lar-in-<u>ji</u>-tis	inflammation of the larynx
laryngotracheo-bronchitis	la-<u>rin</u>-go-<u>tra</u>-ke-o-brong-<u>ki</u>-tis	inflammation of the larynx, trachea, and bronchi
lung abscess	lung <u>ab</u>-sess	pus formed by the destruction of lung tissue and microorganisms by white blood cells that have gone to a localized area to fight infection
orthopnea	or-<u>thop</u>-nee-ah	a clinical condition where the person can only breathe normally and without discomfort in an erect sitting or standing position
pertussis	per-<u>tus</u>-is	acute upper respiratory infectious disease caused by bacterium *Bordetella pertussis*; commonly called whooping cough
pharyngitis	far-in-<u>ji</u>-tis	inflammation of the pharynx
pleural effusion	<u>ploo</u>-ral eh-<u>fyoo</u>-shun	accumulation of fluid in the pleural space, which compresses the underlying portion of the lung, resulting in dyspnea
pleurisy	ploor-<u>i</u>-se	inflammation of the pleura
pneumoconiosis	nu-mo-<u>ko</u>-ne-o-sis	any lung disease, e.g., anthracosis, silicosis, caused by permanent deposition of substantial amounts of particulate matter in the lungs
pneumothorax	nu-moh-<u>thoh</u>-racks	a collection of gas or air in the pleural cavity, resulting from a perforation through the chest wall or the visceral pleura
rhinitis rhinorrhea	ri-<u>ni</u>-tis <u>ri</u>-no-re-ah	inflammation of the nasal membrane; "runny nose"
SIDS	sidz	sudden infant death syndrome, or crib death; cause unknown; associated failure of synapse of nerves to activate the diaphragm
silicosis	sill-ih-<u>koh</u>-sis	a lung disorder caused by inhalation of silica (quartz) dust, resulting in the formation of small nodules
sinusitis	si-<u>nu</u>-si-tis	inflammation of a sinus
sneeze	sneeze	spasmodic contraction of muscles causing air to be expelled forcefully through the nose and mouth
streptococcal throat	strep-to-<u>kok</u>-al	sore throat caused by the spore bacteria *Streptococcus*
tonsillitis	ton-si-<u>li</u>-tis	inflammation of the tonsils, especially the palatine tonsils

(continues)

TABLE 13-2 *(continued)*

Condition	Pronunciation	Definition
tuberculosis (TB)	too-<u>ber</u>-ku-<u>lo</u>-sis	an infectious disease, marked by tubercles and caseous necrosis in tissues of the lung
URI		upper respiratory infection, general term for colds or "flu"
valley fever		see *coccidioidomycosis*
wheezing	wheez-<u>ing</u>	a high-pitched, whistling sound from air movement through narrowed bronchioles during exhalation; symptom of asthma and COPD
whooping cough	<u>hoop</u>-ing kof	a respiratory infection caused by *Bordetella pertussis*, marked by peculiar paroxysms of cough, ending in a prolonged crowing or whooping respiration

DIAGNOSTIC, SURGICAL, AND MEDICAL PROCEDURES AND GENERAL TERMS

The signs and symptoms of respiratory diseases are unique to the system. They provide doctors, nurses, and patients with clues in terms of sight and sound. For example, wheezing (sound), a certain color of phlegm (sight), coughing (sound), sneezing (sight and sound), and so forth. These manifestations are all helpful in diagnosing the problem.

The medical terminology included in Table 13-3 on diagnostics should become part of your vocabulary.

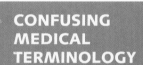

CONFUSING MEDICAL TERMINOLOGY

bronch/o Versus brachi/o

bronch/o (or bronchi/o) = bronchus (one of two branches leading from the trachea); e.g., bronchitis (brong-<u>kahy</u>-tis) refers to inflammation (-itis) or infection of the bronchus; bronchiectasis (brong-<u>kee</u>-ek-tuh-sis) refers to a condition of dilation (-ectasis) of the bronchus

brachi/o (brachio-, brachi-) = arm, e.g., brachialis (brey-kee-uhl-<u>al</u>-is) refers to a muscle of the upper arm

TABLE 13-3

Term	Pronunciation	Definition
aerosol	<u>a</u>-er-o-sol´	a medication that can be sprayed from a container to relieve bronchial distress, especially asthma
anoxia	an-<u>ok</u>-se-ah	without oxygen
apnea	<u>ap</u>-ne-ah	temporary cessation of breathing; asphyxia

TABLE 13-3 *(continued)*

Term	Pronunciation	Definition
bifurcation	bi´-fer-<u>ka</u>-shun	a division into two branches, e.g., bronchi
blood gases	blud <u>gas</u>-iz	oxygen, carbon dioxide, and other gases in the blood
bronchodilator	brong´-ko-di-<u>la</u>-tor	an agent capable of dilating the bronchi
bronchoscope	<u>brong</u>-ko-skop	an instrument for inspecting the bronchi
bronchoscopy	brong-<u>kos</u>-ko-pe	lung examination using a bronchoscope
bronchospasm	<u>brong</u>-ko-spazm	spasmodic contraction of bronchi muscles, as in asthma
Cheyne-Stokes	<u>chan</u>-stokes	breathing characterized by waxing and waning of the depth of respiration: the patient breathes deeply a short time and then breathes slightly or stops altogether; the cycle repeats
CO_2 (carbon dioxide)		an odorless, colorless gas resulting from oxidation of carbon, formed in the tissues and eliminated by the lungs
consolidation	kon-sol´-i-<u>da</u>-shun	solidification of lung tissue, as in pneumonia
CPR		cardiopulmonary resuscitation; artificial means of providing circulation and breathing during cardiac and respiratory arrest
cyanosis	si-ah-<u>no</u>-sis	a bluish discoloration of skin and mucous membranes caused by insufficient oxygen in the blood
dysphonia	dis-<u>fo</u>-ne-ah	voice impairment; difficulty in speaking
dyspnea	<u>disp</u>-ne-ah	labored or difficult breathing
endotracheal (ET) tube	en´-do-<u>tra</u>-ke-al	an airway catheter inserted in the trachea during surgery and for a temporary airway in emergency situations
expectorant	ek-<u>spek</u>-to-rant	an agent that promotes expectoration (loosening of secretions)
hemoptysis	he-<u>mop</u>-ti-sis	the spitting of blood or of blood-stained sputum (from the lungs)
hiatus	hi-<u>a</u>-tus	a gap (opening), especially in the diaphragm
hilus	<u>hi</u>-lus	part of lung where vessels, nerves, and bronchi enter
hypercapnia	hi´-per-<u>kap</u>-ne-ah	an excess of carbon dioxide in the blood
hyperventilation	hi´-per-ven´-ti-<u>la</u>-shun	increased rate and/or depth of respiration, e.g., from anxiety
hyposensitization	hi´-po-sen´-si-ti-<u>za</u>-shun	the process of rendering hyposensitive, e.g., exposing a patient to an offending substance to reduce his or her sensitivity to the substance
hypoxia	hi-<u>pok</u>-see-ah	insufficient oxygen

(continues)

TABLE 13-3	*(continued)*	
Term	**Pronunciation**	**Definition**
IPPB		intermittent positive pressure breathing, used as treatment with ventilation
Kussmaul breathing	<u>koos</u>-mowl	gasping, labored breathing; also called air hunger
laryngectomy	lah-rin-<u>jek</u>-to-me	excision of the larynx
laryngoscopy	lar´-ing-<u>gos</u>-ko-pe	visual examination of the interior larynx with an instrument called a laryngoscope
lavage of sinuses	lah-<u>vahzh</u> si-<u>nus</u>-es	the irrigation or washing out of sinuses
lobectomy	lo-<u>bek</u>-to-me	excision of a lobe of the lung
Mantoux (test)	man-<u>too</u>	tuberculosis skin test
O₂ (oxygen)	<u>ok</u>-si-jen	constitutes about 20% of atmospheric air; inhaled and carried in the blood
orthopnea	or´-thop-<u>ne</u>-ah	difficult breathing, except in the upright position
oximetry	ox-im-e-try	measurement of the oxygen saturation of arterial blood
palpation	<u>pal</u>-pay-shun	application of hands and fingers to external surfaces to detect abnormalities
parenchyma (lung)	pah-<u>reng</u>-ki-mah	the essential elements or "working parts" of an organ, e.g., alveoli in the lung
peak expiratory flow rate	pek ex-pi-<u>ra</u>-tory <u>flo</u>-rat	measurement of how fast a person can exhale using a small handheld device to monitor treatment in asthma or COPD
percussion and auscultation (P & A)	per-<u>kush</u>-un aw´-skul-<u>ta</u>-shun	striking the body (e.g., chest) with short, sharp blows of the fingers, and listening through a stethoscope for the sounds produced; technique used by practitioners
perfusion	per-<u>fu</u>-zhun	the passage of a fluid through the vessels of a specific organ to supply nutrients and oxygen
pneumothorax	nu´-mo-<u>tho</u>-raks	air or gas in the pleural space; from trauma or from deliberate introduction; may be spontaneous
postural drainage	<u>pos</u>-chur-al <u>dran</u>-ij	drainage by placing the patient's head downward so that the trachea will be inclined below the affected area and the secretions mobilized
PPD		purified protein derivative (TB test)
productive cough	pro-<u>duk</u>-tiv kof	cough with spitting of material from the bronchi
pulmonary function	<u>pul</u>-mo-ner´-e <u>fungk</u>-shun	tests to assess ventilatory status
pulmonary parenchyma	<u>pull</u>-mon-air-ee par-<u>en</u>-kih-mah	a structural arrangement of the lungs allowing the alveoli with very thin walls to exchange gases between the lungs and the blood

TABLE 13-3   *(continued)*

Term	Pronunciation	Definition
rales, rhonchi	rahlz, <u>rong</u>-ki	an abnormal respiratory sound heard on auscultation, indicating some pathologic condition
rarefaction	rar´-e-<u>fak</u>-shun	condition of being less dense, e.g., decreased density in x-ray films
residual air	re-<u>zed</u>-u-al	air remaining or left behind after expiration
respirator (ventilator)	<u>res</u>-pi-ra´-tor (ven´-ti-<u>la</u>-tor)	a device for giving artificial respiration or to assist in pulmonary ventilation
rhinoplasty	<u>ri</u>-no-plas´-te	plastic surgery of the nose
scan (lung, pleura)	skan	an image or a "picture" produced using radioactive isotopes, e.g., B-mode ultrasonography
SMR		submucous resection, excision of a portion of the submucous membrane of the nose to correct a defect
SOB		shortness of breath
spirometer (spirometry)	spi-<u>rom</u>-e-ter (spi-<u>rom</u>-e-tre)	an instrument for measuring air taken into and expelled from the lungs; spirometry is the measurement of lung capacity
sputum	<u>spu</u>-tum	matter ejected from the trachea, bronchi, and lungs through the mouth
tachypena	tak´-ip-<u>ne</u>-ah	very rapid respiration
thoracentesis	thor´-rah-sen-<u>te</u>-sis	surgical puncture of the chest wall into the parietal cavity to remove fluid
tine test		TB test
tracheostomy	tra´-ke-<u>os</u>-to-me	creation of an opening into the trachea through the neck, e.g., insertion of a tube to facilitate ventilation
tracheotomy	tra´-ke-<u>ot</u>-o-me	incision of the trachea through the skin and muscles of the neck
ventilator	ven´-ti-<u>la</u>-tor	an apparatus to assist in pulmonary ventilation; see also *respirator*
vital capacity	<u>vi</u>-tal kah-<u>pas</u>-i-te	amount of air that can be expelled from the lungs after deep inspiration (pulmonary function test)
wheeze	hweez	breathing with a raspy or whistling sound; common symptom of asthma
x-ray examination		visual record made using x-rays, for diagnostic examination of the chest; may be AP (anteroposterior) or Lat (side) views

PHARMACOLOGY AND MEDICAL TERMINOLOGY

Drug Classification	antitussive (an-tih-<u>tuss</u>-iv)	bronchodilator (brong-koh-<u>dye</u>-lay-tor)
Function	to reduce cough from various causes	expands the bronchial tubes by relaxing the bronchial muscles
Word Parts	**anti-** = against; **tussive** = pertaining to a cough	**bronch/o** = airway; **dilator** = pertaining to dilate or become wider
Active Ingredients (examples)	dextromethorphan hydrobromide (Benylin DM, Robitussin Pediatric, Vick's Formula 44, Vick's Formula 44 Pediatric Formula); pseudoephedrine hydrochloride and guaifenesin (Novahistex Expectorant with Decongestant, Robitussin PE, Sudafed Expectorant)	theophylline (Bronkodyl, Quibron-T/SR, Theobid Duracaps); aminophylline (Aminophylline, Truphyllin)

LESSON TWO   Progress Check

MATCHING

Match the terms in the left-hand column to their definitions on the right.

1. apnea	**a.** incomplete expansion or collapse of the lung
2. dyspnea	**b.** chronic dilation of the lung
3. orthopnea	**c.** spasm and swelling in the airways
4. tachypnea	**d.** abnormal accumulation of air
5. atelectasis	**e.** difficulty breathing except when sitting up
6. bronchiectasis	**f.** escape of fluid
7. dysphagia	**g.** very rapid breathing
8. emphysema	**h.** difficulty swallowing
9. asthma	**i.** difficult breathing
10. effusion	**j.** temporary cessation of breathing

MULTIPLE CHOICE

Circle the letter of the correct answer:

1. The pulmonary function test is used to
   a. diagnose abnormal lung tissue
   b. demonstrate abnormal pulmonary blood flow
   c. evaluate how a patient breathes
   d. measure obstructions to pulmonary function

2. When the chest wall is punctured with a needle to obtain fluid for diagnosis, the procedure is known as
    a. thoracentesis
    b. bronchoscopy
    c. pleural biopsy
    d. pulmonary angiogram

3. Coccidioidomycosis is
    a. a malignant lung tumor
    b. a disease caused by a fungus
    c. coughing up of blood
    d. a collection of fluid in the pleural cavity

4. Which of the following statements describes eupnea?
    a. shortness of breath
    b. lack of oxygen
    c. difficult breathing
    d. normal breathing

5. Heart failure caused by pulmonary disease is called
    a. coryza
    b. cor pulmonale
    c. COPD
    d. carcinoma

6. A deviated septum is a
    a. malfunctioning alveoli
    b. defect in the wall between nostrils
    c. broken nose
    d. pulmonary obstruction

7. Which of the following terms describes the coughing up of blood?
    a. expectorate
    b. hypoxia
    c. hemoptysis
    d. sputum

8. A hemothorax is a
    a. collection of blood in the chest
    b. collapsed lung
    c. creation of a new opening into the chest
    d. nosebleed

9. When part of the stomach protrudes through the diaphragm into the chest, the medical term is
    a. hyaline membrane disease
    b. hemothorax
    c. hiatal hernia
    d. histoplasmosis

10. The common name for pertussis is
   a.   measles
   b.   hay fever
   c.   hiccups
   d.   whooping cough

DEFINITIONS

Define the following terms:

1. pharynx _____

2. larynx _____

3. trachea _____

4. alveoli _____

5. bronchi _____

6. intercostal _____

7. sinuses _____

8. lungs _____

9. diaphragm _____

10. SIDS _____

11. COPD _____

12. pleurisy _____

13. cystic fibrosis _____

14. influenza _____

15. emphysema _____

16. ARDS _____

17. tachypnea _____

18. rhinoplasty _____

ABBREVIATIONS

Identify the following abbreviations:

1. URI _____

2. SOB _____

3. IPPB _____

4. SMR _____

5. CBC _____

6. TPR _____

7. PPD _____

8. CPR _____

9. ET tube _____

10. A & P _____

NAMING

Name the following respiratory symptoms from their descriptions:

1. excessive amount of carbon dioxide in the blood _____

2. breathing is possible only in an upright position _____

3. difficult breathing _____

4. condition where there is a bluish discoloration of the skin _____

5. spitting up blood _____

6. deficiency of oxygen _____

7. condition of pus in the pleural cavity _____

8. high-pitched, harsh sound heard during inspiration _____

9. inability to make sounds _____

10. blood in the pleural cavity _____

MATCHING: BREATH SOUNDS

Match the following breath sounds on the left with their descriptions on the right.

1. pleural rub   **a.** crackling sounds heard on auscultation, usually during inhalation
2. rales   **b.** loud, coarse, rattling sounds heard on auscultation
3. rhonchi   **c.** abnormally rapid breathing
4. wheeze   **d.** labored or difficult breathing
5. dyspnea   **e.** whistling sound heard without a stethoscope, usually during exhalation
6. tachypnea   **f.** rubbing sound heard on auscultation
                         g. abnormally slow breathing
                         h. high-pitched sound made during inspiration

◆ WORD PUZZLE ON THE RESPIRATORY SYSTEM

Find the 54 words related to the respiratory system by reading forward, backward, up, down, and diagonally. When you have circled the 54 listed words, the remaining letters spell the word AIR.

```
L  O  B  U  L  E  S  A  N  I  R  A  C  I  C  A  R  O  H  T
A  M  U  T  P  E  S  L  A  S  A  N  X  O  B  E  C  I  O  V
R  T  H  R  O  A  T  X  N  Y  R  A  H  P  S  T  I  D  A  L
Y  S  C  A  S  Y  R  A  N  O  M  L  U  P  A  S  S  A  G  E
N  I  N  S  P  I  R  A  T  I  O  N  I  N  H  A  L  E  A  B
X  N  O  I  T  A  R  I  P  S  E  R  C  I  L  I  A  B  S  R
E  E  R  U  S  S  E  R  P  L  A  I  T  R  A  P  T  R  E  O
D  S  H  A  L  L  O  W  C  T  R  A  C  H  E  A  I  O  X  N
I  A  E  R  A  T  E  I  O  E  V  R  E  S  E  R  V  N  C  C
X  H  E  T  A  R  B  R  L  S  U  L  O  E  V  L  A  C  H  H
O  C  S  A  A  O  Y  A  M  U  C  U  S  E  B  O  L  H  A  I
I  N  O  N  R  C  H  E  C  N  A  I  L  P  M  O  C  U  N  O
D  O  N  E  E  X  P  I  R  A  T  I  O  N  I  O  N  S  G  L
N  C  A  N  E  M  G  A  R  H  P  A  I  D  U  C  T  S  E  E
O  Y  T  I  L  I  B  I  S  N  E  T  S  I  D  T  U  B  E  S
B  E  E  R  T  L  A  I  H  C  N  O  R  B  O  X  Y  G  E  N
R  V  E  N  T  I  L  A  T  I  O  N  L  A  U  D  I  S  E  R
A  I  T  R  A  N  S  P  O  R  T  R  C  E  L  L  U  L  A  R
C  A  P  A  C  I  T  Y  T  I  V  A  C  L  A  R  U  E  L  P
G  N  U  L  S  U  R  F  A  C  T  A  N  T  B  R  E  A  T  H
```

Words to Look for in the Word Puzzle

1. aerate	**15.** diaphragm	**29.** nasal septum	**43.** shallow
2. aerobic	**16.** distensibility	**30.** nose	**44.** surfactant
3. alveolus	**17.** ducts	**31.** oxygen	**45.** tidal
4. breath	**18.** exhale	**32.** partial pressure	**46.** thoracic
5. bronchial tree	**19.** expiration	**33.** passage	**47.** throat
6. bronchioles	**20.** gas exchange	**34.** pleural cavity	**48.** trachea
7. bronchus	**21.** inhale	**35.** pulmonary	**49.** transport
8. capacity	**22.** inspiration	**36.** pharynx	**50.** tubes
9. carbon dioxide	**23.** larynx	**37.** rate	**51.** ventilation
10. carina	**24.** lobe	**38.** reserve	**52.** vital
11. cellular	**25.** lobules	**39.** residual	**53.** voice box
12. cilia	**26.** lung	**40.** respiration	**54.** ions
13. compliance	**27.** mucus	**41.** respiratory center	
14. concha	**28.** nare	**42.** sacs	

CHAPTER

14

Cardiovascular System

LESSON ONE: MATERIALS TO BE LEARNED

The Cardiovascular System
  Parts of the Heart
  The Circulatory System
  Types of Blood Vessels
  Blood Components
  Blood Pressure
  Clinical Disorders Affecting the
    Cardiovascular System
  Surgery, Lab, and Medical Tests
  Abbreviations

LESSON TWO: MATERIALS TO BE LEARNED

The Lymphatic System
  Components of the System
  Parts and Functions of the System
  Pathologic Conditions of the Lymph
    System

LESSON THREE: PROGRESS CHECK

Definitions
Naming
Matching: Diagnostic Procedures
Multiple Choice
Abbreviations
Word Puzzle on the Heart

OBJECTIVES

After completion of this chapter and the exercises, the student should be able to:

1. Identify the organs of the cardiovascular system.
2. Describe the location of the structures.
3. List the functions of the cardiovascular system.
4. Identify the structure and functions of the lymphatic system.
5. Name the five blood-forming organs associated with the circulatory system.
6. Identify and describe the types and functions of the blood vessels.
7. Identify and define selected clinical disorders affecting the cardiovascular system.
8. Explain medical tests and lab procedures used in the diagnosis of cardiovascular diseases/disorders.
9. Correctly spell and pronounce new medical terms.

ALLIED HEALTH PROFESSIONS

Cardiovascular Technologists and Technicians, Nuclear Medicine Technologists, Surgical Technologists, Emergency Medical Technicians, and Paramedics

Cardiovascular technologists and technicians assist physicians in diagnosing and treating cardiac (heart) and peripheral vascular (blood vessel) ailments. They schedule appointments, perform ultrasound or cardiovascular procedures, review doctors' interpretations and patient files, and monitor patients' heart rates. They also operate and maintain testing equipment, explain test procedures, and compare test results to a standard to identify problems. Other day-to-day activities vary significantly between specialties.

Surgical technologists, also called scrubs and surgical or operating room technicians, assist in surgical operations under the supervision of surgeons, registered nurses, or other surgical personnel. Surgical technologists are members of operating room teams, which most commonly include surgeons, anesthesiologists, and circulating nurses.

Before an operation, surgical technologists help prepare the operating room by setting up surgical instruments and equipment, sterile drapes, and sterile solutions. They assemble both sterile and nonsterile equipment, as well as check and adjust it to ensure that it is working properly. Technologists also prepare patients for surgery by washing, shaving, and disinfecting incision sites. They transport patients to the operating room, help position them on the operating table, and cover them with sterile surgical drapes. Technologists also observe patients' vital signs, check charts, and help the surgical team put on sterile gowns and gloves.

Nuclear medicine technologists operate cameras that detect and map the radioactive drug in a patient's body to create diagnostic images. After explaining test procedures to patients, technologists prepare a dosage of the radiopharmaceutical and administer it by mouth, injection, inhalation, or other means. They position patients and start a gamma scintillation camera, or "scanner," which creates images of the distribution of a radiopharmaceutical as it localizes in, and emits signals from, the patient's body. The images are produced on a computer screen or on film for a physician to interpret.

Paramedics, or emergency medical technicians (EMTs), have a career that often is very dramatic, calling for immediate, calm application of the EMT's skills amid sometimes dangerous conditions. The September 11, 2001, attack on the World Trade Center was the most dramatic and deadly situation that paramedics, along with teams of firefighters and police, have ever faced, and they lived up to their potential and training with great heroism. If you watched the terrible events unfolding at that scene, you saw many of them in action as their ambulances drove through smoke, fire, and rubble to help rescue and transport the critically injured to hospitals. Their bravery in the face of peril speaks well of the crucial role played by paramedics in times of crisis as well as in everyday life.

INQUIRY

Alliance of Cardiovascular Professionals: www.acp-online.org
American Society of Radiologic Technologists: www.asrt.org
Society of Nuclear Medicine Technologists: www.snm.org

For a list of accredited programs in nuclear medicine technology, visit the following websites:
Joint Review Committee on Educational Programs in Nuclear Medicine Technology: www.jrcnmt.org
National Association of Emergency Medical Technicians: www.naemt.org

Data from Stanfield, Peggy S., Cross, Nanna, and Hui, Y.H. *Introduction to the Health Professions*, 6th ed. Burlington, MA: Jones & Bartlett Learning; 2012.

The cardiovascular system is a subset of the circulatory system. It consists of the heart, blood vessels, and blood. The lymphatic system is also a part of the circulatory system, consisting of lymph vessels and lymph nodes within the larger vessels. Associated with the circulatory system are the blood-forming organs, that is, the spleen, liver, bone marrow, thymus gland, and lymph tissue (see **Figures 14–1** through **14–4**).

The heart is a four-chambered hollow organ that lies between the lungs in the middle of the *thoracic* cavity. Two-thirds of the heart lies left of the *midsternum*. It is about the size of the owner's fist. It is cone-shaped, the base directed toward the right shoulder and the apex pointed toward the left hip.

The heart is covered with a double-walled sac called the *pericardium* that encloses the heart and great blood vessels. It is attached to the *diaphragm*, the *sternum*, and the lung pleura. The tough outer layer of the pericardium protects the heart. The inner *serous* layer contains the visceral membrane (*epicardium*) that covers the heart surface

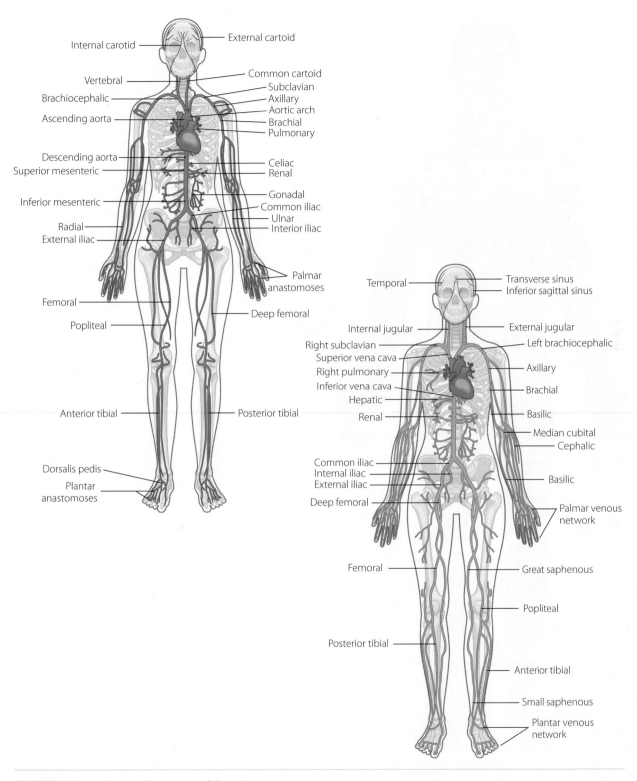

FIGURE 14–1 The arterial system and the venous system

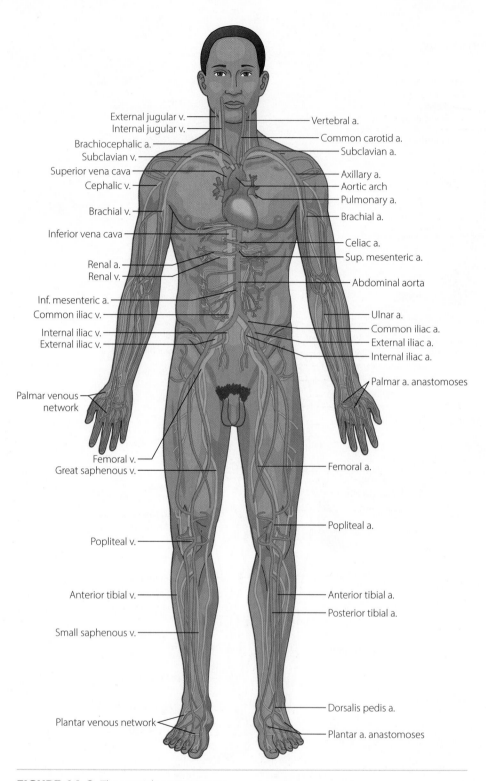

External jugular v.
Internal jugular v.
Brachiocephalic a.
Subclavian v.
Superior vena cava
Cephalic v.
Brachial v.
Inferior vena cava
Renal a.
Renal v.
Inf. mesenteric a.
Common iliac v.
Internal iliac v.
External iliac v.
Palmar venous network
Femoral v.
Great saphenous v.
Popliteal v.
Anterior tibial v.
Small saphenous v.
Plantar venous network

Vertebral a.
Common carotid a.
Subclavian a.
Axillary a.
Aortic arch
Pulmonary a.
Brachial a.
Celiac a.
Sup. mesenteric a.
Abdominal aorta
Ulnar a.
Common iliac a.
External iliac a.
Internal iliac a.
Palmar a. anastomoses
Femoral a.
Popliteal a.
Anterior tibial a.
Posterior tibial a.
Dorsalis pedis a.
Plantar a. anastomoses

FIGURE 14–2 The arterial-venous system

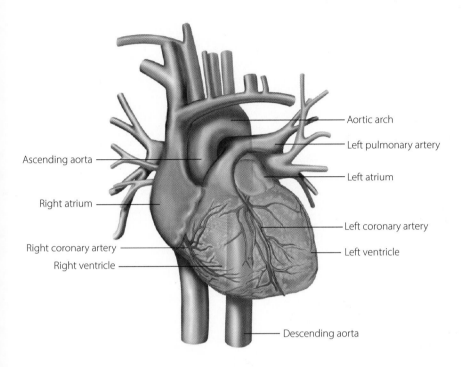

Aortic arch

Left pulmonary artery

Ascending aorta

Left atrium

Right atrium

Left coronary artery

Right coronary artery

Left ventricle

Right ventricle

Descending aorta

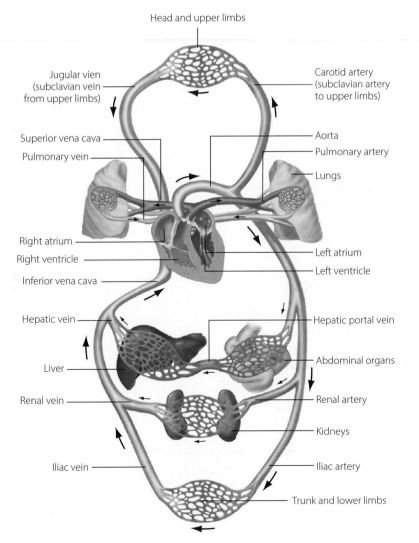

Head and upper limbs

Jugular vien
(subclavian vein
from upper limbs)

Carotid artery
(subclavian artery
to upper limbs)

Superior vena cava

Aorta

Pulmonary vein

Pulmonary artery

Lungs

Right atrium

Left atrium

Right ventricle

Left ventricle

Inferior vena cava

Hepatic vein

Hepatic portal vein

Liver

Abdominal organs

Renal vein

Renal artery

Kidneys

Iliac vein

Iliac artery

Trunk and lower limbs

FIGURE 14–3 The heart and blood circuits

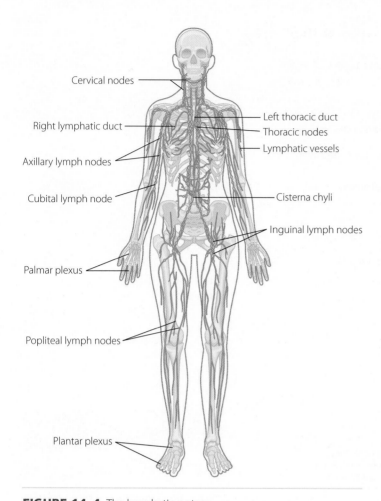

FIGURE 14–4 The lymphatic system

and the parietal membrane that lines the inside of the pericardium. There is fluid in the space between these layers that lubricates the membrane and prevents friction.

There are four heart chambers, upper right and left *atria* and lower right and left *ventricles*. The ventricles are separated by the *interventricular* septum. The *tricuspid* valve lies between the right atrium and right ventricle. Blood flows forward through the valve in one chamber, backward in another. It regulates blood pressure in the heart, sending blood into the right ventricle when the pressure is greater in the right atrium and preventing backflow of blood into the right atrium.

The blood vessels are a series of closed tubes that carry blood from the heart to the tissue and back to the heart. The three major types of vessels are *arteries, capillaries,* and *veins.*

Arteries carry blood from the heart. Elastic arteries are the largest arteries from the heart. Muscular arteries branch into medium-sized and small arteries that contain both muscular and elastic tissue. The smallest, the *arterioles,* deliver blood to capillary beds in the tissues.

Veins carry blood back to the atria of the heart. The venous system holds 75% of total blood volume and returns blood under low pressure. The venous system begins at the *capillary* beds and flows into larger *venules* and then into small, medium, and large veins.

The major arteries of systemic circulation are the *aorta*, the largest vessel in diameter in the body, and the branches from the aorta leading toward the head and neck, and descending into the trunk and lower extremities (see Figures 14–1, 14–2, and 14–3 for complete details).

The circulatory system can be divided into three types of circulation: pulmonary (lung), systemic (whole body), and portal (intestine, liver, and spleen). Functions of the circulatory system are:

1. *Transport:* gases, hormones, minerals, enzymes, and other vital substances are carried in the blood to every cell in the body; all waste materials are carried by the blood to the lungs, skin, or kidneys for elimination from the body (*pulmonary circulation*)
2. *Body temperature:* the blood vessels maintain body temperature by dilating at the skin surface to dissipate heat or by constricting to retain heat
3. *Protection:* the blood and lymphatic systems protect the body against injury and foreign invasion through the immune system; blood clotting mechanisms protect against blood loss
4. *Buffering:* blood proteins provide an acid–base buffer system to maintain optimum pH of the blood

The parts of the heart are defined and illustrated in Lesson One of this chapter.

LESSON ONE	**Materials to Be Learned**

The human circulatory system consists of a pump (the heart) and a network of vessels that transport blood throughout the body. The workhorse of the circulatory system is the heart, propelling blood through approximately 60 miles of blood vessels in the body.

Lesson One explains the parts and functions of the heart and blood vessels and the terminology related to them. It also describes disorders/diseases affecting the system and some means of diagnosis and treatment of them. Blood pressure terminology, blood types, blood components, and other general and related terms are included. The lymphatic system, which is an integral part of the circulatory system, is discussed in Lesson Two.

THE CARDIOVASCULAR SYSTEM

This information should be studied in conjunction with **Figures 14–5** through **14–9**.

Parts of the Heart

The heart is a muscular, cone-shaped organ, about the size of a clenched fist, that pumps blood throughout the body and beats normally about 70 times per minute by coordinated nerve impulses and muscular contractions. *Pulmonary circulation* provides for oxygenation of blood and *systemic circulation* is responsible for transportation of blood to and from body cells. The heart is enclosed in a fibroserous sac and is divided into four chambers.

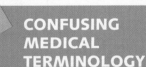

CONFUSING MEDICAL TERMINOLOGY

aort/o Versus atri/o Versus arteri/o Versus arteriol/o

aort/o = aorta, e.g., aortostenosis (a-or-to-<u>steh</u>-no-sis) refers to narrowing of the aorta (a-<u>or</u>-toh)

atri/o = atrium, e.g., atrium (<u>a</u>-tre-um) refers to each of the two (left and right) upper chambers of the heart

arteri/o = artery, e.g., arteriosclerosis (ar-te-re-<u>o</u>-skleh-ro-sis) refers to hardening of an artery

arteriol/o = arteriole, e.g., arteriolitis (ar-ter-i-o-<u>li</u>-tis) refers to inflammation of an arteriole

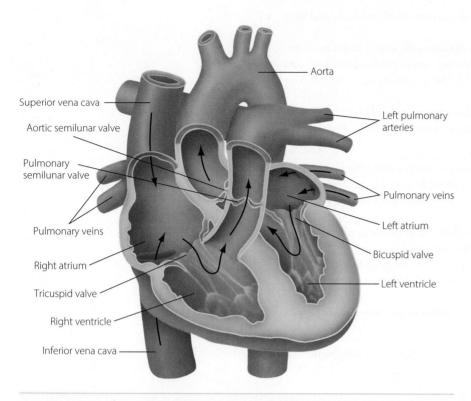

Aorta

Superior vena cava

Aortic semilunar valve

Pulmonary
semilunar valve

Left pulmonary
arteries

Pulmonary veins

Pulmonary veins

Left atrium

Right atrium

Bicuspid valve

Tricuspid valve

Left ventricle

Right ventricle

Inferior vena cava

FIGURE 14–5 Diagram of the heart; arrows indicate direction of blood flow

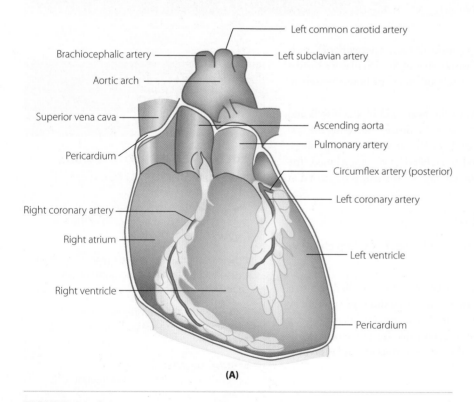

Left common carotid artery

Brachiocephalic artery

Left subclavian artery

Aortic arch

Superior vena cava

Ascending aorta

Pericardium

Pulmonary artery

Circumflex artery (posterior)

Left coronary artery

Right coronary artery

Right atrium

Left ventricle

Right ventricle

Pericardium

(A)

FIGURE 14–6 (A) Anterior structure of the heart.

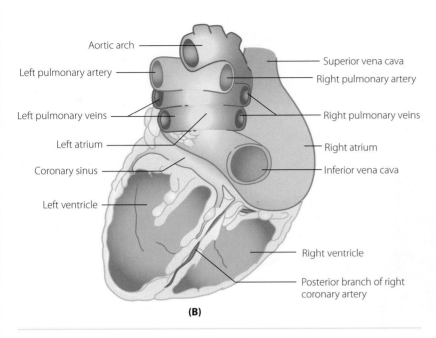

FIGURE 14–6 (B) Posterior structure of the heart.

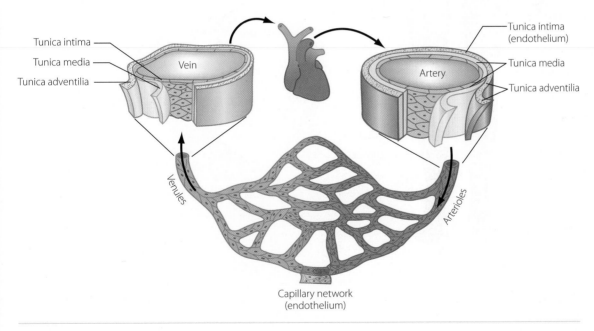

FIGURE 14–7 Blood vessels, showing the single-cell endothelium of all the vessels and the layered muscular coats of arteries and veins

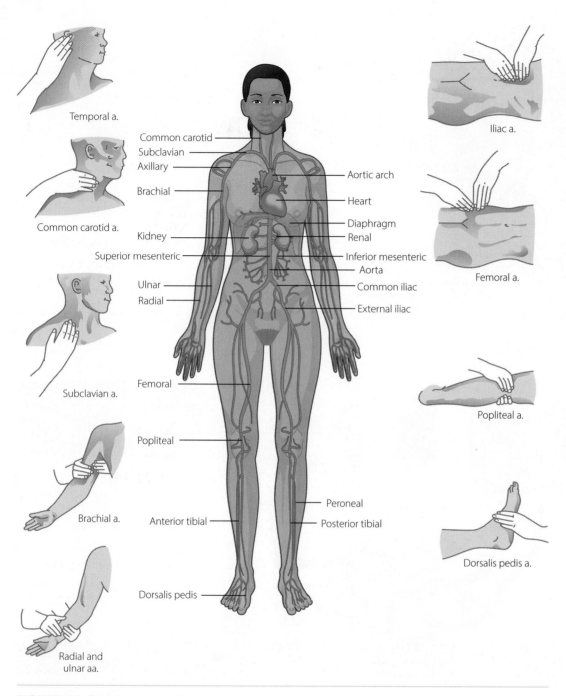

FIGURE 14–8 Major arteries of the body

The Circulatory System

The circulatory system in the body transports oxygen and nutrients *to* and carbon dioxide and wastes *away from* the cells.

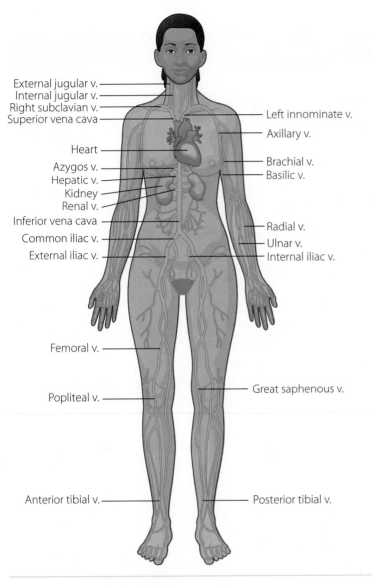

External jugular v.
Internal jugular v.
Right subclavian v.
Superior vena cava
Heart
Azygos v.
Hepatic v.
Kidney
Renal v.
Inferior vena cava
Common iliac v.
External iliac v.

Left innominate v.
Axillary v.
Brachial v.
Basilic v.
Radial v.
Ulnar v.
Internal iliac v.

Femoral v.

Popliteal v.

Great saphenous v.

Anterior tibial v.

Posterior tibial v.

FIGURE 14–9 Major veins of the body

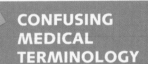

CONFUSING MEDICAL TERMINOLOGY

apheresis Versus -poiesis

apheresis = removal of blood, e.g., therapeutic apheresis (<u>ah</u>-fer-ee-cis) refers to the removal of a component of the blood that contributes to a disease state

-poiesis = formation, e.g., hematopoiesis (hi-mat-oh-poi-<u>ee</u>-sis) refers to formation of blood

CONFUSING MEDICAL TERMINOLOGY

hemostasis Versus homeostasis

hemostasis = control of blood flow (hee-<u>muh</u>-stey-sis)

homeostasis = a steady state (<u>hoh</u>-mee-uh-stey-sis)

TABLE 14-1

Parts of the Heart	Pronunciation	Definition
heart	hart	the organ of circulation of the blood
atrium (pl, atria)	<u>a</u>-tre-um (<u>a</u>-tre-uh)	one of the two (left and right) upper chambers of the heart; also known as the auricle; these upper chambers collect blood
ventricle	<u>ven</u>-tri-kul	one of the two (left and right) lower chambers of the heart; they pump blood from the heart
apex	<u>a</u>-peks	the pointed end (of the heart)

(continues)

TABLE 14-1   (continued)

Parts of the Heart	Pronunciation	Definition
Valves	valvz	a membrane in a passage to prevent backward flow
tricuspid	tri-<u>kus</u>-pid	having three points or cusps, situated between the right atrium and the right ventricle
pulmonary semilunar	<u>pul</u>-mon-ner´-e sem´-i-<u>lu</u>-nar	pertaining to the lung and resembling a crescent valve; located between the right ventricle and the pulmonary artery
mitral	<u>mi</u>-tral	shaped like a miter, also called bicuspid valve; situated between the left atrium and the left ventricle
aortic	a-<u>or</u>-tic	located between the left ventricle and the aorta
septum	<u>sep</u>-tum	a dividing wall between the right and left sides of the heart
Muscle	<u>muhs</u>-uhl	
myocardium	mi´-o-<u>kar</u>-de-um	middle, thickest layer of the heart wall, made of cardiac muscle
Membranes	<u>mem</u>-brânz	
pericardium	per´-i-<u>kar</u>-de-um	the fibroserous sac enclosing the heart
endocardium	en´-do-<u>kar</u>-de-um	lining membrane of the heart's cavities
epicardium	ep´-i-<u>kar</u>-de-um	the visceral pericardium
Conduction System		
sinoatrial node, or SA node	si´-no-<u>a</u>-tre-al nod	atypical muscle fibers at the junction of the superior vena cava and right atrium; it originates the cardiac rhythm and is therefore called pacemaker of the heart
atrioventricular node	a´-tre-o-ven-<u>trik</u>-u-lar nod	Purkinje fibers beneath the endocardium of the right atrium in the septum
bundle of His	<u>bun</u>-d´-l of his	cardiac muscle fibers connecting the atria with the ventricles of the heart

TABLE 14-2

Circulation	Pronunciation	Definition
circulation	ser´-ku-<u>la</u>-shun	movement in circuitous course; as the movement of blood through the heart and blood vessels
pulmonary	<u>pul</u>-mo-ner´-e	movement of blood through the lungs and the pulmonary artery
systemic	sis-<u>tem</u>-ic	pertaining to movement of blood to the body as a whole
portal	<u>por</u>-tal	circulation of blood from the gastrointestinal tract and spleen through the portal vein to the liver

Types of Blood Vessels

Three types of vessels carry blood throughout the body. Each has a unique structure and function.

TABLE 14-3

Blood Vessels	Pronunciation	Definition
Artery	ar-ter-e	a vessel in which blood flows away from the heart, carrying oxygenated blood
aorta	a-or-tah	the great artery arising from the left ventricle; largest artery
coronary arteries	kor-o-ner´-e ar-ter-es	arteries from the base of the aorta that supply the heart muscle with blood
Vein	vân	a vessel in which blood flows toward the heart, carrying blood with little oxygen
vena cava	ve-nah ca-vah	largest vein. *Inferior:* the venous trunk for the lower viscera. *Superior:* the venous trunk draining blood from head, neck, upper limbs, and thorax
Capillary	kap-i-ler´-e	a minute, hairlike vessel connecting arterioles and venules

Blood Components

TABLE 14-4

Component	Pronunciation	Definition
Red Blood Cells (RBCs)	red blud	red corpuscles; one of the formed elements in peripheral blood. They contain hemoglobin and transport oxygen. Also called erythrocytes
White Blood Cells (WBCs)	wahyt blud	colorless blood corpuscles capable of ameboid movement; protect the body against pathogenic microorganisms. There are five types of white blood cells. Also called leukocytes
granulocytes	gran-u-lo-sitz´	any cells containing granules, especially a granular leukocyte; formed in the bone marrow. There are three types: neutrophils, eosinophils, and basophils
neutrophils	nu-tro-filz	having a nucleus with three to five lobes and cytoplasm containing very fine granules. Neutrophils defend the body by ingesting invaders. Type 1 WBC
eosinophils	e´-o-sin-o-filz	having a nucleus with two lobes and cytoplasm containing coarse, round granules. May be associated with allergy. Type 2 WBC
basophils	ba-so-filz	any structure cells staining readily with basic dyes; functions unknown. Type 3 WBC
agranulocytes	ah-gran-u-lo-sitz´	nongranular leukocytes, produced by the spleen and lymph nodes. There are two types
lymphocytes	lim-fo-sitz	participate in immunity; produced by the spleen and lymph nodes. Type 4 WBC
monocytes	mon-o-sitz	destroy foreign invaders in the body. Type 5 WBC

(continues)

TABLE 14-4 *(continued)*

Component	Pronunciation	Definition
Other Components		
fibrinogen	fi-<u>brin</u>-o-jen	promotes blood clotting
thrombocytes	<u>throm</u>-bo-sitz	blood platelets
plasma	<u>plas</u>-mah	the fluid portion of the blood or lymph, without the cells, amber-colored; when whole blood is undisturbed in a tube, clotting cells settle in the bottom, and the clear plasma is on top
serum	<u>se</u>-rum	the clear portion of the blood separated from solid elements; plasma minus fibrinogen
platelet	<u>plât</u>-let	a disk-shaped structure in the blood, for blood coagulation; also called thrombocyte
reticulocytes	re-<u>tik</u>-u-lo´-sitz	immature red blood cells, in the bone marrow
Landsteiner types	<u>land</u>-sti-ner	refers to the type of red blood cell: A, B, AB, and O
universal donor	<u>do</u>-ner	a person with group O blood; frequently used in emergency transfusion
universal recipient	re-<u>sip</u>-e-ent	able to receive blood of any type; group AB
type and crossmatch (x match)		determination of the compatibility of the blood of a donor and that of a recipient before transfusion by placing the donor's cells in the recipient's serum and the recipient's cells in the donor's serum; absence of agglutination, hemolysis, and cytotoxicity indicates compatibility
Rh factors		a genetically determined antigen, present on the surface of erythrocytes. There are at least eight variations. It is named for rhesus monkeys used in early experiments. One Rh factor present in blood means it is Rh positive; if no factor is found, the blood is Rh negative

Blood Pressure

TABLE 14-5

Term	Pronunciation	Definition
hypertension	hi´-per-<u>ten</u>-shun	persistently high arterial blood pressure; causes may or may not be identifiable
sphygmomanometer	sfig´-mo-mah-<u>nom</u>-e-ter	an instrument for measuring arterial blood pressure
systolic pressure	sis-<u>tol</u>-ic <u>presh</u>-ur	the contraction, or period of contraction, of the heart, especially of the ventricles; the top number in a blood pressure reading
diastolic pressure	di-ah-<u>stol</u>-ic <u>presh</u>-ur	the dilation, or the period of dilation of the heart, especially of the ventricles; the bottom number in a blood pressure reading
normal BP		an acceptable range for systolic pressure is ≤ 120, and for diastolic < 80

Clinical Disorders Affecting the Cardiovascular System

TABLE 14-6		
Condition	**Pronunciation**	**Definition**
anemia	ah-<u>ne</u>-me-ah	reduction below normal of red blood cells, hemoglobin, or the volume of packed red cells in the blood; a symptom of various disorders
aneurysm	<u>an</u>-u-rizm	a sac formed by localized dilation of an artery or vein
angina pectoris	an-<u>ji</u>-nah <u>pek</u>-to-ris	pain in the chest, caused by decreased supply of oxygen to the heart muscle; can be precipitated by increased activity or stress
arrhythmia	ah-<u>rith</u>-me-ah	variation from the normal rhythm of the heartbeat
arteriosclerosis	ar-te´re-o-skle-<u>ro</u>-sis	thickening and loss of elasticity of the arterial walls, slowing the flow of blood
asystole	a-<u>sis</u>-to-le	cardiac standstill; no heartbeat
atherosclerosis	ath´-er-o-skle-<u>ro</u>-sis	a form of arteriosclerosis in which fats (e.g., cholesterol) are deposited on arterial walls
cardiac arrest	<u>kar</u>-de-ak ah-<u>rest</u>	cessation of heart function
coarctation	ko´-ark-<u>ta</u>-shun	stricture or narrowing of a vessel
Congenital Defects	kon-<u>jen</u>-i-tal <u>de</u>-fekts	defects present at birth
cyanosis	sigh´-ah-<u>no</u>-sis	dark, slightly bluish discoloration of the skin resulting from reduced hemoglobin in the blood
patent ductus arteriosus	<u>pa</u>-tent <u>duk</u>-tus ar-te-re-<u>o</u>-sus	birth defect; duct with an abnormal open lumen in the ductus arteriosus
tetralogy of Fallot	te-<u>tral</u>-o-je of fah-<u>lo</u>	birth defect consisting of pulmonic stenosis, interventricular septal defect, hypertrophy of right ventricle, and transposition of the aorta
congestive heart failure (CHF)	kon-<u>jes</u>-tiv hart <u>fâl</u>-yer	defective blood-pumping system, marked by breathlessness and abnormal retention of sodium and water (see **Figure 14–10**)
embolism	<u>em</u>-bo-lizm	the sudden blocking of an artery by an embolus
embolus	<u>em</u>-bo-lus	a foreign object (i.e., air, fat, tissue, or blood) brought by the blood and forced into a smaller vessel, thus obstructing the circulation
endocarditis	en´-do-kar-<u>di</u>-tis	exudative and proliferative inflammation of the endocardium
fibrillation	fi´-bri-<u>la</u>-shun	a small, local, involuntary muscular contraction, caused by spontaneous activation of single muscle cells or muscle fibers

(continues)

TABLE	14-6	(continued)

Condition	Pronunciation	Definition
Heart Attack		
coronary thrombosis	<u>kor</u>-o-ner-e throm-<u>bo</u>-sis	thrombosis of a coronary artery, often leading to myocardial infarction
infarction	<u>in</u>-fark-shun	a localized area of ischemic necrosis owing to occlusion of the arterial supply
myocardial infarction	mi-o-kar´-de-al in-<u>fark</u>-shun	gross necrosis of the myocardium, caused by decreased blood supply to the area
occlusion	o-<u>kloo</u>-zhun	obstruction, a closing off of the coronary arteries, leading to a heart attack
heart block	hart blok	impairment of conduction in heart excitation; often applied specifically to arterioventricular heart block
heart murmur	hart <u>mer</u>-mer	an auscultatory sound (soft, blowing); a periodic sound of short duration of cardiac origin; may be the result of an incompetent valve
hemophilia	he´-mo-<u>fil</u>-e-ah	a hereditary hemorrhagic condition caused by lack of one or more clotting factors
Hodgkin's disease	<u>hoj</u>-kinz di-<u>zez</u>	painless progressive enlargement of lymph nodes, spleen, and lymphoid tissue; symptoms include anorexia, lassitude, weight loss, fever, itching, night sweats, and anemia
hypertension	hi´-per-<u>ten</u>-shun	persistently high arterial blood pressure; causes may or may not be identifiable
ischemia	is-<u>ke</u>-me-ah	deficiency of blood in a part; caused by spasm of blood vessel, temporarily reducing blood flow
leukemia	loo-<u>ke</u>-me-ah	a malignant disease of the blood-forming organs, e.g., abnormal proliferation and development of leukocytes and related cells in blood and bone marrow
myocarditis	mi´-o-kar-<u>di</u>-tis	inflammation of the myocardium
pericarditis	per´-i-kar-<u>di</u>-tis	inflammation of the pericardium
plaque	plak	a deposit of fatty material in the artery (atherosclerosis)
rheumatic heart disease	roo-<u>mat</u>-ik	the most important manifestation and sequel to rheumatic fever, consisting chiefly of valvular deformities
stroke (cerebrovascular accident [CVA])	strôk	a sudden and acute vascular lesion of the brain caused by hemorrhage, embolism, thrombosis, or rupturing blood vessels
thrombophlebitis	throm´-bo-fle-<u>bi</u>-tis	inflammation of a vein associated with thrombus formation
transient ischemic attack (TIA)	<u>tran</u>-s-hən is-<u>kem</u>-ik ah-<u>tak</u>	brief interruption of circulation to a portion of the brain owing to vascular spasm, causing temporary loss of function; a precursor to CVA
varicose veins	<u>var</u>-i-kos vânz	a dilated, tortuous vein, usually in the leg, caused by a defective venous valve

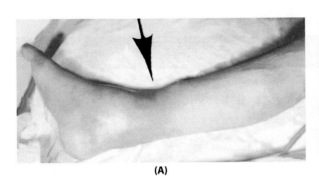
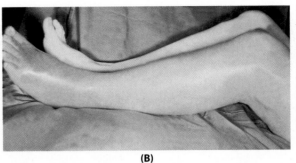

FIGURE 14–10 (A) Marked pitting edema of leg as a result of chronic heart failure. (B) Localized edema of left leg caused by venous obstruction; right leg appears normal.

Surgery, Lab, and Medical Tests

TABLE 14-7

Term	Pronunciation	Definition
angiography	an´-je-<u>og</u>-rah-fe	x-ray technique using an injected contrast medium to visualize the heart and blood vessels
angioplasty	<u>an</u>-je-o-plas´-te	surgical or percutaneous reconstruction of blood vessels
balloon angioplasty		insertion of a balloon to dilate a vessel (see PTCA)
anticoagulant	an´-ti-ko-<u>ag</u>-u-lant	any substance that removes or prevents blood clotting
antihypertensive drug	an´-ti-hi´-per-<u>ten</u>-siv	a drug that reduces or eliminates high blood pressure
auscultation	aws´-kul-<u>ta</u>-shun	the act of listening for sounds within the body chiefly to ascertain the condition of the thoracic or abdominal viscera; may be performed with the unaided ear or with a stethoscope
bradycardia	brad´-e-<u>kar</u>-de-ah	slowness of the heartbeat, as evidenced by a pulse rate of < 60
bypass	<u>bi</u>-pas	a surgically created route to circumvent the normal path
cardiac catheterization	<u>kar</u>-de-ak kath´-e-ter-i-<u>za</u>-tion	a long, fine catheter is navigated through a peripheral blood vessel into the chambers of the heart using x-ray visualization as a guide
cardiac enzyme test	<u>kar</u>-de-ak <u>en</u>-zym test	tests on drawn blood samples to determine if there is damage to the myocardial muscle
collateral circulation	ko-<u>lat</u>-er-al ser´-ku-<u>la</u>-shun	circulation by secondary channels after obstruction of the principal channel supplying the heart
commissurotomy	kom´-i-shur-<u>ot</u>-o-me	surgical incision of a defective heart valve to increase the size of the orifice; commonly done to separate adherent, thickened leaflets of a stenotic mitral valve

(continues)

TABLE 14-7   (continued)

Term	Pronunciation	Definition
computed axial tomography (CAT scan or CT scan)	kuh-m-<u>pyoot</u>-ed <u>ak</u>-see-al toh-<u>mog</u>-rah-fee	diagnostic x-ray technique that uses ionizing radiation to produce cross-section images of the body; the x-ray feeds the images into a computer that produces cross-sectional pictures
coronary artery bypass graft	<u>kor</u>-o-ner-e <u>ar</u>-ter-e <u>bi</u>-pas	use of a leg vein or synthetic material to substitute for an occluded artery in the heart
digitalize	dij´-i-tal-<u>iz</u>	to administer digitalis in a dosage schedule designed to produce and then maintain optimal heart contraction with nominal side effects
diuretic	di´-u-<u>ret</u>-ik	an agent that promotes removal of excess interstitial fluid and results in increased urine secretion
Doppler	<u>dop</u>-ler	a device for measuring blood flow that transmits and reflects sound waves
dyscrasia	dis-<u>kra</u>-ze-ah	any abnormal condition of the blood
echocardiography	ek-oh-car-dee-<u>og</u>-rah-fee	diagnostic procedure using ultrasound waves to study the structure and motion of the heart and to detect changes in some heart disorders
electrocardiogram	e-lek´-tro-<u>kar</u>-de-o-gram´	the record produced by electrocardiography; abbreviated ECG or EKG
endarterectomy	en´-dar-ter-<u>ek</u>-to-me	excision of thickened areas of the innermost coat of an artery to increase blood flow
exercise stress test		test widely used to assess cardiac function by means of subjecting the patient to controlled amounts of physical stress, such as the treadmill, pedaling a stationary bike, or climbing stairs
hemoglobin	he´-mo-<u>glo</u>-bin	the oxygen-carrying pigment of the red blood cells; it contains iron and copper
heparin	<u>hep</u>-ah-rin	a substance that counteracts blood clotting, existing both as a natural substance in the blood and as a drug
Holter monitor	<u>hol</u>-tur	a portable device for monitoring blood pressure or heart/respiratory rate, e.g., ECG
low-salt diet		common term for a diet low in sodium content to reduce body-water level; correctly termed sodium-restricted diet
lumen	<u>loo</u>-men	the cavity or channel within a tube, e.g., a blood vessel
magnetic resonance imaging (MRI)	mag-<u>neh</u>-tic rehz-oh-nans <u>im</u>-uh-jing	noninvasive procedure that uses strong magnetic fields and radiofrequency waves to produce images of soft tissue, heart, blood vessels, and brain; it can also show the heartbeat and blood flow. Used to detect possible tumors and other pericardial conditions
pacemaker	<u>pâs</u>-mâk-er	that which sets the pace at which a phenomenon occurs; often used alone to indicate the natural cardiac pacemaker or an artificial cardiac pacemaker
phlebotomy	fle-<u>bot</u>-o-me	incision of a vein

TABLE 14-7 *(continued)*

Term	Pronunciation	Definition
positron emission tomography (PET)	<u>pawz</u>-ih-tron ee-mish-<u>un</u> toh-<u>mog</u>-rah-fee	computerized x-ray technique using radioactive substances, which are given by injection, to measure blood flow and metabolic activity of the heart and blood vessels; the radiation emitted is measured by the PET camera
percutaneous transluminal coronary angioplasty (PTCA)	per´-ku-<u>ta</u>-ne-us trans-<u>lum</u>-i-nul <u>kor</u>-o-ner-e <u>an</u>-je-o-plas´-te	dilation of a blood vessel by means of a balloon catheter inserted through the skin and into the chosen vessel and then passed through the lumen of the vessel to the site of the lesion, where the balloon is inflated to flatten plaque against the artery wall
serum lipid test	<u>see</u>-rum <u>lip</u>-id test	tests on drawn blood samples to measure the amount of cholesterol, triglyceride, and lipoprotein substances in the blood
sinus rhythm	<u>si</u>-nus <u>rith</u>-uh-m	the normal heart rhythm originating in the sinoatrial (SA) node
tachycardia	tak´-e-<u>kar</u>-de-ah	abnormally rapid heart rate
thallium stress test	thal-<u>ee</u>-um stress test	thallium injections are given intravenously in conjunction with the stress test to determine whether there are changes in coronary blood flow during exercise; changes may be indicative of ischemia, severe coronary narrowing, or infarction
thrombolysis	throm-bo-<u>li</u>-sis	injection of a drug to dissolve a blood clot and restore blood flow in the coronary artery to prevent heart damage during a heart attack
vasodilator	vas´-o-di-<u>la</u>-tor	an agent that dilates blood vessels
vasopressor	vas´-o-<u>pres</u>-or	an agent that constricts blood vessels
venipuncture	ven´-i-<u>pungk</u>-chur	puncture of a vein with a needle to withdraw blood or infuse fluid

Abbreviations

These abbreviations are frequently used when diagnosing and/or charting cardiovascular disorders.

TABLE 14-8

Abbreviation	Definition	Abbreviation	Definition
ALL	acute lymphocytic leukemia	ASHD	arteriosclerotic heart disease
AMI	acute myocardial infarction	BASO	basophil (type of WBC)
AML	acute myeloblastic leukemia (myeloblast: primitive bone marrow WBC)	BBB	bundle branch block
ASD	arterial septal defect	BP	blood pressure

(continues)

TABLE 14-8 *(continued)*

Abbreviation	Definition
CABG	coronary artery bypass graft
CBC	complete blood count
CCU	coronary care unit
CHF	congestive heart failure
CO_2	carbon dioxide
CPR	cardiopulmonary resuscitation
CVA	cerebrovascular accident
DOE	dyspnea on exertion
DVT	deep vein thrombosis
ECG, EKG	electrocardiogram
ECHO	echocardiogram
Eos	eosinophil (type of WBC)
HDL	high-density lipoprotein
LDL	low-density lipoprotein
Lymph	lymphocyte (type of WBC)
MI	myocardial infarction
Mono	monocyte (type of WBC); *mono* also can mean mononucleosis

Abbreviation	Definition
MRI	magnetic resonance imaging
MVP	mitral valve prolapse
O_2	oxygen
PMI	point of maximal impulse (of heart on chest wall)
PMN	polymorphonuclear (leukocyte)
PTCA	percutaneous transluminal coronary angioplasty
PVC	premature ventricular contractions
RBC	red blood cell, red blood (cell) count
SA	sinoatrial
Segs	white blood cells with segmented nuclei
TIA	transient ischemic attack
VSD	ventricular septal defect
VT	ventricular tachycardia
WBC	white blood cell; white blood (cell) count

LESSON TWO   Materials to Be Learned

The lymphatic system is an accessory component of the circulatory system. It produces and stores *lymphocytes* and *lymph fluid* (which is derived from tissue fluid). Lymph vessels return lymph fluid to the circulation. Functions of the lymphatic system are as follows:

1. Returns excess tissue fluid that has leaked from the capillaries. If not removed, this fluid collects in spaces between the cells and results in *edema*.
2. Returns plasma proteins that have leaked out of the capillaries into the circulation. If not returned, these proteins would accumulate, increase the osmotic pressure in the tissue fluid, and upset capillary function.

3. Transports absorbed nutrients. Specialized lymph vessels transport nutrients, especially fats, from the digestive system to the blood.
4. Removes toxic substances and other cellular debris from circulation in tissues after infection or tissue damage.
5. Controls quality of tissue fluid by filtering it through lymph nodes before returning it to the circulation.

THE LYMPHATIC SYSTEM

Components of the System

Components of the lymphatic system include lymph fluid, lymph vessels, and lymph nodes. The functions of this system are as follows:

1. Transporting fluid from the tissues back to the bloodstream.
2. Assisting in controlling infection caused by microorganisms.
3. Transporting fats away from the digestive organs.

Parts and Functions of the System

TABLE 14-9

Term	Pronunciation	Definition
adenoids	add-_eh_-noyds	masses of lymph tissue near the opening into the pharynx
antibodies	an-tih-_bod_-eez	substances produced by the body in response to foreign organisms
Lymphatic	lim-_fat_-ic	
capillaries	cap-_ih_-lair-eez	smallest of the lymph vessels, they transport interstitial fluid back to the blood via large lymph vessels
ducts	ducts	the largest of the lymph vessels, point of entry to blood circulation
fluid	_floo_-id	interstitial fluid in the lymph vessels
nodes	nodes	collections of lymphatic tissue
lymphocytes	lim-_foh_-sights	leukocytes originating from stem cells and developing in the bone marrow
macrophage	_mack_-roh-fayj	large cell involved in defending against infection; found in lymph nodes, liver, spleen, lungs, brain, and spinal cord
phagocytes	_fag_-oh-sights	cells that engulf and destroy bacteria
spleen	spleen	large organ located behind the stomach that filters blood to remove pathogens and serves as a blood reservoir
T cells	t sels	important part of the immune response; provide defense against disease by attacking foreign and abnormal cells
thymus gland	_thigh_-mus	endocrine gland that stimulates red bone marrow to produce T lymphocytes (T cells)
tonsils	_ton_-sills	three masses of lymphatic tissue that help protect against harmful substances gaining entry through the mouth and nose

Pathologic Conditions of the Lymph System

TABLE 14-10

Term	Pronunciation	Definition
carinii pneumonia	<u>kah</u>-rye-nee-eye noo-<u>mon</u>-ia	pneumonia caused by a common worldwide parasite to which most people have a natural immunity
hypersplenism	high´-per-<u>splen</u>-izm	enlargement of the spleen; splenomegaly
Kaposi's sarcoma	<u>kap</u>-oh-seez´ sahr-<u>koh</u>-muh	malignant tumor of the blood vessels associated with AIDS
lymphadenopathy	<u>lim</u>-fad-en-noh-pa-thee	any disorder of the lymph nodes or lymph vessels
lymphoma	<u>lim</u>-foh´-mah	malignant tumor of the lymph nodes and lymph tissue (see **Figure 14–11**)
mononucleosis	moh-oh-noo-<u>klee</u>-oh-sis	benign self-limiting acute infection of B lymphocytes usually caused by Epstein-Barr virus
pneumonocystic pneumonia	<u>noo</u>-moh´-noh-<u>sis</u>-tik <u>noo</u>-mon-ia	a rare form of pneumonia in AIDS patients
sarcoidosis	sar-<u>koyd</u>-oh-sis	a systemic inflammatory disease characterized by small rounded lesions forming on the spleen, lymph nodes, and other organs
sarcoma	<u>sar</u>-kom´-ah	a malignant neoplasm of the connective and supportive tissues of the body

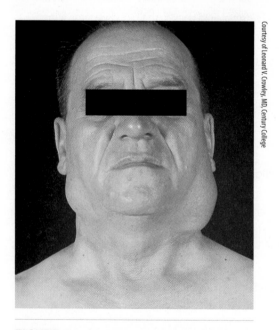

Courtesy of Leonard V. Crowley, MD, Century College

FIGURE 14–11 Marked enlargement of cervical lymph nodes as a result of malignant lymphoma

PHARMACOLOGY AND MEDICAL TERMINOLOGY

Drug Classification	antiarrhythmic (an-tee-ah-<u>rith</u>-mik)	anticoagulant (an-tih-koh-<u>ag</u>-yoo-lant)	antihypertensive (an-tih-high-per-<u>ten</u>-siv)
Function	corrects cardiac arrhythmias (irregular beats)	prevents clot continuation and formation	opposes high pressure (blood)
Word Parts	**anti-** = against; **arrhythm/o** = rhythm; **-ic** = pertaining to	**anti-** = against; **coagul/o** = clotting	**anti-** = against; **hyper-** = excess; **tensive** = pertaining to tension or pressure
Active Ingredients (examples)	digoxin (Lanoxin); propranalol hydrochloride (Inderal)	heparin calcium (Calcilean); warfarin sodium (Coumadin)	nadolol (Corgard); furosemide (Lasix); diltiazem hydrochloride (Cardizem, Cardizem CD)

LESSON THREE   Progress Check

DEFINITIONS

Define these cardiovascular diagnostic, surgical, and treatment terms:

1. angiography _____

2. angioplasty _____

3. anticoagulant _____

4. cardiac catheterization _____

5. commissurotomy _____

6. diuretic _____

7. doppler _____

8. electrocardiogram _____

9. endarterectomy _____

10. hypothermia _____

11. pacemaker _____

12. sinus rhythm _____

13. sodium-restricted diet _____

14. vasodilator _____

15. vasopressor _____

16. venipuncture _____

🔷 NAMING

Name the structure or fluid from the lymphatic system for the definitions given below:

1. large lymph vessel in the chest that drains the lymph from the upper right part of the body _____

_____

2. masses of lymph tissue in the nasopharynx _____

3. organ in the mediastinum that produces T-cell lymphocytes and helps in the immune response _____

_____

4. tiniest lymph vessels _____

5. stationary lymph tissue along the path of lymph vessels all over the body _____

6. large lymph vessel in the chest that drains lymph from the lower part and left side of the body above the diaphragm _____

_____

7. fluid that lies between cells and becomes lymph as it enters lymph capillaries _____

8. organ near the stomach that produces, stores, and eliminates blood cells _____

🔷 MATCHING: DIAGNOSTIC PROCEDURES

Match the following diagnostic procedures to their function:

1. echocardiogram	**a.** complete blood count: Hg, Hct, WBC, RBC, differential
2. Holter monitor	**b.** measurement of O_2, CO_2, and pH
3. treadmill test	**c.** reflected sound waves from the heart
4. angiography	**d.** x-ray record of heart and blood vessels
5. arterial blood gases	**e.** x-ray record of an artery
6. CBC	**f.** blood coagulation test
7. cholesterol	**g.** recording device for ECG activity
8. ECG	**h.** electrical recording of heart activity
9. prothrombin	**i.** a fatlike substance found in vessel walls
10. angiocardiography	**j.** evaluation of heart function by exercise

🔷 MULTIPLE CHOICE

Circle the letter of the correct answer:

1. The function(s) of the spleen is (are) to
    a. build up and destroy blood cells
    b. build bone marrow
    c. form antibodies
    d. manufacture lymph nodes

2. Which of these is *not* a function of circulation?
    a. carry oxygen and nutrients to the cell
    b. carry carbon dioxide and wastes from the cell
    c. carry blood to the heart
    d. carry electrical impulses

3. Erythrocytes are
  a. red blood cells
  b. blood fluids
  c. white blood cells
  d. blood clots

4. Leukocytes are
  a. red blood cells
  b. blood fluids
  c. white blood cells
  d. blood clots

5. Hemoglobin is
  a. an anticoagulant
  b. red blood cell pigment
  c. a protein that produces fibrin
  d. a protein that coagulates like egg white

6. Plasma is
  a. blood solids
  b. blood fluids
  c. blood clotting proteins
  d. blood cell pigments

7. Fibrinogen is
  a. a blood clotting protein
  b. an anticoagulant
  c. a blood platelet
  d. an immature blood cell

8. Serum is
  a. blood solids
  b. blood fluid that does not clot
  c. a blood clotting protein
  d. an immature blood cell

9. Diastolic pressure is
  a. the top number in a blood pressure reading
  b. the measurement of blood viscosity
  c. an abnormal blood pressure reading
  d. the bottom number in a blood pressure reading

10. A sphygmomanometer is
  a. a test for cardiac function
  b. an instrument for performing venipuncture
  c. an instrument for measuring blood pressure
  d. a measuring device for counting white blood cells

ABBREVIATIONS

Define the following commonly used abbreviations:

1. ASD _____

2. BP _____

3. CBC _____

4. CCU _____

5. CHF _____

6. CO_2 _____

7. CPR _____

8. CVA _____

9. ECG, EKG _____

10. MI _____

11. O_2 _____

12. PVC _____

13. RBC _____

14. TIA _____

15. WBC _____

◆ WORD PUZZLE ON THE HEART

Find the 59 words related to the heart by reading forward, backward, up, down, and diagonally. When you have circled the 59 listed words, the remaining letters will spell the word LIFE.

```
M  U  I  D  R  A  C  O  Y  M  U  I  D  R  A  C  I  R  E  P
E  I  M  P  U  L  S  E  S  A  R  D  O  S  L  E  H  N  B  U
D  S  T  S  D  N  U  O  S  V  O  E  P  A  D  Y  D  I  A  R
I  I  C  R  M  U  T  P  E  S  I  S  E  O  T  O  C  A  S  K
A  H  O  L  A  C  I  P  A  R  R  O  N  H  C  U  U  T  E  I
S  F  N  L  V  L  C  A  Y  E  E  L  M  A  S  R  S  R  A  N
T  O  T  A  E  T  A  C  R  B  F  C  R  P  I  R  I  I  E  I
I  E  R  W  N  R  I  E  A  I  N  D  I  C  E  E  N  O  N  E
N  L  A  R  A  I  D  M  N  F  I  D  L  Y  R  P  O  V  I  F
U  D  C  A  C  C  R  A  O  U  W  E  A  S  O  I  A  E  D  I
M  N  T  N  A  U  A  K  M  E  O  L  S  Y  I  C  T  N  N  B
C  U  I  U  V  S  C  E  L  L  E  E  S  R  A  R  T  E  E  E
I  B  F  L  A  P  S  R  U  C  F  L  V  T  E  R  I  R  T  R
L  T  O  I  T  I  I  C  P  I  C  C  L  O  P  D  A  I  E  S
O  R  R  M  F  D  N  I  R  R  U  Y  A  L  U  I  L  C  A  M
T  A  C  E  E  F  U  T  E  T  S  C  V  E  S  U  C  U  D  U
S  E  E  S  L  E  S  R  L  N  P  U  M  P  A  M  A  L  R  I
A  H  R  I  G  H  T  O  A  E  S  E  S  L  U  P  S  A  O  R
I  G  N  I  N  I  L  A  X  V  R  E  C  E  I  V  E  R  H  T
D  E  P  A  H  S  E  N  O  C  O  R  O  N  A  R  Y  X  C  A
```

Words to Look for in the Word Puzzle

1.	aortic	**31.**	mediastinum
2.	apex	**32.**	mitral
3.	apical	**33.**	myocardium
4.	atrioventricular	**34.**	node
5.	atrium	**35.**	open
6.	auricle	**36.**	pacemaker
7.	AV	**37.**	pericardium
8.	base	**38.**	pulmonary
9.	bicuspid	**39.**	pulses
10.	bundle of His	**40.**	pump
11.	cardiac	**41.**	Purkinje fibers
12.	chordae tendineae	**42.**	receive
13.	closed	**43.**	relax
14.	cone-shaped	**44.**	rhythm
15.	contract	**45.**	right
16.	coronary	**46.**	SA
17.	cusps	**47.**	sac
18.	cycle	**48.**	semilunar
19.	diastolic	**49.**	septum
20.	endocardium	**50.**	sinoatrial
21.	epicardium	**51.**	sinus
22.	fibers	**52.**	sounds
23.	flow	**53.**	superior
24.	force	**54.**	systole
25.	heart	**55.**	tricuspid
26.	inferior	**56.**	valves
27.	impulses	**57.**	vena cava
28.	layers	**58.**	ventricle
29.	left	**59.**	wall
30.	lining		

CHAPTER

15

Nervous System

LESSON ONE: MATERIALS TO BE LEARNED

Central Nervous System
Autonomic Nervous System
    (Peripheral Nervous System)
Clinical Disorders
Terms Used in Diagnosis and Surgery
Psychiatric Terms
Special Terms

LESSON TWO: PROGRESS CHECK

Fill-in
Matching: Nerves
Matching: Disease States
True or False
Definitions
Spelling and Definition
Word Puzzle on the Nervous System

OBJECTIVES

After completing this chapter and the exercises, the student should be able to:

1. Identify the organs of the nervous system (NS).
2. List the functions of the NS.
3. Identify and define clinical disorders affecting the NS.
4. List and explain laboratory tests and medical procedures used in diagnosing NS disorders.
5. Create new medical terms using combining forms and give their meanings.
6. Correctly spell and pronounce new medical terms.

ALLIED HEALTH PROFESSIONS

Physical Therapists and Physical Therapist Assistants and Aides

Physical therapists provide services that help restore function, improve mobility, relieve pain, and prevent or limit permanent physical disabilities. They restore, maintain, and promote overall fitness and health. Their patients include accident victims and individuals with disabling conditions such as low-back pain, arthritis, heart disease, fractures, head injuries, and cerebral palsy.

Therapists examine patients' medical histories and then test and measure the patients' strength, range of motion, balance and coordination, posture, muscle performance, respiration, and motor function. Next, physical therapists develop plans describing a treatment strategy and its anticipated outcome.

Physical therapist assistants and aides help physical therapists to provide treatment that improves patient mobility, relieves pain, and prevents or lessens physical disabilities of patients. A physical therapist might ask an assistant to help patients exercise or learn to use crutches, for example, or an aide to gather and prepare therapy equipment. Patients include accident victims and individuals with disabling conditions such as low-back pain, arthritis, heart disease, fractures, head injuries, and cerebral palsy.

Physical therapist assistants perform a variety of tasks. Under the direction and supervision of physical therapists, they provide part of a patient's treatment. This might involve exercises, massages, electrical stimulation, paraffin baths, hot and cold packs, traction, and ultrasound. Physical therapist assistants record the patient's responses to treatment and report the outcome of each treatment to the physical therapist.

Physical therapist aides help make therapy sessions productive, under the direct supervision of a physical therapist or physical therapist assistant. They usually are responsible for keeping the treatment area clean and organized and for preparing for each patient's therapy. When patients need assistance moving to or from a treatment area, aides push them in a wheelchair or provide them with a shoulder to lean on. Physical therapist aides are not licensed and do not perform the clinical tasks of a physical therapist assistant in states where licensure is required.

The duties of aides include some clerical tasks, such as ordering depleted supplies, answering the phone, and filling out insurance forms and other paperwork. The extent to which an aide or an assistant performs clerical tasks depends on the size and location of the facility.

INQUIRY

American Physical Therapy Association: www.apta.org

Data from Stanfield, Peggy S., Cross, Nanna, and Hui, Y.H. *Introduction to the Health Professions*, 6th ed. Burlington, MA: Jones & Bartlett Learning; 2012.

The human NS provides functions not seen in other animal species, for instance, the formation of ideas. We are able to think and reason, that is, judge right from wrong, separate logical from illogical, and plan for the future. Our NS is the center of all mental activity, including thought, learning, and memory (see **Figure 15–1**). It is no wonder, then, that any abnormal condition that affects the NS affects the entire body.

This chapter briefly describes the anatomy and physiology of the NS and its disorders. The study of the NS is called *neurology*. There are two physician specialties for the treatment of NS conditions: the *neurologist* diagnoses and treats diseases and disorders, while a *neurosurgeon* specializes in surgery involving the brain, spinal cord, or peripheral nerves. When studying materials in this chapter, refer to **Figures 15–2, 15–3,** and **15–4**.

The nervous system consists of two main anatomic subdivisions, the central nervous system (CNS) and the peripheral nervous system (PNS). Its three main components are the brain, spinal cord, and nerves. There are 12 pairs of cranial nerves and 31 pairs of spinal nerves in the PNS. The brain and spinal cord constitute the CNS and are housed in the skull and vertebral canal, respectively. The brain and spinal cord receive, store, and process all sensory and motor data and control consciousness.

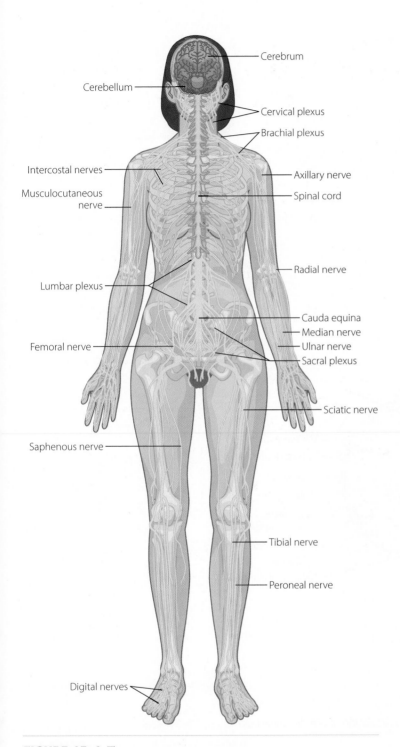

Cerebrum

Cerebellum

Cervical plexus

Brachial plexus

Intercostal nerves

Axillary nerve

Musculocutaneous nerve

Spinal cord

Radial nerve

Lumbar plexus

Cauda equina

Median nerve

Femoral nerve

Ulnar nerve

Sacral plexus

Sciatic nerve

Saphenous nerve

Tibial nerve

Peroneal nerve

Digital nerves

FIGURE 15–1 The nervous system

The PNS transmits sensory and motor information back and forth between the CNS and the rest of the body.

The human brain comprises 2% of the body's total weight, consumes 25% of its oxygen, and receives 15% of its cardiac output (see Figure 15–1). The protective outer coverings of the brain are the bony skull and the *meninges,* the three connective tissue layers. The innermost covering, called the *pia mater,* is thin and delicate and closely adheres to the brain. The *arachnoid* is the middle layer and is separated from the pia

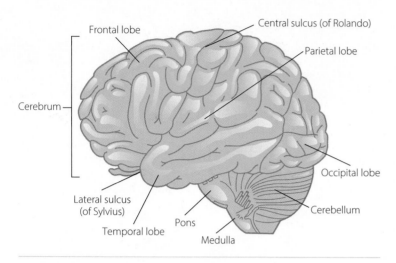

FIGURE 15–2 Surface view of the brain

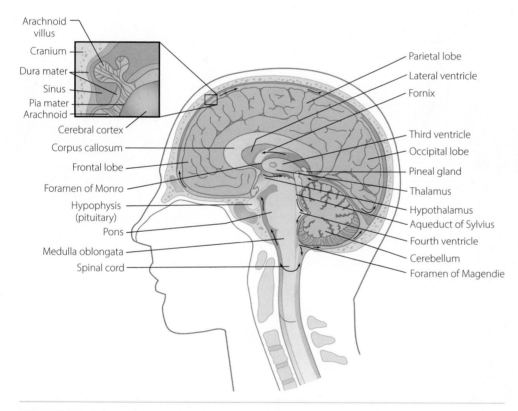

FIGURE 15–3 Midsagittal section of the human brain, showing circulation of cerebrospinal fluid in the brain and spinal cord; inset shows the cranial meninges

mater by *subarachnoid* space. It contains cerebrospinal fluid, blood vessels, and weblike tissue that secure it to the pia mater. The *dura mater* is the thick outermost layer that adheres to the inner surface of the cranium.

Cerebrospinal fluid surrounds the *subarachnoid* spaces around the brain and spinal cord and fills the ventricles within the brain. White and gray matter are contained in the brain and spinal cord.

The *cerebrum* is the largest part of the brain. It has two hemispheres. The functional areas of the *cerebral cortex* include primary motor areas, primary sensory areas, and secondary areas that function at a higher level than the primary areas.

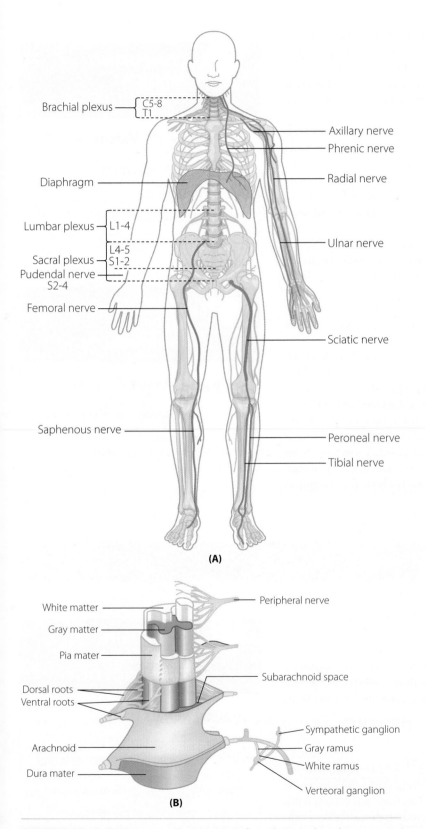

Brachial plexus — C5-8 T1

Axillary nerve
Phrenic nerve
Radial nerve

Diaphragm

Lumbar plexus — L1-4

Ulnar nerve

Sacral plexus — L4-5 S1-2
Pudendal nerve S2-4

Femoral nerve

Sciatic nerve

Saphenous nerve

Peroneal nerve
Tibial nerve

(A)

White matter
Gray matter
Pia mater

Peripheral nerve

Dorsal roots
Ventral roots

Subarachnoid space

Arachnoid

Sympathetic ganglion
Gray ramus
White ramus

Dura mater

Verteoral ganglion

(B)

FIGURE 15–4 (A) Sensory and motor tracts from the spinal cord to the brain. (B) Diagram of spinal cord, showing three meningeal layers and association with sympathetic trunk.

The *hypothalamus* lies inferior to the thalamus and forms the floor and lower part of the side walls of the third *ventricle.* It plays an important role in the regulation of appetite, heart rate, body temperature, water balance, digestion, and sexual activity.

The *cerebellum* lies inferior to the *pons* and is the second largest area of the brain. A cross-section of the cerebellum looks like a tree and is often referred to as *arbor vitae,* or tree of life.

Unconscious functions are housed in the cerebellum, hypothalamus, and brain stem. Although consciousness resides in the cerebral cortex, many body functions, such as heartbeat and breathing, occur at the unconscious level.

This region of the brain controls unconscious actions. It sits below the cerebrum on the brain stem. The cerebellum controls muscle synergy and helps maintain posture. It receives impulses from the sense organs in the ear that detects body position and sends these impulses to the muscles to maintain or correct posture.

Inside the spinal cord is an inner section of gray matter associated with the PNS and an outer section of white matter. The white matter is covered with a myelin sheath and conducts impulses to and from the brain. It carries all the nerves that affect the limbs and lower part of the body.

The cord of nervous tissue enclosed within the vertebral column is the spinal cord. It controls many of the reflex actions of the body and transmits impulses to and from the brain via ascending and descending tracts.

The PNS is all the nervous tissue found outside the brain and spinal cord. As outlined and defined in Lesson One, it includes the *optic, olfactory, trochlear, trigeminal, abducens, facial, vestibulo-ocular, glossopharyngeal, vagus, hypoglossal,* and *spinal accessory* nerves. Those nerves that control the special senses are discussed in the chapter pertaining to their functions and disorders. The PNS has two subsystems, the *somatic* nervous system and the *autonomic* nervous system. In general, the subdivisions of the autonomic nervous system (*sympathetic* and *parasympathetic*) exert opposing actions. Activation of the sympathetic portion causes the rate and intensity of reactions to increase, while the parasympathetic will slowly bring the body back to normal functions.

> **CONFUSING MEDICAL TERMINOLOGY**
>
> ### MS Versus MS Versus MS
>
> **MS** = musculoskeletal system
>
> **MS** = mitral stenosis
>
> **MS** = multiple sclerosis

> **CONFUSING MEDICAL TERMINOLOGY**
>
> ### delusion Versus illusion
>
> **delusion** = a persistent belief in an untruth
>
> **illusion** = an inaccurate sensory perception based on a real stimulus

| LESSON ONE | Materials to Be Learned |

When studying this lesson, refer to Figures 15–2, 15–3, and 15–4.

CENTRAL NERVOUS SYSTEM

The CNS is one of the two main divisions of the nervous system of the body, consisting of the brain and the spinal cord. The CNS processes information to send to and receive from the PNS and is the main network of coordination and control for the entire body.

AUTONOMIC NERVOUS SYSTEM (PERIPHERAL NERVOUS SYSTEM)

The PNS is composed of nerves and ganglia. Ganglia are groups of nerve cells outside of the CNS. The PNS is divided into two subdivisions: the somatic and autonomic portions. The somatic portion (SNS) controls voluntary functions and certain reflex actions, such as knee jerk. The autonomic portion (ANS) controls the rest of the involuntary functions. The PNS contains both the SNS, which provides voluntary control over skeletal muscle, and the ANS, which controls smooth muscle, cardiac muscle, and gland secretions. The ANS is absolutely essential to survival.

> **CONFUSING MEDICAL TERMINOLOGY**
>
> ### mental Versus mental
>
> **mental** = pertaining to the chin, e.g., mental foramen (fo-<u>ra</u>-men) refers to one of two holes (foramina) located on the anterior (front) surface of the mandible (lower jaw)
>
> **mental** = pertaining to the mind, e.g., mental health

TABLE 15-1

Term	Pronunciation	Definition
Brain	brān	comprising the forebrain, midbrain, and hindbrain
cerebrum	ser-e-brum	main (largest) portion of the brain, occupying the upper part of the cranial cavity; its two hemispheres, united by the corpus callosum, form the largest part of the CNS in humans
cerebellum	ser´-e-bel-um	situated on the back of the brain stem; consisting of a median lobe (vermis) and two lateral lobes (the hemispheres)
brain stem	brān stem	the stemlike portion of the brain connecting the cerebral hemispheres with the spinal cord and comprising the pons, medulla oblongata, and midbrain
encephalon	en-sef-al-on	located between the cerebrum and midbrain, it contains the thalamus, hypothalamus, and pineal glands; involved in controlling body temperature, sleep, appetite, blood pressure, and sexual activity
Spinal Cord	spi-nal kord	that part of the central nervous system lodged in the spinal column
meninges	men-in-jez	the three membranes covering the brain and spinal cord: dura mater, arachnoid, and pia mater
dura mater	du-rah ma-ter	the outermost, toughest of the three meninges (membranes) of the brain and spinal cord
arachnoid	ah-rak-noid	the delicate membrane interposed between the dura mater and the pia mater
pia mater	pi-ah ma-ter	the innermost of the three meninges covering the brain and spinal cord
cerebrospinal fluid	ser´-a-bro-spi-nal floo-id	fluid within the ventricles of the brain, the subarachnoid space, and the central canal

TABLE 15-2

Term	Pronunciation	Definition
Cranial Nerves	kra-ne-al nerves	the 12 pairs of nerves emerging from the cranial cavity through various openings in the skull, as follows
olfactory	ol-fak-to-re	sense of smell
optic	op-tic	vision
oculomotor	ok´-u-lo-mo-tor	movements of the eye
trochlear	trock-le-ar	muscles of the eyes
trigeminal	tri-jem-in-al	facial movements

(continues)

TABLE 15-2 *(continued)*

Term	Pronunciation	Definition
abducens	ab-<u>du</u>-sens	muscles of the eye turning the eye outward
facial	<u>fa</u>-shal	muscles of the face, ears, and scalp
auditory	<u>aw</u>-di-to-re	pertaining to the ear or the sense of hearing
glossopharyngeal	glos´-o-fah-<u>rin</u>-je-al	pertaining to the tongue and pharynx
pneumogastric vagus	nu´-mo-<u>gas</u>-tric <u>va</u>-gus	voice and swallowing
spinal	<u>spi</u>-nal	neck muscles
hypoglossal	hi´-po-<u>glos</u>-al	beneath the tongue
Spinal Accessory Nerves		the 31 pairs of nerves without special names that are connected to the spinal cord
Other Components		
sympathetic	sim´-pah-<u>thet</u>-ik	the part of the autonomic nervous system assisting the body in emergencies, defense, and survival
parasympathetic	par´-ah-sim´-pah-<u>thet</u>-ik	the part of the autonomic nervous system bringing body functions back to normal after a stressful situation has ended

CLINICAL DISORDERS

TABLE 15-3

Term	Pronunciation	Definition
abscess (brain)	<u>ab</u>-ses	secondary to infection in the body, e.g., ear, sinuses
Alzheimer's disease (presenile dementia)	<u>alts</u>-hi-merz di-<u>sez</u> (pre-<u>se</u>-nīl de-<u>men</u>-she-ah)	characterized by confusion, restlessness, agnosia, speech disturbances, inability to carry out purposeful movements, and hallucinations; the disease usually begins in later midlife with slight defects in memory and behavior and occurs with equal frequency in men and women. The cause is unknown
amyotrophic lateral sclerosis (ALS)	ah´-mi-o-<u>trof</u>-ic <u>lat</u>-er-al skle-<u>ro</u>-sis	progressive degeneration of the upper and lower motor neurons; usually fatal
anencephaly	an´-en-<u>sef</u>-ah-le	congenital absence of the brain; death occurs in 1–2 days
Bell's palsy	<u>pawl</u>-ze	unilateral facial paralysis of sudden onset caused by lesion of the facial nerve; facial distortion

TABLE 15-3	(continued)	

Term	Pronunciation	Definition
carpal tunnel syndrome	car-pal tun-ell sin-drom	the disorder is largely due to the result of repetitive overuse of the fingers, hands, or wrists, which causes inflammation of the median nerve in the tunnel. Symptoms are intermittent or continuous pain, especially at night; treatment involves anti-inflammatory drugs, splints, physical therapy, and ceasing the overuse. If these measures fail, surgical measures to relieve the pressure may be necessary
cerebral palsy	ser-e-bral pawl-ze	paralysis from developmental defects or trauma; many symptoms; appearing before age 3 years, caused by nonprogressive damage to the brain
cerebrovascular accident (CVA)	ser´-e-bro-vas-ku-lar	a decrease in blood flow supply to the brain, causing death to the specific portion of the brain tissue affected; the three types of CVA are hemorrhagic stroke, which occurs when a cerebral vessel ruptures; thrombotic stroke, which occurs when a blood clot in the arteries leading to the brain becomes occluded (blocked); and embolic stroke, which occurs when an embolus (fragment of blood clot, fat, bacteria, or tumor) lodges in a cerebral vessel and causes occlusion
concussion	kon-kush-un	a violent blow to the head; there may or may not be a loss of consciousness
convulsion (seizure)	kon-vul-shun (se-zhur)	an involuntary contraction or series of contractions of the voluntary muscles; sudden disturbances in mental functions and body movements, some with loss of consciousness
encephalitis	en´-sef-ah-li-tis	inflammation of the brain
epilepsy	ep-i-lep´-se	seizure disorder; cause usually unknown; symptoms can be managed with medication
fracture (skull)	frak-chur	a break in the bones of the skull; cause can be injury, gunshot wounds
grand mal seizure	grand mall seez-yoor	also called tonic-clonic seizures; characterized by a sudden loss of consciousness, falling down, and involuntary muscle contractions; often preceded by an aura, a peculiar sensation such as visual disturbance, numbness, or dizziness, which appears just before more definite symptoms
hematoma	he´-mah-to-mah	blood "tumor" (clot); must be removed if large enough to cause pressure on the brain
herpes zoster	her-peez zos-ter	"shingles"; an acute inflammatory disease of cerebral or spinal nerve caused by viral infection; common in elderly adults
Huntington's chorea	ko-re-ah	ceaseless occurrence of rapid, jerky, involuntary movements; hereditary disease marked by chronic progressive chorea and mental deterioration
hydrocephalus	hi´-dro-sef-ah-lus	"water on the brain"; a congenital or acquired condition marked by dilation of the cerebral ventricles accompanied by an accumulation of cerebrospinal fluid within the skull; typically, there is enlargement of the head, prominence of the forehead, mental deterioration, and convulsions
Korsakoff's syndrome	kor-suh-kufs sin-drom	an alcoholic psychosis with disorientation, progressing to complete amnesia
meningitis	men´-in-ji-tis	inflammation of the meninges caused by bacterial, viral, or fungal infection

(continues)

TABLE 15-3   *(continued)*

Term	Pronunciation	Definition
meningocele (myelomeningocele)	me-<u>ning</u>-go-sel (mi′-e-lo-me-<u>ning</u>-go-sēl)	hernial protrusion of the meninges through a bone defect in the cranium or vertebral column; may be repaired surgically
multiple sclerosis (MS)	<u>mul</u>-te-p′-l skle-<u>ro</u>-sis	brain and cord contain areas of degenerated myelin. Symptoms of lesions include weakness, incoordination, speech disturbances, and visual complaints
myasthenia gravis (MG)	my-ass-<u>thee</u>-nee-ah <u>grav</u>-iss	a progressive neuromuscular disorder characterized by chronic fatigue and muscle weakness; considered to be an autoimmune disease. Antibodies block and destroy receptors at the myoneural junction because of a deficiency of acetylcholine. The onset of symptoms is gradual, with drooping eyelids, difficulty speaking and swallowing, and weakness of the facial muscles; the weakness may then extend to other muscles enervated by cranial nerves, especially the respiratory muscles. The disease occurs more often in women than men, with onset between ages 20 and 40 years in women, and in older men between ages 50 and 60 more often than in younger men
neuropathy	nu-<u>rop</u>-ah-the	disease of cranial and peripheral nervous system; motor, sensory, and reflex impairment
organic brain syndrome (chronic brain syndrome)	or-<u>gan</u>-ik	any mental disorder caused by impairment of brain tissue function; may be acute and reversible, caused by injury, infection, and nutritional deficiency, or chronic, resulting from relatively permanent organic impairment of brain tissue function
Parkinson's disease	<u>par</u>-kin-sunz di-<u>sez</u>	a slowly progressive, degenerative, neurologic disorder characterized by resting tremor
petit mal seizures	pet-<u>ee</u> mall <u>seez</u>-yoorz	also called absence seizure, the petit mal is a minor seizure lasting only a few seconds. The person has a momentary clouding of consciousness, may have a blank facial expression, and blink the eyes rapidly; the duration of the seizure is 5–10 s. The individual may not be aware of the episode. It is more frequent in children
poliomyelitis	po′-le-o-mi′-e-<u>li</u>-tis	an acute viral disease with fever, sore throat, headache, vomiting, and often stiffness of the neck and back; may be minor or major; can be prevented by vaccination
sciatica	si-<u>at</u>-i-kah	severe pain in the leg along the course of the sciatic nerve; also pain radiating into the buttock and lower limb, most commonly caused by herniation of a lumbar disk
shunt	shunt	to bypass, e.g., using a catheter to drain fluid from brain cavities to the spinal cord
spinal cord injuries	<u>spi</u>-nal kord <u>in</u>-ju-rez	a traumatic disruption of the spinal cord, with extensive musculoskeletal involvement; spinal fractures and dislocations are common in car accidents and airplane crashes and can cause varying degrees of paraplegia and quadriplegia
subdural hematoma	sub-<u>doo</u>-ral hee-mah-<u>toh</u>-mah	beneath the dura mater, usually a result of a closed head injury, acceleration-deceleration injury, use of anticoagulants, contusions, or chronic alcoholism; they are largely a result of venous bleeding. An acute subdural hematoma can occur within minutes or hours following an injury; a chronic subdural hematoma takes weeks to months to evolve. Symptoms include drowsiness, headache, confusion, possible seizure, and signs of intracranial pressure and paralysis; treatment involves surgical evacuation of the blood, and in acute subdurals, it may be removed through burr holes in the skull, but chronic ones require a craniotomy because the blood has solidified and cannot be aspirated through burr holes

TABLE 15-3 (continued)

Term	Pronunciation	Definition
Tay-Sach's disease	<u>tay</u>-sacks dih-<u>zeez</u>	an inherited inborn error of metabolism in which there is an enzyme deficiency causing altered lipid metabolism; deficiency of this enzyme results in accumulation of a specific lipid in the brain, which leads to physical and mental retardation. It is a progressive disorder, marked by degeneration of brain tissue, dementia, convulsions, paralysis, blindness, and death. The symptoms begin around 6 months of age; death occurs between 2 and 4 years of age. It is possible to test for this disease in the unborn fetus through amniocentesis. No therapy is available for the disease; supportive and symptomatic care is indicated. Tay-Sach's primarily affects children of the Ashkenazic Jews
tumors (cord, brain)	<u>too</u>-morz	benign or malignant, primary or metastatic; may be classified by location, tissue type, or degree of malignancy, e.g., gliomas, neuromas
whiplash	<u>hwip</u>-lash	a popular term for an acute cervical sprain; acceleration extension injury of the cervical spine

TERMS USED IN DIAGNOSIS AND SURGERY

TABLE 15-4

Term	Pronunciation	Definition
angiogram (arteriogram), cerebral	<u>an</u>-je-o-gram (ar-<u>te</u>-re-o-gram´), <u>ser</u>-e-bral	a radiopaque substance is injected into arteries in the neck, then x-ray films are taken
Babinski's sign	bah-<u>bin</u>-skez	reflex response; when sole of the foot is stroked, the big toe turns up instead of down (normal in newborn, but pathologic later on)
burr holes	ber	holes made with a drill creating openings in bone to permit access for biopsy, insertion of drains for relieving pressure, or for monitoring devices
computerized tomography (CT) brain scan; also called CAT scan		three-dimensional view of brain tissue obtained as x-ray beams pass through layers of the brain. A CT scan will show areas of tumors, hemorrhage, blood clots, aneurysms, MS, and brain abscess; contrast medium may also be injected by IV to better visualize abnormalities
cordotomy	kor-<u>dot</u>-o-me	cutting of nerve fibers to relieve intractable pain
craniotomy	kra´-ne-<u>ot</u>-o-me	any operation on the cranium, e.g., puncture of the skull and removal of its contents to decrease the size of the head of a dead fetus and aid in delivery
echoencephalogram (EEG)	ek´-o-en-<u>sef</u>-ah-lo-gram´	use of ultrasound to show displacement of brain structures

(continues)

TABLE 15-4 *(continued)*

Term	Pronunciation	Definition
electroencephalogram (EKG)	e-lek´-tro-en-<u>sef</u>-ah-lo-gram´	record of electrical activity of the brain
laboratory procedures	<u>lab</u>-o-rah-tor´-e pro-<u>se</u>-jurz	examination of cerebrospinal fluid (cell counts, culture, blood)
laminectomy	lam´-i-<u>nek</u>-to-me	excision of the posterior arch of a vertebra to view the spinal cord or to relieve pressure
lumbar puncture (LP)	<u>lum</u>-bar <u>pungk</u>-chur	spinal tap
lumbar sympathectomy	<u>lum</u>-bar sim´-pah-<u>thek</u>-to-me	a surgical interruption of part of the sympathetic nerve pathways, performed for the relief of chronic pain in vascular diseases, such as arteriosclerosis, claudication, and so on
magnetic resonance imaging (MRI) of the brain		noninvasive technique using magnetic waves to create an image of the brain. The MRI is far more precise and accurate than most diagnostic tools; it provides visualization of fluid, soft tissue, and bony structures. MRI and CT are used to complement each other in diagnosing brain and spinal cord lesions. Persons with any implanted metal devices such as a pacemaker, prosthesis, etc., cannot undergo MRI because the strong magnetic field will dislodge them
myelogram (myelography)	<u>mi</u>-e-lo-gram (mi´-e-<u>log</u>-rah-fe)	the film produced by myelography, e.g., injection of a dye into the subarachnoid space to detect tumors or herniated disks
nerve block	nerv blok	injection of anesthetic into a nerve to produce the loss of sensation
nerve cells (neurons)	nerv selz (<u>new</u>-rons)	conducting cells of the nervous system, consisting of a cell body containing the nucleus and its surrounding cytoplasm, and the axon and dendrites; specialized cells for transmitting impulses
pneumoencephalogram (PEG)	nu´-mo-en-<u>sef</u>-ah-lo-gram´	the radiograph obtained by visualization of the fluid-containing structures of the brain after cerebrospinal fluid is intermittently withdrawn by lumbar puncture and replaced by air, oxygen, or helium
positron emission tomography (PET) scan	pos´-ih-tron ee-miss´-shun toh-mog´-rah-fee	images of various structures show how the brain uses glucose and gives information about brain function; PET scans are used to assess Alzheimer's, stroke, epilepsy, and schizophrenia as well as study and diagnose brain tumors
rhizotomy	ri-<u>zot</u>-o-me	cutting the roots of spinal nerves to relieve incurable pain
Romberg test	<u>rom</u>-berg	a test of the sense of balance, e.g., the patient may lose balance when standing erect, feet together, and eyes closed
trephination	tref´-i-<u>na</u>-shun	drilling a hole in the skull to evacuate clots or inject air for a diagnostic procedure
vagotomy	va-<u>got</u>-o-me	surgical transection of the fibers of the vagus nerve
ventriculography	ven-trik´-u-<u>log</u>-rah-fe	radiography of the cerebral ventricles after introduction of air or other contrast medium

PSYCHIATRIC TERMS

TABLE   15-5

Term	Pronunciation	Definition
affect	af-ekt	the feeling experienced in connection with an emotion
aggression	ah-gresh-un	hostile attitude; may be caused by insecurity or inferiority feeling
ambivalence	am-biv-ah-lens	conflicting emotional attitudes toward a goal, e.g., hate and love
amnesia	am-ne-zhe-ah	loss of memory
autism	aw-tizm	developmental disorder characterized by the inability to form social relationships and communicate with others
bipolar disorder	bahy-poh-ler	brain disorder in which the individual experiences extremes in energy, mood, and behavior between mania and depression that interfere with the ability to carry out day-to-day activities; also called manic-depressive illness
catatonia	kat´-ah-ton-e-ah	excessive violent motor activity or lack of reaction and movement; observed in schizophrenia
delirium	de-lir-e-um	a mental disturbance of relatively short duration, e.g., illusions, hallucinations, and excitement
delusion	de-loo-zhun	a false personal belief
depression	de-presh-un	in psychiatry, a morbid sadness, dejection, or melancholy; a decrease of body functions
echolalia	ek´-o-la-le-ah	automatic repetition by a patient of what is said to him or her
electroconvulsive therapy (ECT, EST)	e-lek´-tro-con-vul-siv	introducing convulsions by means of electricity; used on patients with affective disorders
hallucination	hah-lu´-si-na-shun	hearing or seeing things not really present
hypochondria	hi´-po-kon-dre-ah	imaginary illnesses
hysteria	his-te-re-ah	extremely emotional state
major depression	mey-jer dih-presh-uhn	disabling brain disorder that interferes with normal activities of working, eating, sleeping, and enjoying usual activities; most patients require treatment (medications and/or therapy) to improve after a depressive episode
malingering	mah-ling-ger-ing	make believe, e.g., pretending to be ill
megalomania	meg´-ah-lo-ma-ne-ah	belief in one's own extreme greatness, goodness, or power
neurasthenia	nu´-ras-the-ne-ah	mental and physical exhaustion as a result of psychological stress, conflict, or depression; similar to chronic fatigue syndrome
neurosis	nu-ro-sis	an emotional disorder caused by unresolved conflicts, anxiety being its chief characteristic; person is still in touch with reality

(continues)

TABLE 15-5 (continued)

Term	Pronunciation	Definition
paranoid	<u>par</u>-ah-noid	a person who is overly suspicious with feelings of being persecuted or having delusions of his or her abilities or power that are not consistent with reality
phobia	<u>fo</u>-be-ah	any persistent abnormal dread or fear
psychosis	si-<u>ko</u>-sis	a major mental disorder with a loss of contact with reality; characterized by delusions and hallucinations; often part of schizophrenia and severe depressive disorders
rapid eye movements (REM)		occur during periods of dreaming
schizophrenia	skit´-so-<u>fre</u>-ne-ah	a chronic, severe, and debilitating brain disorder characterized by visual and auditory hallucinations and delusions as well as disordered thoughts. Most individuals with schizophrenia are not able to hold a job or care for themselves

SPECIAL TERMS

TABLE 15-6

Term	Pronunciation	Definition
aphasia	ah-<u>fa</u>-zhe-ah	loss of the ability to speak owing to injury or disease of the brain centers
ataxia	ah-<u>tak</u>-se-ah	failure of muscular coordination
biofeedback	bi´-o-<u>fēd</u>-bak	the process of furnishing a person with information on the state of one or more physiologic variables, such as heart rate, blood pressure, or skin temperature, often enabling the person to gain some voluntary control over the body function
cauda equina	<u>kaw</u>-dah e-<u>kwi</u>-na	the collection of spinal roots descending from the lower spinal cord and supplying the rectal area
comatose	<u>ko</u>-mah-tōs	in a deep stupor; cannot be aroused
contrecoup	kon´-truh-<u>koo</u>	denoting an injury to the brain, occurring at a site opposite to the point of impact
deep tendon reflex (DTR)	<u>ten</u>-don <u>re</u>-fleks	a reflex elicited by a sharp tap on the appropriate tendon or muscle to induce brief stretch of the muscle, followed by contraction
encephalon	en-<u>sef</u>-ah-lon	the brain
fissure	<u>fish</u>-er	many meanings; one refers to a deep furrow in the brain

CHAPTER 16

Genitourinary System

Urinary System
  Reproductive System
  Male Reproductive System
  Female Reproductive System

LESSON ONE: MATERIALS TO BE LEARNED

Urinary System
  Organs and Structures
  Clinical Conditions and Procedures
  Diagnostic Medical Terms
  Reproductive System
  Male Organs
  Female Organs
  Male Clinical Conditions
  Female Clinical Conditions
  Male and Female Conditions
  Pregnancy and Birth

LESSON TWO: PROGRESS CHECK

Lists
Multiple Choice
Compare and Contrast
Matching: Clinical Procedures
Completion
Matching: Male Clinical Conditions
Matching: Female Clinical Conditions
Definitions
Word Puzzle on the Genitourinary
  System

OBJECTIVES

After completing this chapter and the exercises, the student should be able to:

1. Identify the organs and describe the location and functions of the following systems: urinary system (US), male reproductive system (MRS), and female reproductive system (FRS).
2. Identify and define clinical disorders affecting the following systems: urinary system, male reproductive system, and female reproductive system.
3. Explain selected laboratory and medical procedures used in diagnosing diseases and disorders of the genitourinary (GU) system.
4. Identify three secondary sex characteristics that occur in the male and female bodies at the onset of puberty.
5. Identify six sexually transmitted diseases of the male and female reproductive systems.

ALLIED HEALTH PROFESSIONS

Radiologic Technologists and Radiation Therapists

Radiologic technologists take x-rays and administer nonradioactive materials into patients' bloodstreams for diagnostic purposes. They also are referred to as radiographers and produce x-ray films (radiographs) of parts of the human body for use in diagnosing medical problems. They prepare patients for radiologic examinations by explaining the procedure, removing jewelry and other articles through which x-rays cannot pass, and positioning patients so that the parts of the body can be appropriately radiographed. To prevent unnecessary exposure to radiation, these workers surround the exposed area with radiation protection devices, such as lead shields, or they limit the size of the x-ray beam. Radiographers position radiographic equipment at the correct angle and height over the appropriate area of a patient's body. Using instruments similar to a measuring tape, they may measure the thickness of the section to be radiographed and set controls on the x-ray machine to produce radiographs of the appropriate density, detail, and contrast. They place the x-ray film under the part of the patient's body to be examined and make the exposure. They then remove the film and develop it.

Treating cancer in the human body is the principal use of radiation therapy. As part of a medical radiation oncology team, radiation therapists use machines—called linear accelerators—to administer radiation treatment to patients. Linear accelerators, used in a procedure called external beam therapy, project high-energy x-rays at targeted cancer cells. As the x-rays collide with human tissue, they produce highly energized ions that can shrink and eliminate cancerous tumors. Radiation therapy is sometimes used as the sole treatment for cancer but is usually used in conjunction with chemotherapy or surgery.

INQUIRY

American Society of Radiologic Technologists: www.asrt.org

Data from Stanfield, Peggy S., Cross, Nanna, and Hui, Y.H. *Introduction to the Health Professions*, 6th ed. Burlington, MA: Jones & Bartlett Learning; 2012.

This chapter discusses together the urinary system and the reproductive system. To acquaint the student with the specifics of each system, this brief introduction considers them separately.

URINARY SYSTEM

All living things produce waste, and humans are no exception. Waste cannot accumulate in an organism without causing harm. Waste excretion occurs by several avenues. In humans, excretion of waste occurs in the lungs, skin, liver, intestines, and kidneys. Of all the organs that participate in removing waste, the kidneys are one of the most important because they relieve the body of the greatest variety of dissolved wastes.

If the kidneys fail, there is no way for all the waste products to be eliminated from the body. Death will follow unless a kidney transplant replaces the failing kidney or the impurities are filtered out by dialysis (artificial kidney).

The urinary system consists of the organs that produce urine and eliminate it from the body. It is a major organ system in the maintenance of homeostasis.

The *urinary system* consists of two *kidneys,* which produce urine; two *ureters,* which carry urine to the urinary bladder for temporary storage; and the *urethra,* which carries urine to the outside of the body through an external *urethral orifice* (see **Figure 16–1** for details). Lesson One defines and illustrates the system along with associated structures.

The kidney has many important functions. Among them are the following:

1. Elimination of organic wastes
2. Regulation of concentration of important ions
3. Regulation of acid–base balance
4. Regulation of red blood cell (RBC) production
5. Regulation of blood pressure

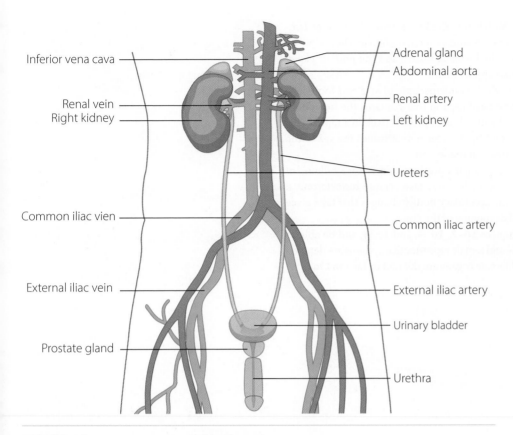

Inferior vena cava

Renal vein
Right kidney

Common iliac vien

External iliac vein

Prostate gland

Adrenal gland
Abdominal aorta

Renal artery
Left kidney

Ureters

Common iliac artery

External iliac artery

Urinary bladder

Urethra

FIGURE 16–1 Urinary system with blood vessels

6. Some control of blood glucose and blood amino acids
7. Elimination of toxic substances
8. Acts as an endocrine gland

The kidneys are bean-shaped, dark red organs approximately 5 in. long and 1 in. thick (about the size of a clenched fist). They are located high on the posterior abdominal wall adjacent to the last two pairs of ribs. They are *retroperitoneal*. Each is capped by an *adrenal* gland. Each kidney is surrounded by three layers of connective tissue. The *renal fascia* (outside covering) anchors the kidney to the surrounding structures and maintains its position. The *perirenal* fat is adipose tissue inside the renal fascia to cushion the kidney. The *renal capsule* is the smooth, transparent membrane that directly covers the kidney and can be easily stripped from it.

For a detailed explanation of the internal structure of the kidney, the structure of a nephron, and blood supply to the kidney, the student is referred to anatomy and physiology texts.

REPRODUCTIVE SYSTEM

The *reproductive* systems in males and females are concerned primarily with perpetuation of the species. In that respect, they differ from all other organ systems of the body, which are concerned with *homeostasis* and survival of the human body. Reproduction begins when the germ cells unite in a process called fertilization. In the female, the germ cell is the *ovum* (pl., *ova*); in the male, it is the *spermatozoon* (pl., *spermatozoa*).

Male Reproductive System
The male reproductive system function is to produce, nourish, and transport sperm from the penis into the female vagina during intercourse (*copulation*) and to produce the male hormone testosterone.

The primary male organs are the *gonads*, which are called *testes* (singular *testis* or *testicle*). They are responsible for production of *spermatozoa* and *testosterone*. The accessory organs of the MRS are a series of ducts, called *seminal vessels*, and the *prostate gland*. The *scrotum*, *penis*, and two *spermatic cords* support them.

The spermatozoon is a mature germ cell. It is microscopic in size and looks like a translucent tadpole. It has a flat elliptical head section that contains the hereditary material, the chromosomes, and a long tail with which it propels itself in a rapid, lashing movement. The sex chromosome carried by the sperm determines the sex of the offspring. When mature, the sperm are carried in the semen.

From puberty on, the male reproductive organs produce and release billions of spermatozoa throughout the lifetime of the male. They also secrete testosterone, a male hormone, which is responsible for the secondary bodily changes that take place at puberty, such as pubic hair, beard, and deepening of the voice.

As you study this chapter, refer to **Figures 16–2**, **16–3**, and **16–4**, and be able to identify and label the structures. The male and female reproductive systems are detailed in Figures 16–3 and 16–4. The male and female organs are defined in Lesson One.

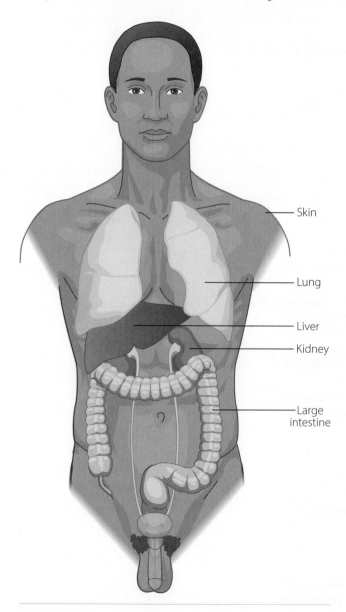

Skin

Lung

Liver

Kidney

Large intestine

FIGURE 16–2 Organs of the excretory system

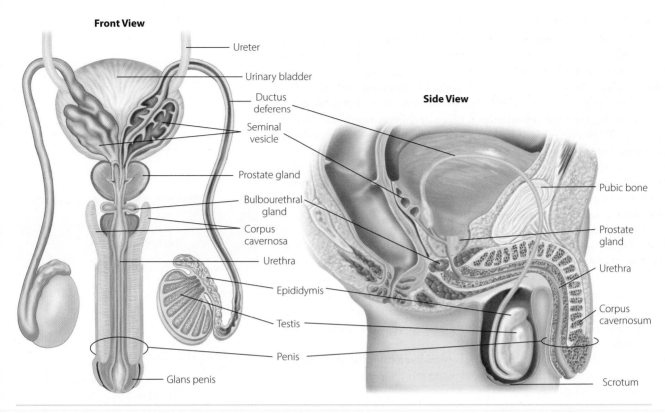

Front View

Ureter

Urinary bladder

Ductus
deferens

Side View

Seminal
vesicle

Prostate gland

Bulbourethral
gland

Corpus
cavernosa

Pubic bone

Urethra

Prostate
gland

Epididymis

Urethra

Testis

Corpus
cavernosum

Penis

Glans penis

Scrotum

FIGURE 16–3 Midsagittal section of the male reproductive system

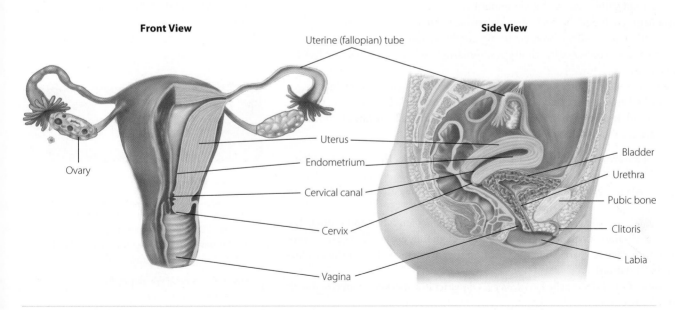

Front View

Side View

Uterine (fallopian) tube

Uterus

Ovary

Endometrium

Bladder

Urethra

Cervical canal

Pubic bone

Cervix

Clitoris

Labia

Vagina

FIGURE 16–4 Midsagittal section of the female reproductive system

Female Reproductive System

Reproduction can only begin when the germ cells from the male (spermatozoa) unite with the germ cells from the female (ova). The reproductive role of the female is to produce eggs (ova) capable of being fertilized and to provide a safe, nutrient-filled environment in which the fetus develops for 9 months if fertilization takes place. The ability to reproduce begins at puberty when mature ova can be released from the ovary and secondary sex characteristics appear, such as breast development, growth of pubic hair, widening of the pelvis ("developing hips," a sight not always welcome to young girls), and menstruation. Body build and stature difference between the male and female become pronounced. The hormones from the ovaries that play important roles in these processes are *estrogen* and *progesterone*. Other sex hormones are secreted by the pituitary gland and adrenal glands.

If fertilization occurs any time between puberty and cessation of the menses (menopause), the fertilized egg will grow and develop in the uterus. If fertilization does not occur, the uterine lining will shed through a bloody discharge, which is menstruation. The female has all of the eggs at birth she will produce in her lifetime, so this cycle repeats itself monthly throughout the childbearing years. At the end of her reproduction cycle, menstruation stops and she no longer discharges eggs from the ovaries. This is known as menopause or climacteric. She also has a decrease in hormone production. Medical terminology in relation to menopause is not given in the chapter. A brief explanation of this condition follows:

Menopause is cessation of menstrual cycles. It is considered complete after *amenorrhea* (absence of menstruation) for 1 year. The *climacteric* is the period during which the cycles are irregular before they stop.

The symptoms of menopause are related to decreased levels of estrogen and progesterone, which affect a number of organ systems and body chemistry:

1. Mammary glands, reproductive organs, and external genitalia decrease in size.
2. Vaginal lining thins and vaginal secretions become alkaline.
3. Vasodilation of blood vessels in the skin results in hot flashes and excessive perspiration in 75–80% of women during the climacteric.
4. Some women experience irritability, insomnia, headache, joint pains, and heart palpitations.
5. In approximately 25% of women, the accelerated loss of bone mass owing to diminished estrogen leads to osteoporosis. This is more likely to occur in small women with less bone mass. Diets low in calcium, especially during childbearing years, are another risk factor that promotes osteoporosis.

Female anatomy consists of external and internal genitalia. The external genitalia are the *mons pubis, labia majora, clitoris, labia minora, vestibule, urinary meatus, vaginal orifice, Bartholin's glands,* and *peritoneum*. Collectively, they are called the *vulva* or *pudendum*.

The internal genitalia consist of the *vagina, uterus, fallopian tubes,* and *ovaries*. The female also has mammary glands (breasts), and although they are not part of the reproductive process, they are part of the FRS because they are responsible for the production of milk (lactation).

The study of the FRS is called *gynecology*. *Obstetrics* is a specialty concerned with pregnancy and delivery.

CONFUSING MEDICAL TERMINOLOGY

ureter/o Versus uter/o Versus urethr/o

ureter/o = ureter, e.g., ureterotomy (u-re-ter-<u>ot</u>-to-me) refers to incision of a ureter

uter/o = uterus, e.g., uterus (yoo-ter-<u>uhs</u>) refers part of the reproductive organ of a woman

urethr/o = urethra, e.g., urethrocystitis (u-re-thro-sis-<u>ti</u>-tis) refers to inflammation of the bladder and urethra

---

CONFUSING MEDICAL TERMINOLOGY

-uria Versus urea

-uria = urinary condition, urination, urine, e.g., polyuria (poly-ee-yoo-r-<u>ee</u>-uh) refers to the passing of an excessive quantity of urine, as in diabetes; also a suffix

urea = chemical waste product, e.g., urea in urine; a medical noun

LESSON ONE	Materials to Be Learned

URINARY SYSTEM

Organs and Structures

TABLE 16-1

Organ or Structure	Pronunciation	Definition
Bowman's capsule (renal capsule)	boh-muhnz cap-suhl	cup-shaped end of renal tubule containing the glomerulus
calyx	ka-liks	cup-shaped part of the renal pelvis through which urine passes from the renal tubules
catheter	cath-eh-ter	a hollow, flexible tube that can be inserted into a body cavity or vessel to allow instilling or withdrawing fluid
cortex	kawr-teks	the outer layer of the kidney
glomerulus	gloh-mer-yah-luhs	collection of coiled intertwined capillaries located in the kidney cortex
kidneys	kid-nez	two organs on the posterior abdominal wall that filter the blood, excreting the end products of body metabolism in the form of urine, and regulating body mineral levels
meatus	mee-ay-tus	an opening or tunnel through any part of the body, as in the urinary meatus, which is the external opening of the urethra
medulla	me-dul-ah	the inner layer of the kidney
nephron	nef-ron	the structural and functional unit of the kidney, the parenchyma, numbering about a million and capable of forming urine
renal artery	ree-nal ar-teh-ree	one of a pair of large arteries branching from the abdominal aorta to supply blood to the kidneys, adrenal glands, and the ureters
renal pelvis	ree-nal pel-vis	the funnel-shaped expansion of the upper end of the ureter
renal tubule	ree-nal toob-yool	long, twisted tube leading from glomerulus to collecting tubules
renal vein	ree-nal vain	one of two large veins that carries blood from the kidneys to the inferior vena cava

(continues)

TABLE 16-1 *(continued)*

Organ or Structure	Pronunciation	Definition
ureter	u-<u>re</u>-ter	the tubular structure through which urine passes from the kidney to the bladder
urethra	yoo-<u>ree</u>-thruh	the passage through which urine is discharged from the bladder to the body exterior
urinary bladder	<u>yoor</u>-uh-ner-ee <u>blad</u>-er	musculomembranous sac that stores urine, receiving it through the ureters and discharging it through the urethra
urinary meatus	<u>yoor</u>-uh-ner-ee me-<u>a</u>-tus	opening of the urethra to the exterior

Clinical Conditions and Procedures

TABLE 16-2

Clinical Condition	Pronunciation	Definition
azoturia	az'-o-tu-<u>re</u>-ah	excess urea (or other nitrogen compounds) in urine
calculus (renal) (pl., calculi)	<u>kal</u>-ku-lus (<u>re</u>-nal)	kidney stone(s)
cystitis	sis-<u>ti</u>-tis	inflammation of the urinary bladder
dialysate	dye-al-ih-<u>sayt</u>	a solution of water and electrolytes that passes through the artificial kidney to remove excess fluids and wastes from the blood; also called "bath"
dialysis	di-<u>al</u>-i-sis	the process of using an artificial kidney to filter waste materials from the body
"floating kidney"	<u>flot</u>-ing <u>kid</u>-ne	a kidney not securely fixed in the usual location because of birth defect or injury
glomerulonephritis	glo-mer'-u-lo-ne-<u>fri</u>-tis	nephritis with inflammation of the capillary loops in the renal glomeruli
hydronephrosis	hi-dro-ne-<u>fro</u>-sis	distention of the renal pelvis with urine, caused by obstruction of the ureter
nephrolithiasis	nef'-ro-li-<u>thi</u>-ah-sis	a condition marked by the presence of renal calculi (stones)
nephroptosis	nef'-rop-<u>to</u>-sis	downward displacement of a kidney
nephrorrhaphy	nef-<u>ror</u>-ah-fe	suture of the kidney
peritonitis	pair-ih-ton-<u>eye</u>-tis	inflammation of the peritoneum (the membrane lining the abdominal cavity)

TABLE   16-2   *(continued)*

Clinical Condition	Pronunciation	Definition
pyelitis	pi'-e-<u>li</u>-tis	inflammation of the renal pelvis
renal failure	<u>re</u>-nal <u>fāl</u>-yer	kidney fails to function normally, e.g., in excretion of body waste
renal transplant	<u>re</u>-nal <u>trans</u>-plant	transferring a kidney surgically from one person to another to replace a diseased structure
uremia	u-<u>re</u>-me-ah	the retention of toxic body waste in blood
ureterostomy	u-re'-ter-<u>os</u>-to-me	creation of a new outlet for a ureter through the abdominal wall to the outside
urethritis	u'-re-<u>thri</u>-tis	inflammation of the urethra
urinary tract infection (UTI)	<u>yoor</u>-uh-ner-ee trakt in-<u>fek</u>-shun	an infection of the urinary tract
Wilms' tumor	vilmz <u>too</u>-mor	a malignant tumor of the kidney, usually affecting children under age 5 years

Diagnostic Medical Terms

TABLE   16-3

Term	Pronunciation	Definition
albuminuria	al-bu'-mi-<u>nu</u>-re-ah	abnormal presence of serum albumin (protein) in the urine
anuria	ah-<u>nu</u>-re-ah	no urine produced
bacteriuria	back-tee-ree-<u>yoo</u>-ree-ah	bacteria in the urine
bladder distention	<u>blad</u>-der dis-<u>ten</u>-shun	full urinary bladder
blood chemistries	blud <u>kem</u>-is-treez	blood tests for kidney function, especially blood urea nitrogen (BUN) and creatinine
blood urea nitrogen (BUN)	blud u-<u>re</u>-ah <u>ni</u>-tro-jin	the urea (in terms of nitrogen) concentration of serum or plasma; an important indicator of renal function
catheterization	kath'-e-ter-i-<u>za</u>-shun	passage of a catheter (tube) into the bladder to relieve bladder distention or for other purposes

(continues)

TABLE 16-3 *(continued)*

Term	Pronunciation	Definition
Clinitest	klin-i-test	popular test for urine glucose or other substances
continent	kon-ti-nent	able to control urination (and/or defecation)
cystoscopy	sis-tos-ko-pe	visual examination of the urinary tract with a cystoscope
diuresis	di'-u-re-sis	increased excretion of urine
dysuria	dis-u-re-ah	painful or difficult urination
enuresis	en'-u-re-sis	uncontrolled urination while sleeping (bed-wetting)
frequency (urgency)	fre-kwen-se (ur-jen-se)	desire to urinate at short intervals, but discharging small amounts because of reduced bladder capacity
glycosuria	glye-kohs-yoo-ree-ah	high level of sugar, especially glucose, in the urine
hematuria	hem'-ah-tu-re-ah	the presence of blood in the urine
incontinent	in-kon-ti-nent	inability to control urination (and/or defecation)
intravenous pyelogram (IVP)	in'-trah-ve-nus pi-e-lo-gram	a technique in radiology for examining the structures and evaluating the function of the urinary system
I & O		intake and output; the amount of fluids (usually) ingested and excreted in a given period of time, measured and charted
ketonuria	kee-toh-noo-ree-ah	excessive amounts of ketone bodies in the urine
KUB		abbreviation for kidney, ureter, and bladder
micturate	mik-tu-rāt	urinate
nocturia, nycturia	nok-tu-re-ah, nik-tu-re-ah	excessive urination at night
oliguria	ol'-i-gu-re-ah	excreting a small amount of urine
polydipsia	pol-ee-dip-see-ah	excessive thirst
pyuria	pi-u-re-ah	pus in the urine
retrograde pyelogram	re-tro-grād pi-e-lo-gram'	a technique in radiology for examining the structures of the collecting system of the kidneys that is especially useful in locating an obstruction in the urinary tract
scan (renal)	skan (re-nal)	an image produced after the patient is injected with a radioactive substance; it determines kidney shape and function
Testape	tes-tap	special paper that changes color when dipped in urine
ultrasonography	ul'-trah-son-og-rah-fe	imaging body structures by recording the echoes of high-frequency sound waves reflected by body tissues on a paper or other device

TABLE 16-3 (continued)

Term	Pronunciation	Definition
urinalysis (UA)	u'-ri-nal-i-sis	analysis of the urine, e.g., acidity, sugar level
urinary retention	yoor-uh-ner-ee re-ten-shun	inability to urinate for various reasons; body retains urine waste
vesico-	ves-i-ko	a combining form meaning "pertaining to the bladder"
void	void	to empty the bladder, urinate

REPRODUCTIVE SYSTEM

Male Organs

TABLE 16-4

Organ	Pronunciation	Definition
Cowper's glands	ku-pers glandz	pea-sized glands that secrete lubricating fluid during intercourse; also called bulbourethral glands
glans penis	glanz pee-nis	tip of the penis (see **Figure 16–5**)
gonad	goh-nad	the male sex glands called the testes (plural) or testicle (singular)
penis	pee-nis	the organ of copulation
perineum	per-uh-nee-uhm	area between the scrotum and anus
prepuce	pree-pyoos	fold of skin covering the glans penis at birth; foreskin
prostate gland	pross-tayt gland	gland surrounding the neck of the bladder and urethra; contributes secretions that enhance sperm motility and neutralizes acidic vaginal secretions
scrotum	scrow-tum	two-compartment sac outside the body that houses the testes
seminal vesicles	sem-in-al vess-ih-kls	glands that secrete a thick, yellowish fluid, known as seminal fluid, into the vas deferens
testis (pl., testes)	tes-tis (tes-tez)	one of the pair of male gonads that produce semen

(continues)

TABLE 16-4 *(continued)*

Organ	Pronunciation	Definition
Ducts	duks	narrow tubular structures for excretion of semen and spermatozoa
epididymis	ep'-i-<u>did</u>-i-mis	a duct bordering the testes for storage, transit, and maturation of spermatozoa
vas deferens	vas <u>def</u>-er-enz	extension of the epididymis that joins the seminal vesicle to form the ejaculatory duct
seminal duct	<u>sem</u>-in-al duk	the passages for conveyance of spermatozoa and semen
ejaculatory duct vesicle	e-<u>jak</u>-u-<u>la</u>-tor'-e duk <u>ves</u>-i-cul	the duct formed by union of the vas deferens and the duct of the seminal vesicle
urethra	yoo-<u>ree</u>-thruh	opening for sperm and urine passage to the outside of the body
accessory glands	ak-<u>ses</u>-o-re glandz	their secretions mix with sperm to form seminal fluid
external genitalia	eks-<u>ter</u>-nal jen'-i-<u>ta</u>-le-ah	scrotum and penis

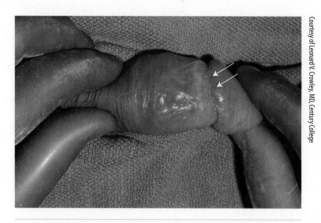

Courtesy of Leonard V. Crowley, MD, Century College

FIGURE 16–5 Several small superficial herpetic ulcers on shaft of penis behind the glans

CONFUSING MEDICAL TERMINOLOGY

vesic/o Versus vesicul/o

vesic/o = urinary bladder, e.g., vesicotomy (ves-ih-<u>kot</u>-o-me) refers to incision of the bladder

vesicul/o = seminal vesicle, blister, little bladder, e.g., vesiculectomy (veh-sik-u-<u>lek</u>-to-me) refers to excision or surgical removal of a vesicle (in this case, the seminal vesicle)

Female Organs

TABLE 16-5

Organ	Pronunciation	Definition
Bartholin's glands	bar-teh-linz glandz	small mucus-secreting glands located near the vagina
clitoris	klit'-or-is	erectile tissue at junction of labia majora and labia minora; equivalent to male penis
hymen	high-men'	thin elastic connective tissue covering the vaginal opening
Internal Genitalia		
cervix	ser-viks	necklike section at lower end of uterus
fallopian tubes (oviducts)	fah-loh-pee-an toobs (oh-vih-duks)	ducts in which fertilization occurs and passageway for ova to the uterus
ovary	oh-vay-ree	the female gonad: either of the paired female sex glands in which ova are formed and released, and which produce the female hormones
uterus	yoo'-ter-us	cavity opening into the vagina below and into a fallopian tube on either side; organ for nourishing the fetus
vagina	vaj-in-nah	birth canal and receptacle for copulation
External Genitalia		
adnexa	ad-nek-sah	structures in the uterus that are next to or near another, including the fallopian tubes, ovaries, and ligaments of the uterus
areola	ah-ree-oh-lah	The darker pigmented, circular area surrounding the nipple of each breast; also known as the "areola mammae" or the "areola papillaris"
labia majora	lay-bee-ah mah-jor-ah	two outer folds of skin on either side of the vaginal orifice
labia minora	lay-bee-ah mih-nor-ah	two thin folds of skin within the folds of the labia majora
mammary glands	mam-oh-ree glandz	female breasts; considered accessory glands to the FRS, they are necessary for breastfeeding the infant (lactation)
mons pubis	monz pew-biss	mound of fatty tissue over the pubis
perineum	par-ih-nee-um	area between vaginal orifice and anus
vulva	vull-vah	the external genitalia including the mons pubis, labia majora, clitoris, labia minora, vestibule, urinary meatus, vaginal orifice, Bartholin's glands, and the perineum collectively referred to as the vulva; also known as the pudendum

Male Clinical Conditions

TABLE 16-6

Clinical Condition	Pronunciation	Definition
balanoplasty	<u>bal</u>-ah-noh-plas-tee	surgical repair of the glans penis
benign prostatic hypertrophy (BPH)	bi-<u>nīn</u> pros-<u>tat</u>-ic hi-<u>per</u>-tro-fe	enlargement of the prostate gland, common among men by the age of 50 years
circumcision	ser'-kum-<u>sizh</u>-un	removing foreskin, or prepuce
cryptorchidism	krip'-<u>tor</u>-ki-dizm	undescended testicle(s)
epididymitis	ep'-i-did'-i-<u>mi</u>-tis	inflammation of the epididymis; from venereal disease
hydrocele	<u>hi</u>-dro-sel'	fluid collected in the testes
opportunistic infections	op-or-<u>toon</u>-is-tik in-<u>fek</u>-shuns	an infection occurring in a patient with decreased immunity resulting from, e.g., surgery, illnesses, and disorders such as AIDS. The organisms that cause the infection are normally non-disease-producing ones
orchiectomy	or'-ke-<u>ek</u>-to'-me	castration
orchiopexy	<u>or</u>-ke-o-pek'-se	fixation of an undescended testis in the scrotum
orchitis	or-<u>ki</u>-tis	inflammation of a testis
prostatectomy	pros'-tah-<u>tek</u>-to'-me	excision of all or part of the prostate
varicocele	<u>var</u>-i-ko-sel'	varicose veins near the testes
vasectomy	vah-<u>sek</u>-to-me	male sterilization by cutting or tying the vas deferens

Female Clinical Conditions

TABLE 16-7

Clinical Condition	Pronunciation	Definition
abortion (AB)	ah'-<u>bor</u>-shun	expulsion from the uterus of the products of conception before the fetus is viable
Bartholin's cyst or abscess	<u>bar</u>-tel-inz sist or <u>ab</u>-ses	chronic or acute inflammation of Bartholin's gland

TABLE 16-7 *(continued)*

Clinical Condition	Pronunciation	Definition
colporrhaphy	kol-<u>por</u>-ah-fe	suture of the vagina; to correct cystocele and rectocele
colposcopy	kol-<u>pos</u>-ko-pe	examination of the cervix by means of a colposcope
cystocele	<u>sis</u>-to-sel	hernia of the bladder into the vagina
dilatation and curettage (D&C)	dil'-ah-<u>ta</u>-shun ku'-re-<u>tahzh</u>	dilating the uterine cervix and using a curette to scrape the endometrium of the uterus; to diagnose disease, to correct vaginal bleeding, or to produce abortion
endometriosis	en'-do-me'-tre-<u>o</u>-sis	cells of the lining of the uterus spreading into the pelvis (peritoneal cavity)
fibroids	<u>fi</u>-broidz	colloquial term for benign tumor (leiomyoma) of the uterus
fistula	<u>fis</u>-tu-lah	an abnormal passage between two internal organs, e.g., vesicovaginal (between bladder and vagina) fistula
hydrosalpinx	hi'-dro-<u>sal</u>-pinks	fluid collecting in the uterine tube, causing distention
hysterectomy	his'-te-<u>rek</u>-to-me	excision of the uterus
hysterosalpingogram	his'-ter-o-sal-<u>ping</u>-go-gram	an x-ray film of the uterus and the fallopian tubes to allow visualization of the cavity of the uterus and the passageway of the tubes
laparoscopy	lap'-ah-<u>ro</u>-sko'-pe	laparoscopic visualization of the peritoneal cavity
leukorrhea	loo-ko-<u>re</u>-ah	a whitish, viscid discharge from the vagina
miscarriage	mis'-<u>kar</u>-ij	spontaneous abortion
monilia (moniliasis)	mo'-<u>nil</u>-e-ah (mon'-i-<u>li</u>-ah-sis)	yeastlike fungus infection of the vagina and other body parts
oophorectomy	o'-of-o-<u>rek</u>-to-me	excision of one or both ovaries; female castration
pelvic examination	<u>pel</u>-vic eg'-zam'i-<u>na</u>-tion	a diagnostic procedure in which the external and internal genitalia are physically examined using inspection, palpation, etc.
pelvic inflammatory disease (PID)	<u>pel</u>-vic in-<u>flam</u>-a-to-ry di-<u>sez</u>	any inflammatory condition of the female pelvic organs, especially one caused by bacterial infection
prolapse of uterus	<u>pro</u>-laps of <u>u</u>-ter-us	downward displacement of the uterus into the vagina
salpingectomy	sal'-pin-<u>jek</u>-to-me	excision of one or both fallopian tubes
salpingitis	sal'-pin-<u>ji</u>-tis	inflammation of one or both fallopian tubes
trichomonas infection	trik'-o-<u>mo</u>-nas in-<u>fek</u>-shun	inflammation of the vagina by a parasite, with itching and foul discharge
tubal ligation	<u>tu</u>-bal li-<u>ga</u>-shun	sterilization by "tying" both fallopian tubes
vaginal speculum	<u>vaj</u>-i-nal <u>spek</u>-u-lum	an instrument used to dilate the vagina during a pelvic examination

Male and Female Conditions

Sexually Transmitted Diseases (STDs)

The following conditions occur in both men and women and are the most communicable diseases in the world. They are spread through sexual contact with body fluids such as blood, semen, and vaginal secretions. STDs may be contracted during vaginal, oral, or anal intercourse or by direct contact with infected skin. AIDS can also be transmitted through sharing of needles by drug users, from the placenta of the infected mother to the baby during birth, and through breast milk of an infected mother when nursing the baby. The incidence of STDs in the United States is extremely high and may reach epidemic proportions because the latest figures indicate that AIDS is again on the rise after a period of decline.

TABLE 16-8

Term	Pronunciation	Definition
acquired immunodeficiency syndrome (AIDS)		a fatal disease caused by the human immunodeficiency virus (HIV), which destroys the body's immune system by invading the helper T cells (T lymphocytes). HIV replicates itself in the T cell, destroying the cell, and then invades other T cells
chlamydia	klah′-<u>mid</u>-ee-ah	a widespread sexually transmitted bacterial infection that invades the urethra of men and the vagina and cervix of women; the disease is asymptomatic in the early stages, which makes possible the spread of chlamydia as the partners are unaware that they have it
genital herpes	<u>jen</u>-ih′-tal <u>her</u>-peez	a highly contagious venereal disease caused by the type 2 herpes simplex virus (HSV-2), although it may be caused by HSV-1, the virus associated with oral infections (cold sores). Genital herpes is transmitted by direct contact with infected body secretions; remissions and relapses occur and no drug is known to be effective as a cure (see **Figure 16–6** for herpes of the female exterior genitalia)
genital warts	<u>jen</u>-ih′-tal warts	small, fleshy growths on the external genitalia; genital warts are transmitted from person to person through sexual intercourse. They are caused by the human papillomavirus (HPV) and appear from 1 to 6 months after the initial contact
gonorrhea	<u>gon</u>-oh′-ree-ah	inflammation of the mucous membranes of the genital tract, affecting both males and females, caused by gonococci (berry-shaped) bacteria; gonorrhea is spread by intercourse with an infected partner or is passed from an infected mother to her infant during birth
syphilis	<u>sif</u>-ih′-lis	a chronic, infectious disease caused by spirochete bacteria and transmitted by sexual intercourse with an infected partner; this is a highly infectious disease that can affect any body organ. A chancre (hard ulcer) appears on the external genitalia a few weeks after exposure; it usually develops on the penis of the male and on the labia of the female

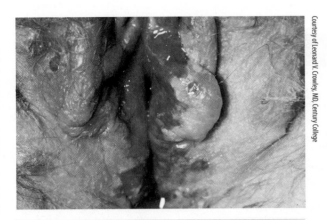

Courtesy of Leonard V. Crowley, MD, Century College

FIGURE 16–6 Multiple confluent ulcers of vulva (female external genitalia) as a result of herpes

Pregnancy and Birth

TABLE	16-9

Term	Pronunciation	Definition
amniocentesis	am'-ne-o-sen-<u>te</u>-sis	taking a sample of amniotic fluid during pregnancy for various reasons
amnion (BOW)	<u>am</u>-ne-on	amniotic sac; bag of waters
amniotic fluid	am-nee-<u>ot</u>-ik fluid	a liquid produced by and contained within the fetal membranes during pregnancy that protects the fetus from trauma and temperature variations and helps maintain fetal oxygen supply. The fluid also permits freedom of fetal movement
anesthesia (OB)	an'-es-<u>the</u>-ze-ah	loss of feeling or sensation, especially the loss of pain sensation induced to permit the performance of surgery or other painful procedures
antepartum	an-te-<u>par</u>-tum	period from conception to onset of labor
Apgar	<u>ap</u>-gar	the evaluation of an infant's physical condition, usually performed 1 and 5 min after birth, based on a rating of five factors that reflect the infant's ability to adjust to extrauterine life
bloody show	<u>blud</u>-e sho	appearance of blood forerunning labor
caesarean (C-section)	si-<u>zar</u>-i-en	a surgical procedure in which the abdomen and uterus are incised and a baby is delivered
cephalopelvic disproportion (CPD)	sef'-ah-lo-<u>pel</u>-vik dis-pruh-<u>pawr</u>-shuhn	a condition in which the fetal head is too large for the mother's pelvis

(continues)

TABLE 16-9	(continued)	
Term	**Pronunciation**	**Definition**
Coombs' test	kumz test	a blood test to diagnose hemolytic anemias in a newborn
culdocentesis	kull-doh-sen-<u>tee</u>-sis	a clinical process using a needle to aspirate, through the vagina into the cul-de-sac area (area immediately behind the vagina), fluid for examination or diagnosis
dystocia	dis-<u>to</u>-se-ah	abnormal labor or childbirth
ectopic pregnancy (extrauterine)	ek-<u>top</u>-ik (eks'-trah-<u>u</u>-ter-in)	pregnancy outside the uterus, usually in the fallopian tube
EDC		expected date of confinement (due date)
effacement	eh-<u>face</u>-ment	the thinning of the cervix to enlarge the diameter of its opening during childbirth in the normal processes of labor
episiotomy	e-piz'-e-<u>ot</u>-o-me	surgical incision into the perineum and/or vagina for obstetric purposes
fetal heart tones (FHT, fht)	<u>fe</u>-tal hart tonz	the fetal heart sounds heard through the mother's abdomen in pregnancy
forceps delivery	<u>for</u>-seps de-<u>liv</u>-er-e	applying forceps to fetal head; *low* or *midforceps* delivery according to the degree of engagement of the fetal head and *high* when engagement has not occurred
gestation	jes-<u>ta</u>-shun	period from conception to birth
Goodell's sign	<u>goo</u>-dels	the softening of the uterine cervix, a probable sign of pregnancy
gravida	<u>grav</u>-i-dah	a pregnant woman; *gravid* means "pregnant"
ICN		intensive care nursery
induction	in-<u>duk</u>-shun	labor is initiated artificially, e.g., by a drug
insemination	in-sem'-i-<u>na</u>-shun	the depositing of seminal fluid within the vagina or cervix
intrapartum	in-tra-<u>par</u>-tum	period from onset of labor through first hour after delivery
linea nigra	<u>lin</u>-ee-ah <u>nig</u>-rah	a darkened vertical midline appearing on the abdomen of a pregnant woman, connecting the distance between the umbilicus and the symphysis pubis
LMP		last menstrual period (due date)
lochia	<u>lo</u>-ke-ah	a vaginal discharge during the first week or two after childbirth
meconium	me-<u>ko</u>-ne-um	dark green mucilaginous material in the intestine of the full-term fetus, expelled as first stool
multigravida	mul-ti-<u>grav</u>-i-dah	a woman who has had more than one pregnancy
multipara	mul-<u>tip</u>-ah-rah	a woman who has borne more than one viable infant

TABLE 16-9 *(continued)*

Term	Pronunciation	Definition
Nagele's rule	nay-geh-leez	a formula for calculating when the baby is due or the date of birth: Subtract 3 months from the first day of the last normal menstrual period and add 7 days to that date to arrive at the estimated due date
neonatal period	ne'-o-na-tal	the first 4 weeks after birth
obstetrical index (OB index)	ob-stet-ri-cal in-deks	the number of pregnancies, term deliveries, abortions, and stillbirths a woman has experienced
pelvimeter (pelvimetry)	pel-vim-e-ter (pel-vim-e-tre)	an instrument used to measure the capacity and diameter of the pelvis for delivery
placenta	plah-sen-tah	organ for exchange of nutrients and wastes between mother and fetus; called the afterbirth
postpartum	post-par-tum	6-week period following childbirth
prenatal	pre-na-tal	before birth
presentation	prez'-en-ta-shun	the position of a baby in utero with reference to the part of the baby that is directed toward or into the birth canal
primipara	pri-mip-ah-rah	a woman bearing her first viable child
quickening	kwik-en-ing	the first movement of the fetus felt by the woman, usually between 18 and 20 weeks' gestation
stillborn (sb)	stil-born	born dead
test-tube baby		the fertilization of an ovum outside of the uterus
toxemia	tok-se-me-ah	a group of pathologic conditions, essentially metabolic disturbances, occurring in pregnant women, manifested by hypertension, edema, etc.; may be preeclampsia or eclampsia
trimester	tri-mes-ter	a period of 12 weeks
ultrasonography	ull-trah-son-og-rah-fee	a noninvasive method using reflected sound waves to detect the presence of the embryo or fetus
vernix caseosa	ver-niks ca-see-o-suh	a "cheesy" white substance on the skin of the newborn

PHARMACOLOGY AND MEDICAL TERMINOLOGY

Drug Classification	antifungal (an-tih-<u>fung</u>-gal)	anti-infective (antibiotic) (an-tih-in-<u>fek</u>-tiv)	diuretic (dye-yoor-<u>ret</u>-ik)
Function	destroys or inhibits the growth of fungi	stops or controls the growth of infection-causing microorganisms	increases urine secretion
Word Parts	**anti-** = against; **fung/o** = fungus; **-al** = pertaining to	**hyper-** = excess; **infective** = pertaining to infection	pertaining to an increase in urination
Active Ingredients (examples)	miconazole (Monistat); nystatin (Mycostatin); clotrimazole (Gyne-Lotrimin)	amoxycillin (Amoxil, Polymox); doxycycline hyclate (Vibramycin)	furosemide (Lasix); hydrochlorothiazide (Hydro-Diuril)

LESSON TWO   Progress Check

LISTS

1. List the organs of the urinary system:

    a.   two _____

    b.   two _____

    c.   one _____

    d.   one _____

2. List three important functions of the urinary system:

    a.   _____

    b.   _____

    c.   _____

3. List the important function of the reproductive system: _____

4. List the sex organs of male reproduction:

    a.   two _____

    b.   three _____

    c.   four _____

    d.   one _____

    e.   one _____

    f.   one _____

5. List the sex organs of female reproduction:

a. two _____

b. two _____

c. two _____

d. one _____

e. one _____

f. one _____

MULTIPLE CHOICE

Circle the letter of the correct answer:

1. Which of the following statements describes the cortex?
   a. membranous sac containing urine
   b. outer layer of the kidney
   c. upper end of the ureter
   d. the renal pelvis

2. The medulla is:
   a. the inner part of the kidney
   b. the outer layer of the kidney
   c. the renal pelvis
   d. the urinary meatus

3. The functional unit of the kidney that produces urine is called a
   a. ureter
   b. bladder
   c. nephron
   d. urethra

4. The urinary bladder receives urine through the _____ and discharges it through the _____.
   a. ureter, nephron
   b. bladder, urethra
   c. medulla, meatus
   d. ureter, urethra

COMPARE AND CONTRAST

Explain the *differences* in the following conditions of the urinary tract:
Example: calculi/cystitis   calculi are kidney stones, but cystitis is inflammation of the urinary bladder

1. albuminuria/anuria _____

2. enuresis/diuresis _____

3. incontinence/urinary retention _____

4. hydronephrosis/nephrolithiasis _____

5. nycturia/oliguria/dysuria _____

6. pyelitis/glomerulonephritis _____

◆ MATCHING: CLINICAL PROCEDURES

Match the procedure with its definition:

1. catheterization	**a.** imaging with sound waves
2. Clinitest	**b.** radiologic examination of the kidneys' collecting system
3. cystoscopy	**c.** determination of acidity and sugar levels of urine
4. IVP	**d.** measure of the amount of glucose in the urine
5. I & O	**e.** tube in the bladder for urine drainage
6. UA	**f.** visual examination of the bladder
7. ultrasonography	**g.** measuring and charting all ingested and excreted fluids
8. retrograde pyelogram	**h.** radiologic technique for examining kidney function

◆ COMPLETION

Write in the medical term for each of the following meanings:

1. _____ a male gonad that supplies sperm to the semen

2. _____ the scrotum, penis, vulva, clitoris, and urethra

3. _____ extension of the epididymis and part of the ejaculatory duct

4. _____ gland surrounding the neck of the bladder in males

5. _____ the gland that is used for storage and maturation of spermatozoa

6. _____ passage for spermatozoa and semen

7. _____ a female gonad that produces eggs

8. _____ duct where fertilization occurs

9. _____ female organ that nourishes the fetus

10. _____ birth canal and receptacle for coitus

11. _____ abnormal labor or childbirth

12. _____ fluid collecting in the uterine tube, causing distension

◆ MATCHING: MALE CLINICAL CONDITIONS

Match these clinical conditions that occur in the *male* to their best definition:

1. circumcision	**a.** sterilization
2. cryptorchidism	**b.** excision of the prostate gland
3. orchiectomy	**c.** removal of the prepuce
4. prostatectomy	**d.** undescended testicle(s)
5. vasectomy	**e.** castration

◆ MATCHING: FEMALE CLINICAL CONDITIONS

Match these clinical conditions that occur in the *female* to their best definition:

1. cystocele	**a.** castration
2. endometriosis	**b.** sterilization
3. hysterectomy	**c.** hernia of the bladder into the vagina
4. oophorectomy	**d.** excision of the uterus
5. tubal ligation	**e.** endometrial tissue spread into the peritoneal cavity

◆ DEFINITIONS

These medical terms are specific to pregnancy and childbirth. Name the term that means:

1. taking a sample of amniotic fluid _____

2. evaluation of an infant's condition at birth _____

3. the fetal head is too large for the mother's pelvis _____

4. abnormal labor or childbirth _____

5. a pregnancy outside the uterus _____

6. period from conception to birth _____

7. a pregnant woman _____

8. first 4 weeks after birth (infant) _____

9. six-week period after birth (mother) _____

10. the afterbirth _____

◆ WORD PUZZLE ON THE GENITOURINARY SYSTEM

Find the 50 words related to the genitourinary system by reading forward, backward, up, down, and diagonally. When you have circled the 50 listed words, the remaining letters will spell the words URINARY SYSTEM.

```
R  E  D  D  A  L  B  Y  R  A  N  I  R  U  C  O  R  T  E  X
S  E  T  Y  L  O  R  T  C  E  L  E  D  I  C  A  C  I  R  U
U  G  T  R  A  M  S  P  O  R  T  C  I  T  O  M  S  O  E  R
T  L  F  R  A  L  U  B  U  T  I  R  E  P  L  U  D  R  A  I
A  O  I  B  O  W  M  A  N  S  C  A  P  S  U  L  E  P  B  N
E  M  L  A  C  P  A  F  F  E  R  E  N  T  M  O  S  O  S  A
M  E  T  R  R  U  E  Y  E  N  D  I  K  E  N  O  C  O  O  T
N  R  R  T  E  R  U  R  E  T  E  R  T  T  N  P  E  L  R  I
O  U  A  E  A  E  N  I  R  U  S  S  E  O  O  N  G  P  O
I  L  T  R  T  T  A  D  H  T  Y  V  E  R  R  F  D  N  T  N
T  U  E  I  I  H  I  N  T  S  O  C  C  C  H  H  I  I  I  O
A  S  N  O  N  R  A  N  Y  L  A  N  R  X  P  E  N  D  O  I
R  R  I  L  I  A  E  R  U  L  E  S  E  E  E  N  G  N  N  T
T  E  N  E  N  R  A  M  Y  R  R  I  T  A  N  L  L  E  R  I
N  N  E  S  E  L  E  X  Y  S  U  V  E  Y  L  E  O  C  E  R
E  A  R  F  L  T  U  B  U  L  E  L  C  E  L  L  O  S  T  U
C  L  F  I  S  D  I  U  L  F  S  E  T  S  A  W  P  A  L  T
N  E  P  P  R  O  X  I  M  A  L  P  D  I  S  T  A  L  I  C
O  A  S  T  D  I  M  A  R  Y  P  M  E  D  U  L  L  A  F  I
C  O  N  V  O  L  U  T  E  D  E  M  E  N  O  G  I  R  T  M
```

Words to Look for in the Word Puzzle

1. ADH	**14.** descending loop	**27.** micturition	**40.** trigone
2. afferent	**15.** distal	**28.** nephron	**41.** tubule
3. arterioles	**16.** efferent	**29.** osmotic	**42.** urea
4. ascending loop	**17.** electrolytes	**30.** pelvis	**43.** ureter
5. Bowman's capsule	**18.** excrete	**31.** peritubular	**44.** urethra
6. calyx	**19.** filter	**32.** proximal	**45.** uric acid
7. capillary system	**20.** filtrate	**33.** pyramid	**46.** urinary bladder
8. cell	**21.** fluids	**34.** reabsorption	**47.** urination
9. column	**22.** glomerulus	**35.** renal	**48.** urine
10. concentration	**23.** kidney	**36.** renin	**49.** volume
11. convoluted	**24.** Loop of Henle	**37.** retroperitoneal	**50.** wastes
12. cortex	**25.** meatus	**38.** secrete	
13. creatinine	**26.** medulla	**39.** transport	

CHAPTER 17

Musculoskeletal System

LESSON ONE: MATERIALS TO BE LEARNED

The Skeletal System
  Division
  Body Bones
  Head Bones
  Joints and Accessory Parts
  Bone Processes, Depressions, and Holes
The Muscular System
  Muscles of the Body
  Motion
  Physiological Status of Muscles
  Injuries
  Clinical Disorders
  Medical Management
  Abbreviations (Musculoskeletal System)

LESSON TWO: PROGRESS CHECK

List the Function
Matching: Locations
Multiple Choice
Name the Structure
Matching; Muscles
Compare and Contrast
Word Puzzle on the Musculoskeletal System

OBJECTIVES

After completing this chapter and the exercises, the student should be able to:

1. Locate and name the major bones of the body by labeling the diagram provided.
2. Locate and name the major muscles of the body by labeling the diagram provided.
3. Classify the joints found in the musculoskeletal system (MSS).
4. Identify the types of bone fractures.
5. Identify and describe the types of muscles.
6. Define and explain various pathologic conditions of the musculoskeletal system.
7. Identify important laboratory tests and procedures relating to the musculoskeletal system.

ALLIED HEALTH PROFESSIONS

Clinical Laboratory (Medical) Technologists and Technicians and Medical, Dental, and Ophthalmic Laboratory Technicians

Changes in body fluids, tissues, and cells are often a sign that something is wrong. Clinical laboratory testing plays a crucial role in the detection and diagnosis of disease. Clinical laboratory and medical technologists perform laboratory testing in conjunction with pathologists (physicians who diagnose the cause and nature of disease) and other physicians or scientists who specialize in clinical chemistry, microbiology, or the other biological sciences. Medical technologists develop data on the blood, tissues, and fluids in the human body by using a variety of precision instruments.

Medical appliance technicians construct, fit, maintain, and repair braces, artificial limbs, joints, arch supports, and other surgical and medical appliances. They follow prescriptions or detailed instructions from podiatrists or orthotists, who request braces, supports, corrective shoes, or other devices. They also follow the instructions of prosthetists in constructing replacement limbs—arms, legs, hands, or feet—for patients who need them because of a birth defect, accident, or amputation. Other health professionals may also order medical appliances to be produced by medical appliance technicians. Medical appliance technicians who work with orthotic and prosthetic devices are called orthotic and prosthetic technicians. Other medical appliance technicians work with medical appliances that help correct other medical problems, such as aids to correct hearing loss.

Dental laboratory technicians fill prescriptions from dentists for crowns, bridges, dentures, and other dental prosthetics. First, dentists send a specification of the item to be manufactured, along with an impression or mold of the patient's mouth or teeth. Then dental laboratory technicians, also called dental technicians, create a model of the patient's mouth by pouring plaster into the impression and allowing it to set. They place the model on an apparatus that mimics the bite and movement of the patient's jaw. The model serves as the basis of the prosthetic device.

Ophthalmic laboratory technicians should not be confused with workers in other vision care occupations. Ophthalmologists are "eye doctors" who examine eyes, diagnose and treat vision problems, and prescribe corrective lenses. They are physicians who also perform eye surgery. Ophthalmic laboratory technicians read prescription specifications, select standard glass or plastic lens blanks, and then mark them to indicate where the curves specified on the prescription should be ground. They place the lens in the lens grinder, set the dials for the prescribed curvature, and start the machine. After a minute or so, the lens is ready to be "finished" by a machine that rotates it against a fine abrasive, to grind it and smooth out rough edges. The lens is then placed in a polishing machine with an even finer abrasive, to polish it to a smooth, bright finish.

INQUIRY

American Medical Technologists: www.amt1.com
American Society for Clinical Laboratory Science: www.ascls.org
American Academy of Orthotists and Prosthetists: www.opcareers.org
National Association of Dental Laboratories: www.nadl.org
Commission on Opticianry Accreditation: www.coaccreditation.com

Data from Stanfield, Peggy S., Cross, Nanna, and Hui, Y.H. *Introduction to the Health Professions*, 6th ed. Burlington, MA: Jones & Bartlett Learning; 2012.

The musculoskeletal system includes the bones, muscles, and joints. All have important functions in the body. The human skeleton consists of 206 bones. Bones provide internal structural support, giving shape to our bodies and enabling us to stand upright. Some bones protect internal organs. The rib cage, for example, protects the lungs and heart, and the skull protects the brain. The skeleton plays an important role in purposeful movement as the site of attachment for tendons of many skeletal muscles. The skeletal muscles' action on bones results in movement or stabilizes the skeleton. Bones are home to cells that give rise to red blood cells, white blood cells, and platelets (hematopoiesis). They are a storage depot for fat, which is necessary for cellular energy production, and they are a reservoir for minerals, especially calcium and phosphorus. Bones release and absorb calcium as needed to help maintain normal blood levels. Calcium is essential to muscle contraction, and disturbances in calcium levels can impair their function.

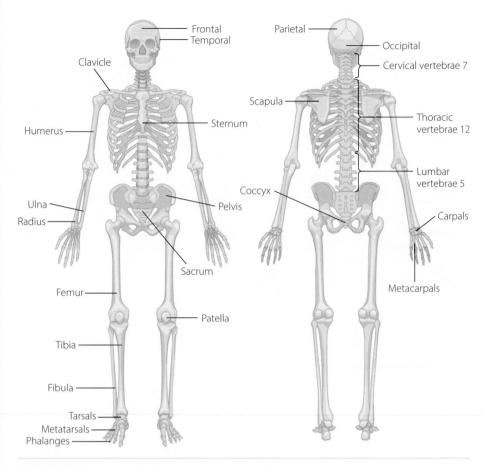

FIGURE 17–1 Skeletal system

The adult human skeleton contains about 206 bones that make up the solid framework of the body. The skeleton is completed in certain areas by cartilage. The skeleton is organized into the *axial* skeleton, the *appendicular* skeleton, and the joints between bones (see **Figures 17–1** and **17–2**). *Axis* and *appendicular* are defined in the first table in Lesson One.

The axial skeleton is composed of 80 bones that make the long axis of the body and protect the organs of the heart, neck, and torso.

1. The *vertebral column* has 26 vertebrae separated by intervertebral disks.
2. The *skull* is balanced on the vertebral column.

    a. *Cranial* bones enclose and protect the brain.
    b. *Facial* bones give shape to the face or contain teeth.
    c. Six *auditory* (ear) *ossicles* transmit sound.
    d. The *hyoid* supports the tongue and larynx.

3. The *thoracic* cage includes the ribs and sternum.

The appendicular skeleton is composed of 126 bones that make up arms, legs, and the pectoral and pelvic girdles that anchor them to the axial skeleton.

Joints are *articulations* between two or more bones. They connect the bones of the skeleton and are classified by the degree of movement they permit. Immovable joints permit no movement. Skull bones, for example, are held together by immovable joints, as is the pubic symphysis that is formed by the two pubic bones. Freely movable joints allow movement, such as the vertebrae. The joints between vertebrae allow

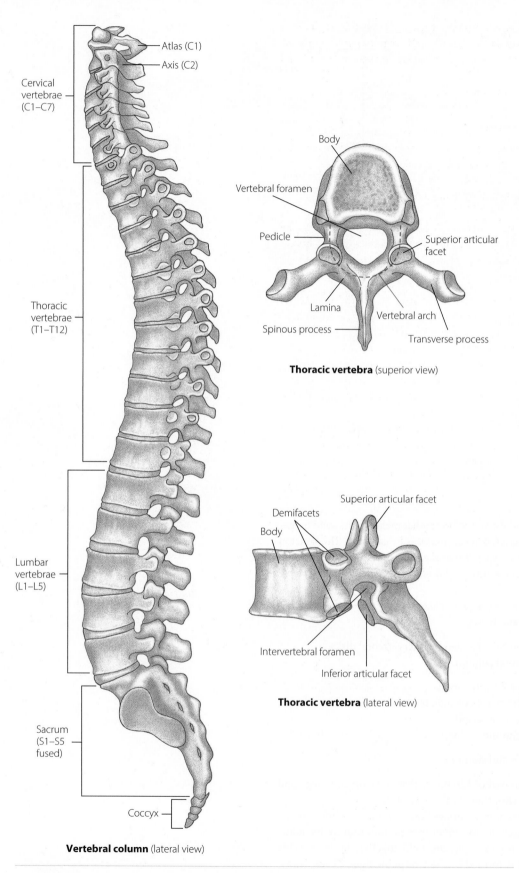

Thoracic vertebra (superior view)

Thoracic vertebra (lateral view)

Vertebral column (lateral view)

FIGURE 17–2 The vertebral column and features of selected vertebrae

some movement so that we can bend or curl up in our beds. The most freely moving joint is the *synovial* joint. This is the ball and socket hip joint or the joint between the pelvis and the femur. Synovial joints differ in structure but share many features. It is a complex joint.

The functions of the skeletal system are the following:

1. To support and shape the body.
2. To provide movement. Bones and joints act as levers. As the muscles that are anchored to bones contract, the force applied to the levers results in movement.
3. For protection. The skeletal system protects soft delicate organs of the body.
4. For blood cell formation (*hematopoiesis*). The red bone marrow is the site of production of red blood cells (*erythrocytes*), white blood cells (*leukocytes*), and *platelets* of the blood.
5. For storage of minerals, primarily calcium phosphate and calcium carbonate. The bones contain 99% of the body's calcium. Calcium and phosphorus in the bone are withdrawn as needed for other body functions. They must be replenished through nutrition.

Muscles, whether attached to bones or to internal organs and blood vessels, are responsible for movement. Most muscles cross one or more joints, and when they contract they cause movement. Internal movement is the contraction and relaxation of visceral muscles. Some muscles steady the joints, helping to maintain upright posture against the pull of gravity. Other muscles anchored to the bones of the skull and face allow us to frown, smile, open and close our eyes, and move our lips. Muscles also produce enormous amounts of heat as a by-product of metabolism. A physician who specializes in bone and joint diseases is called an *orthopedist*.

Muscle tissue constitutes 40–50% of body weight. It consists predominantly of contractile cells called muscle fibers. Through contraction, muscles produce movement and do work (see **Figures 17–3, 17–4,** and **17–5**).

Muscles have these properties: *contractility, excitability* (response when stimulated by nerve impulses), *extensibility* (stretch beyond their relaxed length), and elasticity (return to their original length). Mammals are the only animals with facial muscles, and the human body contains the same number of muscles from birth to death.

There is special classification and terminology related to muscles. These are explained and defined in Lesson One.

The functions of the muscular system are the following:

1. Movement
2. Body support and maintenance of posture
3. Heat production

The energy sources for muscle contraction are an interesting part of muscle physiology involving the citric acid cycle. Additional energy sources are formed by the metabolism of glucose and fatty acids through anaerobic (glycolytic pathway) and aerobic reactions. The value of exercise in weight control can be verified with these facts.

Many injuries, diseases, and disorders affect the musculoskeletal system. These are defined in Lesson One. Lessons to be learned are separated into sections for better identification and clarity:

1. Head and body bones, joints, and accessories
2. Body muscles
3. Pathologic conditions of MSS and the procedures and tests used to diagnose and treat them (medical management)

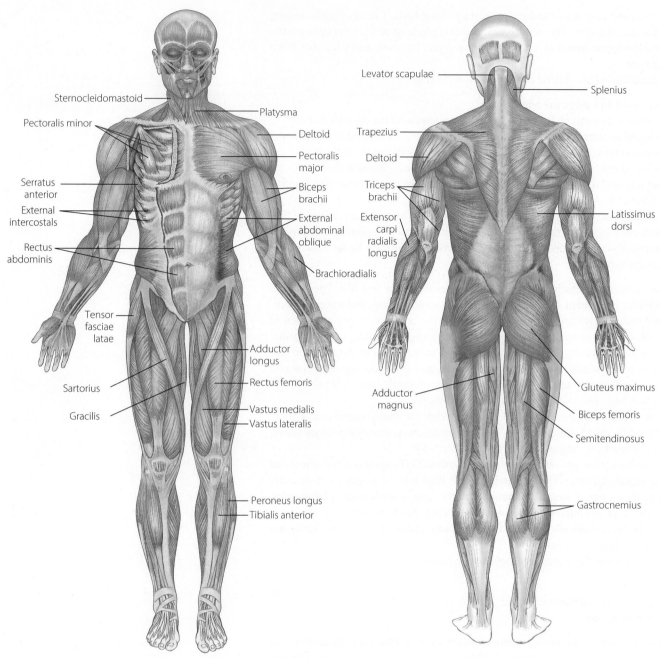

FIGURE 17–3 The muscular system, side and back views

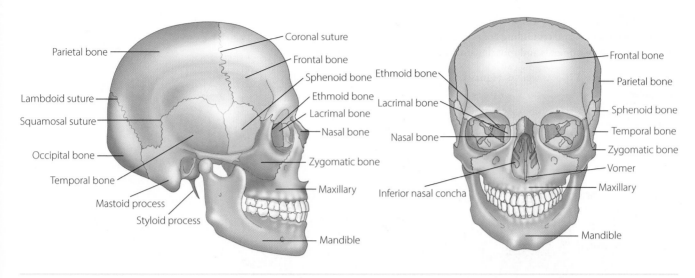

FIGURE 17–4 The skull

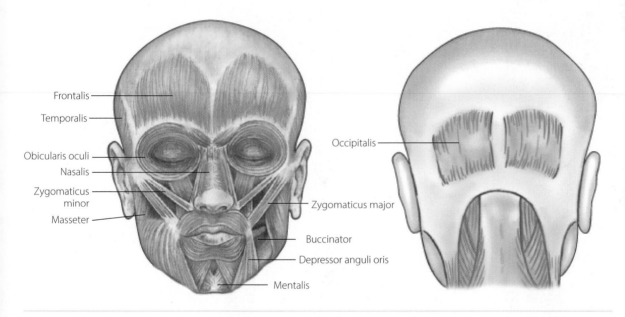

FIGURE 17–5 Muscles of the head

LESSON ONE	Materials to Be Learned

The musculoskeletal system serves the following functions in the body:

1. *Support and protection:* the forms and shapes of the body are maintained and vital organs are protected from injury
2. *Movement:* body movement is made possible by a coordination of different components of the musculoskeletal system

3. *Red blood cell turnover:* marrow from the large bones serves as the site for turnover (destruction and rebuilding) of red blood cells

4. *Storage:* bones store minerals and muscles store nutrients for energy production

Refer to Figures 17–1 to 17–5 as well as **Figures 17–6** and **17–7** when studying the following tables.

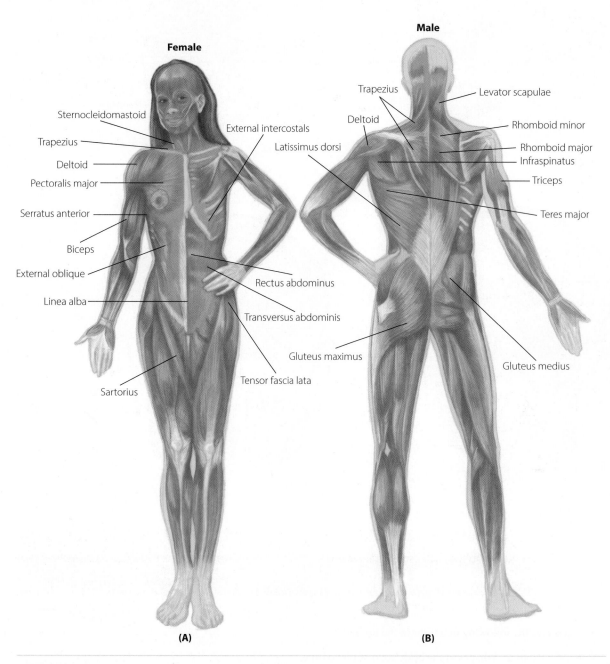

FIGURE 17–6 (A) Anterior aspect of the muscles of the neck, thorax, and arm. (B) Posterior aspect of the muscles of the neck, thorax, and arm.

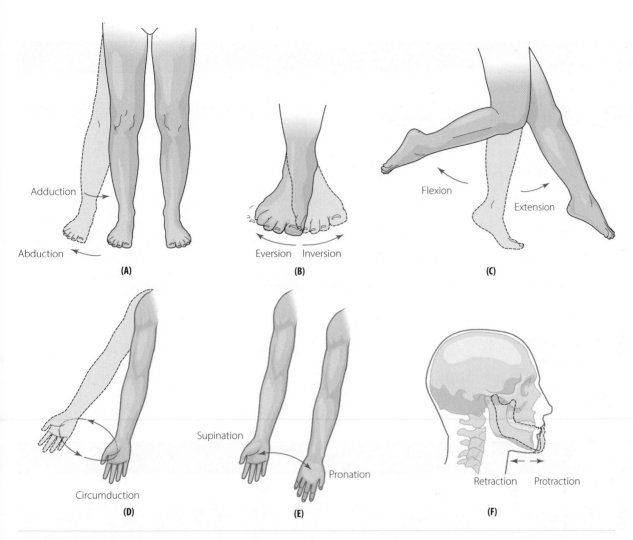

FIGURE 17–7 Movements of diarthrodial joints. (A) Abduction–adduction. (B) Eversion–inversion. (C) Flexion–extension. (D) Circumduction. (E) Supination–pronation. (F) Protraction–retraction.

THE SKELETAL SYSTEM

Division

TABLE   17-1

Main Division	Pronunciation	Definition
appendicular	ap´-en-<u>dik</u>-u-lar	an appendage; limbs
axis (n.) (axial [adj.])	<u>ak</u>-sis (<u>ak</u>-si-el)	a line that passes through the center of the body traversing skull, thorax, and vertebral column
ethmoid	<u>eth</u>-moid	the light and spongy bone at the base of the cranium; the upper nasal bone between the eyes

(continues)

TABLE 17-1 (continued)

Main Division	Pronunciation	Definition
frontal	<u>frun</u>-tal	forehead
mandible	<u>man</u>-di-b´-l	large bone constituting the lower jaw
maxilla	mak-<u>sil</u>-ah	one of a pair of large bones forming the upper jaw
occipital	ok-<u>sip</u>-i-tal	the cuplike bone at the back of the skull
parietal	pah-<u>ri</u>-e-tal	bone of the skull (top of the head)
sphenoid	<u>sfe</u>-noid	bone at the base of the skull, anterior to the temporal bones
temporal	<u>tem</u>-po-ral	large bones forming part of the temples
turbinate	<u>ter</u>-bi-nat	cone-shaped nasal bone

Body Bones

TABLE 17-2

Part	Pronunciation	Definition
clavicle	<u>klav</u>-i-k´-l	a long, curved, horizontal bone just above the first rib (collar bone)
femur	<u>fe</u>-mur	the thigh bone, extending from the pelvis to the knee
fibula and tibia	<u>fib</u>-u-lah and <u>tib</u>-e-ah	the fibula is the smallest of the bones of the leg; the tibia is the second longest bone of the skeleton, located at the medial side of the leg
humerus	<u>hu</u>-mer-us	upper-arm bone, consisting of a body, a head, and the condyle
radius and ulna	<u>ra</u>-de-us and <u>ul</u>-nah	the radius is the larger of the two bones of the forearm; the ulna is the bone on the medial or little-finger side of the forearm, lying parallel with the radius
scapula	<u>skap</u>-u-lah	shoulder blade
sternum	<u>ster</u>-num	the elongated, flattened bone forming the middle portion of the thorax (breastbone)
vertebral column	<u>ver</u>-te-bral <u>kol</u>-em	the flexible structure that forms the longitudinal axis (backbone) of the skeleton; it consists of 26 separate vertebrae arranged vertically from the base of the skull to the coccyx (tailbone)

Head Bones

TABLE 17-3

Part	Pronunciation	Definition
ethmoid	<u>eth</u>-moid	a very light and spongy bone at the base of the cranium; the upper nasal bone between the eyes
frontal	<u>frun</u>-tal	forehead
hyoid	<u>hahy</u>-oid	point of attachment for muscles of head and throat
lachrymal	<u>lak</u>-ruh-muhl	two bones that house the tear ducts
mandible	<u>man</u>-dih-bel	large bone constituting the lower jaw
maxilla	mak-<u>sil</u>-ah	one of a pair of large bones forming the upper jaw
nasal	<u>ney</u>-zuhl	two bones that shape the nose
occipital	ock-<u>sip</u>-it-al	the cuplike bone at the back of the skull
palatine	<u>pal</u>-uh-tahyn	forms the hard palate (roof of the mouth)
parietal	pah-<u>ri</u>-et-al	parietal bone of the skull (top of the head)
sphenoid	<u>sfne</u>-noid	bone at the base of the skull, anterior to the temporal bones
temporal	<u>tem</u>-poor-al	large bones forming part of the temples
turbinate	<u>ter</u>-beh-nate	cone-shaped nasal bone
vomer	<u>voh</u>-mer	lower part of the nasal septum
zygomatic	zahy-guh-<u>mat</u>-ik	two bones, one on each side of the face, that form the high part of the cheek bones and outer eye socket

Joints and Accessory Parts

TABLE 17-4

Part	Pronunciation	Definition
ball and socket	bawl and <u>sok</u>-et	a joint in which the globular head of an articulating bone is received into a cuplike cavity, e.g., the hip and shoulder
hinge	hinj	hinge joint, e.g., elbow, knees, and fingers
sutures	<u>su</u>-cherz	lines of junction between the bones of the skull

(continues)

Part	Pronunciation	Definition
intervertebral	in-ter-<u>ver</u>-te-bral	the fibrous substance between the disks of the spinal vertebrae
aponeurosis	ap´-o-nu-<u>ro</u>-sis	a flattened tendon, connecting a muscle with the parts it moves
bursa (pl., bursae)	<u>ber</u>-sah (<u>ber</u>-see)	a fluid-filled sac located in tissues to reduce friction
fascia (pl., fasciae)	<u>fash</u>-e-ah (<u>fash</u>-shee-ee)	a sheet of fibrous tissue holding muscle fibers together
interphalangeal	in´-ter-fah-<u>lan</u>-je-al	between two contiguous joints and phalanges, e.g., between the fingers and toes
lamina (pl., laminae)	<u>lam</u>-i-nah <u>lam</u>-i-nee	the flattened part of the vertebral arch (thinnest part of a vertebra)
ligament	<u>lig</u>-ah-ment	a band of fibrous tissue connecting bones or cartilages
meniscus (pl., menisci)	me-<u>nis</u>-kus (me-<u>nis</u>-ki)	a crescent-shaped fibrocartilage in the knee joint
synovial fluid	si-<u>no</u>-ve-al	the transparent, viscid fluid found in joint cavities, bursae, and tendon sheaths
tendon	<u>ten</u>-don	a fibrous cord of connective tissue attaching the muscle to bone or cartilage
theca	<u>the</u>-kah	a case or sheath of a tendon

TABLE 17-4 *(continued)*

Bone Processes, Depressions, and Holes

Bone processes are enlarged tissues that extend out from the bones to serve as attachments for muscles and tendons. The bone head is the rounded end of a bone separated from the body of the bone by a neck. Many bones have a small rounded process called a tubercle for attachment of tendons or muscles. Below the neck of the femur is a large bony process called a trochanter, and at the end of the bone is a rounded knuckle-like projection that fits into the fossa (bone depression) of another bone to form a joint.

Bone depressions are the openings or cavities in a bone that help to join one bone to another and are the passageway for the blood vessels and nerves. As noted previously, the fossa is a shallow cavity in or on a bone. The foramen is an opening for blood vessels and nerves. A fissure, or suture, is a deep, narrow, slitlike opening. A sinus is a hollow space in a bone, for example, the paranasal sinuses.

CONFUSING MEDICAL TERMINOLOGY

-metry Versus metr/o

-metry = the process of measurement, e.g., osteometry (os-<u>teo</u>-met-re) refers to measurement of bone

metr/o = uterus, e.g., menometrorrhagia (men-o-me-<u>tro</u>-ra-je-a) refers to excessive menstrual uterine bleeding

TABLE 17-5

Structure	Pronunciation	Definition
acetabulum	as´-e-<u>tab</u>-u-lum	the cup-shaped cavity (socket) receiving the head of the femur
foramen (pl., foramina)	fo-<u>ra</u>-men (fo-<u>ram</u>-i-nah)	holes in a bone for large vessels and nerves to pass through
fossa (pl., fossae)	<u>fos</u>-ah (<u>fos</u>-ee)	a hollow or depressed area
groove	groov	a narrow, linear hollow or depression in bone
malleolus	mah-<u>le</u>-o-lus	a rounded process, such as the protuberance on either side of the ankle joint, at the lower end of the fibula or the tibia
olecranon	o-<u>lek</u>-rah-non	bony projection of the ulna at the elbow
prominence	<u>prom</u>-i-nens	protrusion or projection
sinus	<u>si</u>-nus	one definition is a recess, cavity, or channel, such as one in bone
tuberosity	too´-be-<u>ros</u>-i-te	an elevation or protuberance, especially of a bone

THE MUSCULAR SYSTEM

Basically, there are three categories of muscles in the body:

1. Heart or cardiac muscle.
2. Striated or striped muscles, e.g., skeletal muscles. These muscles are voluntary muscles that a person has control over.
3. Nonstriated or nonstriped muscles, e.g., smooth muscles. These muscles are involuntary and there is no way to have control over them, e.g., movement of the stomach and intestine.

Body muscles are identified in the following manner:

1. *Function:* a muscle name has two parts: The first part is a word root, ending in a suffix (-or or -ens); the second part is the name of the affected body structure. An example is extensor carpi, or extension of the wrist.
2. *Points of origin and attachment:* the muscle name joins the names of points of origin and attachment with a word terminal (-eus or -is). An example is sternoclavicularis, for sternum and clavicle.
3. *Form or position:* the muscle name contains a descriptive word and the name of the muscle location. An example is pectoralis minor, for small chest muscle.
4. *Resemblance to an object for which the muscle is used:* an example is buccinator. This refers to the cheek muscle, which is used in blowing a trumpet.

When studying the following information refer to Figures 17–6, 17–7, and **17–8**.

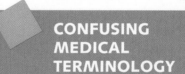

CONFUSING MEDICAL TERMINOLOGY

myel/o Versus myel/o

myel/o = bone marrow, e.g., myeloma (<u>mi</u>-el-o-mah) refers to tumor of the bone marrow (its cells) of the spinal cord

myel/o = spinal cord, e.g., polioencephalomeningomyelitis (<u>po</u>-le-o-en-sef-al-o-men-in-jo-mi-<u>el</u>-i-tis) refers to inflammation of the gray matter of the brain, the membrane, and the spinal cord

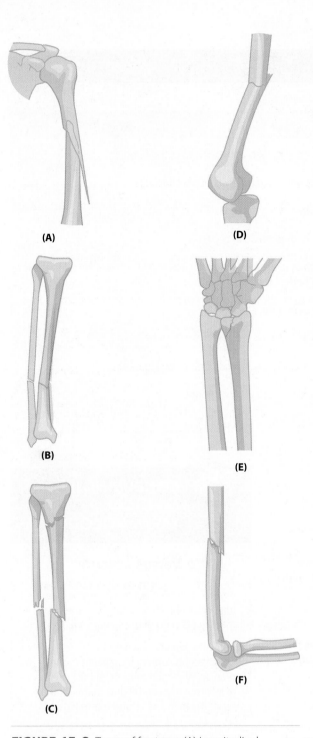

FIGURE 17–8 Types of fractures. (A) Longitudinal, through upper shaft of right humerus. (B) Spiral, of tibia and fibula. (C) Comminuted, of tibia and fibula. (D) Transverse, through lower shaft of femur. (E) Impacted. (F) Pathologin, through area of destruction secondary to metastatic carcinoma.

Muscles of the Body

TABLE	17-6	

Medical Term	Pronunciation	Definition
biceps brachii	bye-<u>seps</u> bray-kee-eye	muscle extending from scapula to radius.; used to flex lower arm and turn palm of hand upward
buccinator	buck-sin-<u>ay</u>-tor	fleshy part of the cheek; used to smile, blow outward, and whistle
cardiac muscle	<u>kar</u>-de-ac <u>muhs</u>-uhl	specialized muscle found in the walls of the heart; involuntary muscles, controlled by the autonomic nervous system
deltoid	<u>dell</u>-toyd	muscle covering the shoulder joint; extends from clavicle and scapula to humerus, and abducts the shoulder
gastrocnemius	gas-trok-<u>nee</u>-mus	main calf muscle; attaches to heel bone
gluteus maximus	gloo-tee-us <u>max</u>-ih-mus	fleshy part of the buttocks; extends from ilium to femur. Extends and rotates hip laterally
hamstring	<u>ham</u>-string	muscle in posterior thigh used for flexing knee, as in kneeling, and for hip extension
latissimus dorsi	lah-<u>tis</u>-ih-mus <u>dor</u>-see	muscle extending from lower vertebrae to humerus; used for adduction of the shoulder joint
masseter	mass-<u>see</u>-ter	muscle at angle of jaw; used for biting and chewing
orbicularis occuli	or-<u>bick</u>-yoo-<u>lar</u>-iss <u>ock</u>-yool-eye	body of the eyelid, opens and closes the eye, wrinkles forehead
orbicularis oris	or-<u>bick</u>-yoo-<u>lar</u>-iss <u>or</u>-iss	muscle surrounding the mouth; closes and purses the lips
pectoralis major	peck-tor-<u>ray</u>-lis	large, fan-shaped muscle across front of the chest; adducts, flexes, and rotates the shoulder joint inward
quadriceps femoris	<u>kwod</u>-rih-seps fem-<u>or</u>-is	anterior thigh muscle; part of a five-muscle group that extends the knee and flexes the hip
skeletal muscle	<u>skel</u>-i-tl <u>muhs</u>-uhl	also called striated (striped) or voluntary muscles; muscles attached to skeletal bones except for face, eyes, tongue, and throat. Under conscious control
smooth muscle	smooth <u>muhs</u>-uhl	muscles found in the wall of the stomach, intestine, blood vessels, and respiratory tract; also called involuntary or visceral muscle (not under conscious control)
sternomastoid	stir-no-<u>mass</u>-toyd	muscle extending from sternum to side of the neck; used for turning the head
temporal	<u>tem</u>-por-al	muscle above the ear; used for opening and closing the jaw
trapezius	trap-<u>pee</u>-zee-us	triangular muscle extending from back of shoulder to clavicle; used to raise shoulders
triceps brachii	<u>tri</u>-seps bray-<u>kee</u>-eye	muscle extending from scapula to ulna; responsible for extending the elbow

Motion

TABLE	17-7

Movement	Pronunciation	Definition
flexion	flek-shun	bending
extension	ek-sten-shun	the movement by which the two ends of any jointed part are drawn away from each other; straightening
adduction	ad-duk-shun	to draw toward the axial (median) line
abduction	ab-duk-shun	to draw away from the axial (median) line
pronation	pro-na-shun	the prone position (palm down, face down)
supination	su´-pi-na-shun	palm or face upward
proximal	prok-si-mal	nearest to a point of reference or origin
distal	dis-tal	farthest from any point of reference or origin

Physiologic Status of Muscles

TABLE	17-8

Condition	Pronunciation	Definition
contracture	kon-trak-chur	permanent contraction of a muscle
muscle atrophy	muhs-uhl at-ro-fe	wasting away of muscle from disuse
muscle hypertrophy	muhs-uhl hi-per-tro-fe	muscle enlargement from overuse
muscle tone	muhs-uhl tōn	normal degree of vigor and tension in a muscle; muscles partially contracted
paralysis	pah-ral-i-sis	loss of muscular contraction because of nerve damage
paresis	pah-re-sis	slight or incomplete paralysis

Injuries

TABLE	17-9	
Type	**Pronunciation**	**Definition**
fracture	<u>frak</u>-chur	the breaking of a bone; there are many types
skull fracture	skul <u>frak</u>-chur	a fracture of the bony structure of the head
torn ligament, tendon, or cartilage	<u>lig</u>-ah-ment, <u>ten</u>-don, <u>kar</u>-ti-lij	a complete or partial tear of a ligament, tendon, or cartilage; common sports injuries
subluxation	sub´-luk-<u>sa</u>-shun	partial dislocation
spondylolisthesis	spon´-di-lo-lis-<u>the</u>-sis	forward displacement of a vertebra over a lower segment; a type of dislocation

Clinical Disorders

TABLE	17-10	
Disorder	**Pronunciation**	**Definition**
arthritis	ar-<u>thri</u>-tis	inflammation of a joint; there are four common types (see **Figures 17–9** and **17–10**)
bursitis	ber-<u>si</u>-tis	inflammation of a bursa
carpal tunnel syndrome	<u>kar</u>-pal <u>tun</u>-el <u>sin</u>-drom	a common painful disorder of the wrist and hand, caused by pressure on the median nerve in the wrist
collagen disease	<u>kol</u>-ah-jen di-<u>zez</u>	a group of diseases with widespread pathologic changes in connective tissue, e.g., lupus erythematosus, dermatomyositis
gout	<u>g</u>owt	a hereditary form of arthritis caused by accumulation of uric acid crystals, especially in the great toe (see **Figure 17–11**)
herniated nucleus pulposus	<u>her</u>-ne-at´-ed <u>nu</u>-kle-us pul-<u>po</u>-sus	a rupture of the fibrocartilage surrounding an intervertebral disk, releasing the nucleus pulposus that cushions the vertebrae above and below
kyphosis	ki-<u>fo</u>-sis	humpback or hunchback; a spinal deformity
Legg-Calvé-Perthes disease	leg-kal-<u>vay</u>-<u>per</u>-tes di-<u>zez</u>	osteochondrosis of the head of the femur in children
lordosis	lor-<u>do</u>-sis	exaggerated forward curvature of the lumbar spine
lupus erythematosus (LE)	<u>loo</u>-pus er-i´-the-ma-<u>to</u>-sus	see systemic lupus erythematosus (SLE)

(continues)

TABLE 17-10 *(continued)*

Disorder	Pronunciation	Definition
muscular dystrophy	<u>mus</u>-ku-lar <u>dis</u>-tro-fe	genetic diseases with progressive atrophy of skeletal muscles
myasthenia gravis	mi-as-<u>the</u>-ne-ah <u>gra</u>-vis	lack of muscle strength
myositis	mi´-o-<u>si</u>-tis	inflammation of a voluntary muscle
Osgood-Schlatter disease	<u>oz</u>-good-<u>shlat</u>-er di-<u>zez</u>	inflammation of the tibial tubercle caused by chronic irritation and seen primarily in muscular, athletic adolescents; characterized by swelling and tenderness over the tibial tubercle that increases with exercise
osteochondritis	os´-te-o-kon-<u>dri</u>-tis	inflammation of the bone and cartilage
osteochondrosis	os´-te-o-kon-<u>dro</u>-sis	disease of the bone and cartilage
osteomalacia	os´-te-o-mah-<u>la</u>-she-ah	softening of the bones resulting from vitamin D deficiency
osteomyelitis	os´-te-o-mi´-e-<u>li</u>-tis	inflammation of bone and marrow caused by bacterial invasion
osteoporosis	os´-te-o-po-<u>ro</u>-sis	porous condition of bones; occurs primarily in postmenopausal women
rheumatism	<u>roo</u>-ma-tizm	disorders marked by inflammation, degeneration, or metabolic derangement of the connective tissue structures, especially the joints and related structures, and attended by pain, stiffness, or limitation of motion (see Figures 17–9 and 17–10)
rickets	<u>rik</u>-ets	vitamin D deficiency, especially in infancy and childhood, marked by bending and distortion of the bones
sarcoma (osteogenic)	sar´-<u>ko</u>-mah (os´-te-o-<u>jen</u>-ik)	a malignant tumor of bone
scoliosis	sko´-le-<u>o</u>-sis	lateral curvature of the spine (see **Figure 17–12**)
spina bifida	<u>spi</u>-nah <u>bi</u>-fid-a	a congenital defect in the spine
spondylitis (ankylosing)	spon´-di-<u>li</u>-tis (ang´-ki-<u>lo</u>-sing)	inflammation of the vertebrae, commonly progressing to eventual fusion of the involved joints
systemic lupus erythematosus (SLE)	sis-<u>tem</u>-ik <u>loo</u>-pus er-i´-the-ma-<u>to</u>-sus	a chronic inflammatory disease affecting many systems of the body
tendinitis	ten´-di-<u>ni</u>-tis	inflammation of a tendon

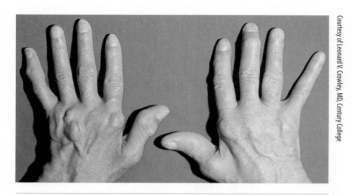

Courtesy of Leonard V. Crowley, MD, Century College

FIGURE 17–9 Rheumatoid arthritis; early manifestations, illustrating swelling of knuckle joints (metacarpophalangeal joints) as a result of inflammation and ulnar deviation of fingers

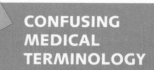

CONFUSING MEDICAL TERMINOLOGY

ile/o Versus ili/o (ileum versus ilium)

ile/o = part of intestine, e.g., ileum (il-<u>ee</u>-uhm) refers to part of the small intestine; e.g., ileorectal (il-<u>e</u>-o-rek-tal) refers to pertaining to the ileum and the rectum

ili/o = part of the hipbone, e.g., ilium (il-<u>ee</u>-uhm) refers to pertaining to the hip bone (pelvic); iliofemoral (il-e-o-<u>fem</u>-or-al) refers to pertaining to the large thigh bone (femur) and the hip bone

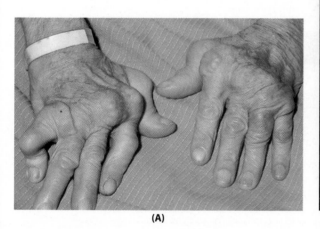

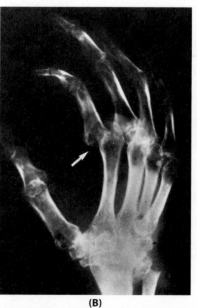

Courtesy of Leonard V. Crowley, MD, Century College

(A) (B)

FIGURE 17–10 (A) Advanced joint deformities caused by rheumatoid arthritis. (B) Radiograph illustrating destruction of articular surfaces and anterior dislocation of base of index finger as a result of joint instability.

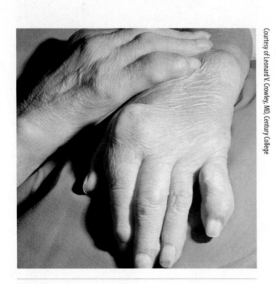

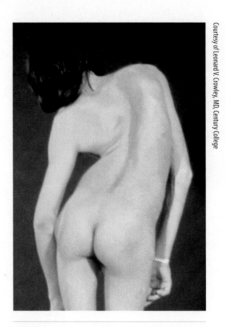

Courtesy of Leonard V. Crowley, MD, Century College

Courtesy of Leonard V. Crowley, MD, Century College

FIGURE 17–11 Deformities of hands caused by accumulation of uric acid crystals (tophi) in and around finger joints

FIGURE 17–12 Severe scoliosis, which caused marked asymmetry of trunk and greatly reduced the size of the thoracic cavities, interfering with pulmonary function

Medical Management

TABLE 17-11

Procedure	Pronunciation	Definition
amputation	am-pu-<u>ta</u>-shun	removal of a limb or other appendage of the body
arthrocentesis	ar-thro-sen-<u>te</u>-sis	puncture of a joint cavity to remove fluid
arthroscopy	ahr-thros-<u>kuh</u>-pe	examination of the interior of a joint with an endoscope
arthrotomy	ar-throt-<u>o</u>-me	surgical creation of an opening into a joint, such as for drainage
electrical stimulation	e-<u>lek</u>-tri-kal stim-u-<u>la</u>-shun	a process used to heal fractures more quickly
electromyogram (electromyography)	e-lek-tro-<u>mi</u>-o-gram (e-lek´-tro-mi-<u>og</u>-rah-fe)	the film record made and the study of muscular contraction
external fixation	eks-<u>ter</u>-nal fik-<u>sa</u>-shun	the process of making a bone immovable
fracture reduction	<u>frak</u>-chur re-<u>duk</u>-shun	the correction of a fracture, luxation, or hernia
laminectomy with diskectomy	lam-i-<u>nek</u>-to-me dis-<u>kek</u>-to-me	excision of the posterior arch of a vertebra; excision of an intervertebral disk
meniscectomy	men-i-<u>sek</u>-to-me	excision of a meniscus, e.g., of the knee joint

CHAPTER

18

Eyes and Ears

LESSON ONE: MATERIALS TO BE LEARNED

Eyes
- Structure of the Eye
- Eye Disorders
- Eye Diagnosis and Surgery
- Common Medical Eye Terms

Ears
- Structure of the Ear
- Ear Disorders
- Ear Surgery
- Common Medical Ear Terms

LESSON TWO: PROGRESS CHECK

Matching: Eye Structures
Multiple Choice: Eye
Identification
Multiple Choice: Ear
Word Puzzle on the Sensory System

OBJECTIVES

After completing this chapter and the exercises, the student should be able to:

1. Identify and label the structures of the eyes and ears.
2. Describe the functions of the eyes and ears.
3. Define and explain various pathologic conditions affecting the eyes and ears.
4. Identify important laboratory tests and procedures related to the diagnosis and treatment for conditions of these special sense organs.
5. Use correctly spelled terminology to build medical words related to structure, function, and pathologic conditions of these special sense organs.
6. Define commonly used abbreviations.

ALLIED HEALTH PROFESSIONS

Dispensing Opticians, Pharmacy Technicians, Pharmacy Aides, and Medical Assistants

Dispensing opticians fit eyeglasses and contact lenses, following prescriptions written by ophthalmologists or optometrists. They examine written prescriptions to determine corrective lens specifications. They recommend eyeglass frames, lenses, and lens coatings after considering the prescription and the customer's occupation, habits, and facial features. Dispensing opticians measure clients' eyes, including the distance between the centers of the pupils and the distance between the eye surface and the lens. Dispensing opticians prepare work orders that give ophthalmic laboratory technicians the information needed to grind and insert lenses into a frame.

Pharmacy technicians, assistants, and/or aides help licensed pharmacists provide medication and other healthcare products to patients. Pharmacy technicians usually perform more complex tasks than assistants do, although in some states their duties and job titles overlap. Technicians typically perform routine tasks, such as counting and labeling, to help prepare prescribed medication for patients. A pharmacist must check every prescription before it can be given to a patient, however. Technicians refer any questions regarding prescriptions, drug information, or health matters to the pharmacist. Pharmacy assistants or aides usually have fewer, less complex responsibilities than pharmacy technicians do. Aides and assistants are often clerks or cashiers who primarily answer telephones, handle money, stock shelves, and perform other clerical duties.

Pharmacy aides also perform administrative duties in pharmacies. They work closely with pharmacy technicians. Aides refer any questions regarding prescriptions, drug information, or health matters to a pharmacist.

Medical assistants perform administrative and clinical tasks to keep the offices of physicians, podiatrists, chiropractors, and other health practitioners running smoothly. They should not be confused with physician assistants, who examine, diagnose, and treat patients under the direct supervision of a physician. The duties of medical assistants vary from office to office, depending on the location and size of the practice and the practitioner's specialty.

INQUIRY

American Board of Opticianry: www.abo.org
National Contact Lens Examiners: www.abo-ncle.org
Pharmacy Technician Certification Board: www.ptcb.org
Institute for the Certification of Pharmacy Technicians: www.nationaltechexam.org
American Society of Health-System Pharmacists: www.ashp.org
National Pharmacy Technician Association: www.pharmacytechnician.org
American Association of Medical Assistants: www.aama-ntl.org

Data from Stanfield, Peggy S., Cross, Nanna, and Hui, Y.H. *Introduction to the Health Professions*, 6th ed. Burlington, MA: Jones & Bartlett Learning; 2012.

The eyes and ears are part of special senses that stem from the peripheral nervous system (PNS). When studying this chapter, refer to **Figures 18–1** and **18–2**.

The eye is an optical system that focuses light rays on photoreceptors, which change light energy to nerve impulses. Human eyes are spherical organs located in bony orbits, or eye sockets, cavities formed by the bones of the skull. The eye is embedded in orbital fat for insulation and protection. It is attached to the orbit by six muscles, the extrinsic eye muscles, which control eye movement. Small tendons connect these muscles to the outermost layer of the eye. Structures of the eye include the following:

1. The *sclera* is the tough, white outer layer of the eyeball that protects the interior of the eye. At the front of the eye, the sclera forms a domed transparent orb called the *cornea*. The cornea has a curved surface that focuses light coming into the eye.

2. The *uvea* is the vascular layer below the sclera. It supplies blood to muscles and nerves within the eye and gives the eye its color. It contains three structures: the choroid, the ciliary body, and the iris.

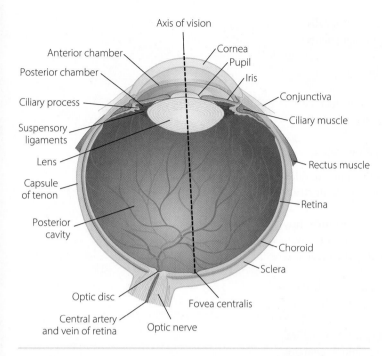

FIGURE 18–1 Transverse section showing the structure of the eye

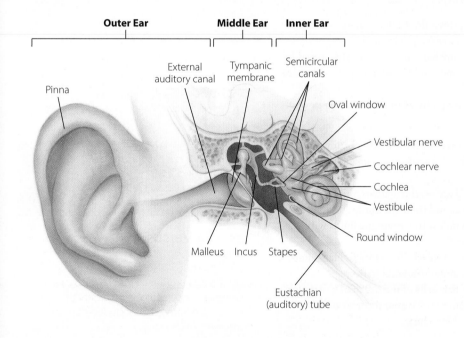

FIGURE 18–2 Frontal diagram of the outer ear, middle ear, and inner ear

3. The *choroid*, a darkly pigmented layer of tissue, houses many tiny blood vessels and acts to absorb light within the eye. This prevents blurring of visual images. The *ciliary body*, an extension of the choroid, enables the eye to focus on objects of varying distances. Another extension of the choroid is the *iris*. The pigmentation of the iris is what determines eye color. At the center of the iris is an opening called the *pupil*. The pupil of the eye expands and contracts, regulating the amount of light entering the eye.

4. On the inner surface of the choroid is the *retina,* light-sensitive receptor cells. The retina contains rods and cones that detect color stimuli (photopigments), which it sends to the brain for interpretation.

5. The *optic nerve* carries impulses from the retina to areas of the brain that are responsible for processing visual information.

6. Although not involved in vision directly, the eyelids and eyelashes protect the eyeball from physical trauma. A thin membrane known as *conjunctiva* lines the inside of each eyelid.

7. The *lacrimal* glands of the eye produce tears, which keep the eye lubricated.

The ear has three distinct and anatomically separate sections—the outer, middle, and inner ears. Please refer to Figure 18–2 to visualize each as we discuss their structure and functions.

The middle ear lies within the temporal bones of the skull. It contains three tiny bones, the auditory ossicles. They are named for their shapes. Starting from the outside, they are the *malleus* (hammer), *incus* (anvil), and *stapes* (stirrup). The malleus is connected to the *tympanic membrane.*

The middle ear cavity opens to the pharynx via the *Eustachian tube,* also called the auditory tube. The Eustachian tube serves as a pressure valve. Yawning and swallowing open the tube to equalize pressure within the middle ear.

The inner ear is a mazelike structure that occupies a large cavity in the temporal bone. It consists of bony and membranous structures surrounded by fluid. It contains two sensory organs—the *cochlea,* a snail-shell-shaped bony structure that houses the organs of hearing, and the *vestibular apparatus.*

The *cochlea* is a hollow, bony spiral containing three fluid-filled canals—the *upper vestibular canal,* the *middle cochlear canal,* and the *lower tympanic canal.*

The *organ of Corti* contains the receptor cells, tiny hair cells that are stimulated by sound vibrations. The sound vibrations are then converted to nerve impulses that are transmitted to the brain for interpretation.

To summarize briefly how we hear, let us create a pathway of sound waves through the ear by structure and function:

1. The outer ear auricle (*pinna*) funnels sound waves into the external auditory canal, which directs it to the tympanic membrane (eardrum), causing it to vibrate.

2. The middle ear, which contains the eardrum ossicles, the malleus, incus, and stapes, vibrate when struck by the sound waves and transmit the sound to the cochlea in the inner ear by causing the oval window to vibrate the fluids within the canals.

3. The cochlea converts the fluid waves to nerve impulses. The semicircular canals, the *sacculi* and *utricle,* detect head movement and linear acceleration.

4. The auditory nerve fibers that lie close to the hair cells of the organ of Corti pick up the sound wave impulses and transmit them to the cerebral cortex of the brain, where they are interpreted and we are able to hear.

All the structures and functions pertaining to the eyes and ears are defined and illustrated throughout the chapter. Major disorders and diseases are also defined and discussed.

CONFUSING MEDICAL TERMINOLOGY

core/o Versus corne/o

core/o = pupil (also, pupill/o), e.g., coreoplasty (<u>kor</u>-ree-o-plas-te), also called coroplasty, refers to plastic surgery to correct a deformed or occluded pupil of the eye

corne/o = cornea, e.g., corneal (<u>kor</u>-ne-al) refers to pertaining to the cornea of the eye

Figures 18–1 and 18–2 describe the anatomic parts of the eyes and ears.

EYES

Structure of the Eye

TABLE 18-1

Structure	Pronunciation	Definition
sclera	skle-rah	tough white outer coat of the eyeball
conjunctiva	kon´-junk-ti-vah	membrane lining the eyelids and covering the eyeball
cornea	kor-ne-ah	transparent anterior part of the eye
choroid	ko-roid	the middle, vascular coat of the eye, between the sclera and the retina
iris	i-ris	pigmented membrane behind the cornea, perforated by the pupil
pupil	pu-pil	opening in the center through which light enters the eye
lens	lenz	transparent body separating the posterior chamber and constituting the refracting mechanism of the eye
ciliary muscle	sil-e-er´-e mus-el	eye muscle capable of changing lens shape during contraction and relaxation
aqueous humor	a-kwe-us hu-mor	watery liquid in chamber in the front of the lens; it circulates through the anterior chamber of the eye
vitreous humor	vit-re-us hu-mor	jellylike transparent substance in the posterior chamber
retina	ret-i-nah	innermost layer of the eyeball, containing elements for reception and transmission of visual stimuli

Eye Disorders

TABLE 18-2

Disorder	Pronunciation	Definition
amblyopia	am´-ble-<u>o</u>-pe-ah	dimness of vision without a detectable organic lesion of the eye; related to absence, weakness, or paralysis of an eye muscle
astigmatism	ah-<u>stig</u>-mah-tism	condition characterized by irregular cornea and lens of the eye; corrected with lenses
blepharitis	blef´-ah-<u>ri</u>-tis	inflammation of the eyelids
blepharoptosis	blef´-ar-op-<u>to</u>-sis	drooping of upper eyelid
cataract	<u>kat</u>-ah-rakt	opaque (not clear) lens of the eye
chalazion	kah-<u>la</u>-ze-on	a small eyelid mass resulting from chronic inflammation of a meibomian gland
color blindness	<u>kul</u>-er <u>blind</u>-nes	popular term for any deviation from normal perception of color
conjunctivitis	kon-junk´-ti-<u>vi</u>-tis	inflammation of the conjunctiva
corneal ulcer	<u>kor</u>-ne-al <u>ul</u>-ser	a local inflammation of the cornea caused by injury or inflammation
dacryoadenitis	dak´-re-o-ad´-e-<u>ni</u>-tis	inflammation of a lacrimal gland
dacryocystitis	dak-re-o-sis-<u>ti</u>-tis	inflammation of the lacrimal sac
dacryolith	<u>dak</u>-re-o-lith´	a lacrimal calculus (stone)
detached retina	de-<u>tacht</u> <u>ret</u>-i-nah	separation of the inner layers of the retina from the pigment epithelium
diabetic retinopathy	<u>dye</u>-ah´-bet-ic´ <u>reh</u>-tin-op´-ah-thee´	scarring of the capillaries of the retina as a consequence of diabetes mellitus (DM) of long duration; retinal effects of DM include abnormal dilation of the retinal veins, hemorrhage, microaneurysms, and neovascularization (new blood vessels forming near the optic disk causing leakage of blood). These effects cause a permanent decline in vision and will lead to blindness; diabetic retinopathy is a leading cause of blindness in the United States
floaters (in vitreous)	<u>flo</u>-ters	"spots before the eyes"; these deposits in the vitreous of the eye usually move about and are probably a benign degenerative change. Also seen in hypertension
foreign body in the eye	<u>for</u>-in <u>bod</u>-e	any object not belonging to the eye; hazards depending on circumstances
glaucoma	glaw-<u>ko</u>-mah	eye disease characterized by an increase in intraocular pressure related to alterations in circulation of vitreous humor, causing pathologic changes and visual defects
hemorrhage (subconjunctival)	<u>hem</u>-o-rij (sub´-kon-junk-<u>ti</u>-val)	blood escaping from the vessels, and bleeding from beneath the conjunctiva
herpes zoster (ophthalmic)	<u>her</u>-pez <u>zos</u>-ter (of-<u>thal</u>-mic)	involving the fifth cranial nerve (forehead, eyelid, and cornea), this infection by a herpes virus can be serious
hyperopia	hi´-per-<u>o</u>-pe-ah	farsightedness, e.g., the person cannot read a book
injury	<u>in</u>-ju-re	eye injuries include foreign bodies, contusions, lacerations, burns, etc.

TABLE 18-2 (continued)

Disorder	Pronunciation	Definition
iritis	i-<u>ri</u>-tis	inflammation of the iris
keratoconus	ker-ah-to-<u>ko</u>-nus	conical protrusion of the central part of the cornea
macular degeneration	mah´-<u>cull</u>-lar de-<u>jen</u>-er-aye-<u>shun</u>	deterioration of the macula of the eye, resulting in a severe loss of central vision in the affected eye
meibomian cyst	mi-<u>bo</u>-me-an	a small localized swelling of the eyelid resulting from obstruction and retained secretions of the meibomian glands; a nonmalignant condition; often requires surgery for correction
nystagmus	nis-<u>tag</u>-mus	involuntary rapid movement (horizontal, vertical, rotary, or mixed, i.e., of two types) of the eyeball
papilledema	pap´-il-e-<u>de</u>-mah	edema of the optic disk
presbyopia	pres-be-<u>o</u>-pe-ah	diminution of accommodation of the lens of the eye caused by loss of elasticity, normally occurring with aging; farsightedness
ptosis	<u>to</u>-sis	drooping of upper eyelid
retinitis	ret´-i-<u>ni</u>-tis	inflammation of the retina
retinoblastoma	ret´-i-no-blas-<u>to</u>-mah	a tumor arising from the retinal cells (see **Figure 18–3**)
retinopathy	ret´-i-<u>nop</u>-ah-the	any disease of the retina
strabismus	strah-<u>biz</u>-mus	squint; deviation of the eye from normal; crossed eyes; usually correctable
stye (or hordeolum)	sti (hor-<u>de</u>-o-lum)	inflammation of the sebaceous glands of the eyelid
trachoma	trah-<u>ko</u>-mah	a contagious disease of the conjunctiva and cornea, producing photophobia, pain, and lacrimation; uncommon
uveitis	u´-ve-<u>i</u>-tis	inflammation of the uvea (iris and blood vessels)

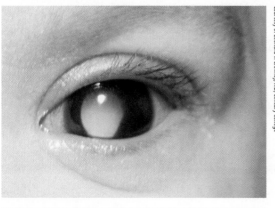

Courtesy of Leonard V. Crowley, MD, Century College

FIGURE 18–3 Retinoblastoma of an eye that appears as a pale mass of tissue seen through the dilated pupil

CONFUSING MEDICAL TERMINOLOGY

oral Versus aural

oral = pertaining to the mouth

aural = pertaining to the ear

Eye Diagnosis and Surgery

TABLE 18-3

Diagnosis or Surgery	Pronunciation	Definition
cataract extraction	<u>kat</u>-ah-rakt eks-<u>trak</u>-shun	a surgical excision of the lens of the eye; special lenses or glasses are prescribed
cryoextraction	kri´-o-eks-<u>trak</u>-shun	application of extremely low temperature for the removal of a cataractous lens
cryoretinopexy	kri´-o-<u>ret</u>-i-no-pex-ee	fixation of a detached retina using extremely low temperature instead of the laser beam
dacryocystotomy	dak´-re-o-sis-<u>tot</u>-o-me	incision of the lacrimal sac and duct
enucleation	e-nu´-kle-<u>a</u>-shun	surgical removal of the eye
fundoscopy	fun-<u>dus</u>-ko-pe	examination and study of the fundus of the eye by means of an ophthalmoscope
gonioscopy	go´-ne-<u>os</u>-ko-pe	instrument for demonstrating ocular motility and rotation
iridectomy	ir´-i-<u>dek</u>-to-me	excision of part of the iris
iridencleisis	ir´-i-den-<u>kli</u>-sis	excision of part of the iris in glaucoma
keratoplasty	<u>ker</u>-ah-to-plas´-te	plastic surgery of the cornea; corneal grafting
laser photocoagulation	<u>la</u>-zer fo´-to-ko-ag´-u-<u>la</u>-shun	using the laser beam to treat retinal detachment
pterygium surgery	te-<u>rig</u>-e-um <u>ser</u>-jer-e	growth of the conjunctiva: neovascularization that invades the cornea; it can be removed surgically
slit lamp		an instrument used in ophthalmology for examining the conjunctiva, lens, vitreous humor, iris, and cornea; a high-intensity beam of light is projected through a narrow slit and a cross-section of the illuminated part of the eye is examined through a magnifying lens
tonometer	to-<u>nom</u>-e-ter	instrument for measuring tension or pressure, especially intraocular pressure
tonometry	to-<u>nom</u>-e-tre	measurement of tension or pressure, e.g., intraocular pressure
trabeculectomy	trah-bek´-u-<u>lec</u>-to-me	excision of fibrous bands or connective tissue
vitrectomy	vi-<u>trek</u>-to-me	aspiration of vitreous fluid and replacement with saline solution

Common Medical Eye Terms

TABLE 18-4

Term	Pronunciation	Definition
accommodation	ah-kom´-o-<u>da</u>-tion	adjustment of the eye for seeing objects at various distances
anisocoria	an´-i-so-<u>ko</u>-re-ah	inequality in size of the pupils of the eyes
Braille	brāl	a system of printing for the blind consisting of raised dots and prints that can be read by touch
canal of Schlemm	kah-<u>nal</u> of shlem	opening through which aqueous humor must flow out or pressure in the eye increases, resulting in glaucoma
canthus (pl., canthi)	<u>kan</u>-thus	the angle at either end of the fissure between the eyelids
CC		with correction (glasses or lenses)
cryoprobe	<u>kri</u>-o-prob	an instrument for applying extreme cold to tissue
cystitome	<u>sis</u>-ti-tome	an instrument for opening the lens capsule
diopter	di-<u>op</u>-ter	unit of measure for lenses
electronystagmography	e-lek´-tro-nis´-tag-<u>mog</u>-rah-fe	recordings of eye movements to provide objective documentation of induced and spontaneous nystagmus
emmetropia	em´-e-<u>tro</u>-pe-ah	normal vision
eye bank		storage for donor organs
fundus	<u>fun</u>-dus	the back portion of the interior of the eyeball, visible through the pupil by use of the ophthalmoscope
fundoscope (or ophthalmoscope)	<u>fun</u>-dus-skōp (of-<u>thal</u>-mo-skōp)	an instrument containing a perforated mirror and lenses used to examine the interior of the eye
guide dogs		trained dogs for the blind; also called seeing-eye dogs
lacrimation	lak´-ri-<u>ma</u>-shun	secretion and discharge of tears
laser	<u>la</u>-zer	a device that transfers light of various frequencies into an extremely intense, small beam of radiation; it is used as a tool in surgery, in diagnosis, and in physiologic studies
lensometer	lenz-<u>om</u>-e-ter	device for obtaining eyeglass prescriptions
miotic (or myotic)	mi-<u>ot</u>-ik	a drug that causes contraction of the pupil
mydriatic	mid´-re-<u>at</u>-ik	a drug that dilates the pupil
OD		abbreviation for oculus dexter (right eye)

(continues)

TABLE 18-4 *(continued)*

Term	Pronunciation	Definition
ophthalmoscope	of´-<u>thal</u>-mo-skop	instrument containing a perforated mirror and lenses, used to examine the interior of the eye; also called fundoscope
OS		abbreviation for oculus sinister (left eye)
OU		abbreviation for oculus uterque (each eye) or oculus unitas (both eyes)
peripheral vision	pe-<u>rif</u>-er-al <u>vizh</u>-un	vision at the outer edges when the eyes are looking straight ahead
PERRLA (or PERLA)		acronym for pupils equal, round, react to light, accommodation
refractive error	re-<u>frak</u>-tiv	the determination of the refractive errors of the eye and their correction with glasses or lenses
SC		without correction (glasses or lenses)
Snellen eye chart		one of several charts used in testing visual acuity; letters, numbers, or symbols are arranged on the chart in decreasing size from top to bottom
visual acuity (VA)	vizh´-<u>u</u>-al ah-<u>ku</u>-i-te	clarity or clearness of vision
20/20 vision		a person who can read what the average person can read at 20 feet has 20/20 vision

EARS

Structure of the Ear

TABLE 18-5

Structure	Pronunciation	Definition
external ear		auricle (or pinna) or ear canal
middle ear		separated from the external ear by the tympanic membrane; consists of three bones: malleus, incus, and stapes
inner ear		the complex inner structure of the ear: vestibule, semicircular canals, and cochlea, composing the membranous labyrinth
tympanic membrane	tim-<u>pan</u>-ik <u>mem</u>-brane	the thin partition between the external acoustic meatus and the middle ear
tympanum	<u>tim</u>-pan-um	eardrum (middle ear)
cerumen	se-<u>roo</u>-men	earwax
Eustachian tube	u-<u>stay</u>-shen	a tube, lined with mucous membrane, that joins the nasopharynx and the tympanic cavity; accomplishes equalization of air pressure

Ear Disorders

TABLE 18-6		

Disorder	Pronunciation	Definition
acoustic neuroma	ah-koos-tic new-rom-ah	a benign tumor arising from the acoustic nerve in the brain that causes tinnitus, vertigo, and decreased hearing; small tumors may be surgically resected or removed by radiation therapy
cholesteatoma	koh-les-tee´-ah-toh-mah	a collection of skin cells and cholesterol in a sac within the middle ear; these cystlike masses are most often the result of chronic otitis media but may also be a congenital defect. Cholesteatoma can lead to conductive hearing loss, occlusion of the middle ear, destruction of ossicles, and inner ear erosion; symptoms include weakness of facial muscles, drainage from the affected ear, vertigo, and earache
conduction deafness	kon-duk-shun def-nes	hearing loss that occurs when the conduction of sound waves through the external and middle ear to the inner ear is impaired
deafness	def-nes	lacking the sense of hearing; hearing impairment
Eustachian salpingitis	u-stay-shen sal´-pin-ji-tis	inflammation of the Eustachian tubes
furunculosis	fu-rung´-ku-lo-sis	a skin infection affecting the ear canal
impacted cerumen	im-pak-ted se-roo-men	cerumen (earwax) impacted firmly into the ear
labyrinthitis	lab´-i-rin-thi-tis	inflammation of the labyrinth (inner ear); otitis interna
mastoiditis	mas´-toi-di-tis	inflammation of the mastoid antrum and cells (of the temporal bone)
Meniere's disease	men´-e-ārz di-zez	deafness, tinnitus, and dizziness; causes unknown
myringitis	mir´-in-ji-tis	inflammation of the tympanic membrane (eardrum)
otitis externa	o-ti-tis ex-ter-na	inflammation of the external ear
otitis media	o-ti-tis me-di-a	inflammation of the middle ear
otosclerosis	o´-to-skle-ro-sis	ankylosis of the stapes, resulting in conductive hearing loss
presbycusis	pres´-bĭ-ku-sis	progressive hearing loss in some elderly persons
sensorineural deafness	sen-soh´-ree-noo-ral def-nes	also called nerve deafness, this type of hearing loss results from physical damage to the hair cells, the vestibulocochlear nerve, or the auditory cortex; this condition may occur because of aging. Explosions, extremely loud noises, such as from machinery or loud music, and some antibiotics can damage the hair cells in the organ of Corti, creating partial to complete deafness; other causes include brain tumors, strokes, infections, trauma, vascular disorders, and degenerative diseases

Ear Surgery

TABLE 18-7		
Surgery	**Pronunciation**	**Definition**
fenestration	fen´-es-<u>tra</u>-shun	the surgical creation of a new opening in the labyrinth of the ear for restoration of hearing in otosclerosis
mastoidectomy	mas´-toi-<u>dek</u>-to-me	excision of the mastoid cells or the mastoid process
myringotomy	mir´-ing-<u>got</u>-o-me	incision of the tympanic membrane; tympanotomy with placement of tubes to maintain drainage
otoplasty	<u>o</u>-to-plas´-te	plastic surgery of the ear (pinna)
stapedectomy	sta´-pe-<u>dek</u>-to-me	excision of the stapes
tympanoplasty	tim´-pah-no-<u>plas</u>-te	plastic surgery on the eardrum
tympanotomy	tim´-pah-<u>not</u>-o-me	myringotomy; incision of the tympanic membrane

Common Medical Ear Terms

TABLE 18-8		
Term	**Pronunciation**	**Definition**
acoustic meatus	ah-<u>koos</u>-tik me-<u>a</u>-tus	opening or passage in the ear
AD		auris dextra, right ear
AS		auris sinistra, left ear
AU		aures unitas (both ears) or auris uterque (each ear)
audiometer	aw´-de-<u>om</u>-e-ter	a device for testing the hearing
audiometrist	aw´-de-<u>om</u>-e-trist	person who performs hearing tests
auditory (or acoustic)	<u>aw</u>-di-to´-re (ah-<u>koos</u>-tik)	pertaining to the ear; sense of hearing
decibel	<u>des</u>-i-bel	a unit of measure of the intensity of sound
hearing aid	<u>hēr</u>-ing	a device used to increase the intensity of sound
hearing-ear dogs		dogs trained to respond to sounds and alert the person with hearing impairment

TABLE 18-8 *(continued)*

Term	Pronunciation	Definition
otoscope	o-to-skōp	an instrument used for inspecting the ear
otoscopy	o-tos-ko-pe	examination of the ear by means of the otoscope
sign language	sine lan-gwij	communication by means of manual signs and gestures
tinnitus	ti-ni-tus	a noise (ringing) in the ears
tuning fork	too-ning	a small metal instrument consisting of a stem and two prongs used to test hearing
vertigo	ver-ti-go	a sensation of rotation or dizziness

CONFUSING MEDICAL TERMINOLOGY

dysarthria Versus dysarthrosis

dysarthria (dis-ahr-three-uh) = difficulty with speech, as in stammering or stuttering

dysarthrosis (dis-ahr-thro-sis) = any disorder of a joint

PHARMACOLOGY AND MEDICAL TERMINOLOGY

Drug Classification	antiviral agent (an-tih-vye-ral)	vitamin (vigh-tah-min)
Function	treats various viral conditions such as serious herpes virus infection, chickenpox, and influenza A	prevents and treats vitamin deficiencies and used as dietary supplement
Word Parts	**anti-** = against; **viral** = pertaining to a virus	pertaining to vital nutrient in the body
Active Ingredients (examples)	acyclovir (Zovirax); vidarabine (Vira-A)	vitamins A, D, E, etc.; ascorbic acid (vitamin C); cyanocobalamin (vitamin B$_{12}$)

| LESSON TWO | Progress Check |

◆ MATCHING: EYE STRUCTURES

For the list of terms on the left, select the correct definition on the right:

1. sclera
2. conjunctiva
3. cornea
4. iris
5. pupil
6. lens
7. aqueous humor
8. vitreous humor
9. retina

a. watery liquid in front of the lens
b. jellylike substance behind the lens
c. innermost layer of the eyeball
d. refracting mechanism of the eye
e. white outer coating of the eye
f. membrane lining the eyelids
g. transparent anterior part of the eye
h. pigmented membrane behind the cornea
i. opening through which light enters

◆ MULTIPLE CHOICE: EYE

Circle the letter of the correct answer:

1. Impairment of vision with aging, caused by loss of elasticity, is a condition known as
   a. strabismus
   b. nystagmus
   c. presbyopia
   d. trachoma

2. Which of the following conditions describes the drooping of the lower eyelid?
   a. chalazion
   b. blepharoptosis
   c. dacrycystoptosis
   d. hyperopia

3. Deviation from normal color perception is a condition of
   a. herpes zoster
   b. floaters
   c. cataracts
   d. color blindness

4. Foreign bodies, contusions, lacerations, and burns to the eye are conditions of
   a. detached retinas
   b. blepharoptosis
   c. injuries
   d. retinopathies

5. A small hard mass on the eyelid formed by sebaceous gland enlargement is a
   a. chalazion
   b. sty
   c. corneal ulcer
   d. foreign body in the eye

6. Astigmatism is a condition in which
   a. the eyeball is too long
   b. there is an increase in intraocular pressure
   c. there is a defective curvature in the eye cornea
   d. there is dilation of the retinal veins

7. The transparent anterior part of the eye is the
   a. cornea
   b. iris
   c. lens
   d. pupil

8. An enucleation is a (an)
   a. cataract removal
   b. excision of the iris
   c. removal of the eye
   d. examination of the conjunctiva

9. A tonometer measures
   a. intraocular pressure
   b. amount of light entering the eye
   c. adjustments for various distances
   d. inequality of size of the pupils

IDENTIFICATION: STRUCTURES OF THE EAR

Identify the location of the following structures of the ears.

1. external ear _____

2. middle ear _____

3. inner ear _____

4. tympanic membrane _____

5. Eustachian tube _____

6. cerumen _____

MULTIPLE CHOICE: EAR

Circle the letter of the correct answer:

1. Which of the following terms denotes the creation of a new opening in the labyrinth of the ear?
   a. fenestration
   b. acoustic meatus
   c. otoplasty
   d. myringotomy

2. Plastic surgery on an eardrum is called
   a. tympanotomy
   b. tympanoplasty
   c. otoplasty
   d. stapedectomy

3. The unit of measure of the intensity of sound is called a (an)
   a. electronystagnometry
   b. audiometry
   c. decibel
   d. tuning fork

4. Which of the following terms describes tinnitus?
   a. dizziness
   b. nausea
   c. intense sound
   d. ringing of the ears

5. *Vertigo* is the term used for
   a. a sensation of rotation
   b. ringing of the ears
   c. intense sound
   d. sign communication

ABBREVIATIONS

Write in the medical terms for the following abbreviations:

1. PNS _____

2. CC _____

3. OS _____

4. OD _____

5. OU _____

6. PERRLA _____

7. VA _____

8. AD _____

9. AS _____

10. AU _____

● WORD PUZZLE ON THE SENSORY SYSTEM

Find the 69 words related to the senses by reading forward, backward, up, down, and diagonally. When you have circled the 69 words, the remaining letters will spell SENSES.

```
L  A  C  R  I  M  A  L  A  P  P  A  R  A  T  U  S  C  I  N  U  T
L  S  E  B  U  T  N  A  I  H  C  A  T  S  U  E  U  A  T  L  A  Y
E  E  Q  U  I  L  I  B  R  I  U  M  L  A  V  O  O  V  H  O  E  M
M  I  E  O  T  O  N  O  I  T  A  T  P  A  D  A  E  I  G  B  L  P
S  T  L  O  C  I  L  I  A  R  Y  B  O  D  Y  E  U  T  I  E  H  A
L  R  D  T  E  E  N  O  I  T  A  S  N  E  S  T  Q  Y  S  S  C  H
A  O  D  O  A  H  A  M  M  E  R  D  U  C  T  S  A  A  S  I  O  I
N  C  I  H  R  L  A  N  R  E  T  X  E  N  N  A  L  D  N  S  C  C
A  F  M  P  S  S  W  E  E  T  S  P  N  S  O  T  O  N  J  F  X  M
C  O  W  C  H  C  O  N  E  S  R  A  O  M  I  R  E  C  O  E  S  E
R  N  I  H  E  U  S  E  Y  E  E  I  I  A  T  R  N  C  V  T  O  M
A  A  N  S  T  R  M  E  S  S  B  N  T  C  A  I  U  M  A  P  S  B
L  G  D  D  T  N  U  O  I  N  M  S  C  U  D  S  O  P  T  S  E  R
U  R  O  S  I  I  I  M  R  E  A  R  A  L  O  C  E  I  S  U  V  A
C  O  W  D  C  O  R  R  I  L  H  A  R  A  M  S  C  E  U  O  A  N
R  S  S  N  L  R  R  Y  N  C  E  F  L  M  S  A  L  E  E  W  E
I  S  L  U  V  U  E  O  V  B  O  T  E  U  O  H  N  C  L  R  D  V
C  I  I  O  I  L  O  R  H  P  A  U  R  T  C  C  I  I  L  T  N  A
I  C  P  E  S  I  S  R  A  C  S  L  S  E  C  U  T  R  A  I  U  C
M  L  U  S  I  V  O  P  H  T  H  A  L  A  A  O  E  U  M  V  O  N
E  E  P  S  O  N  U  F  O  V  E  A  C  E  N  T  R  A  L  I  S  O
S  S  U  O  N  A  R  B  M  E  M  V  I  T  C  N  U  J  N  O  C  A
```

Words to Look for in the Word Puzzle

1. accommodation	13. cones	25. humor	37. ophthal-
2. adaptation	14. conjunctiva	26. incus	38. optic
3. anvil	15. convex	27. inner	39. organ of Corti
4. aqueous	16. ducts	28. iris	40. osseous
5. auricle	17. ears	29. labyrinth	41. ossicles
6. cavity	18. equilibrium	30. lacrimal apparatus	42. oto
7. ceruminous	19. Eustachian tube	31. lens	43. oval
8. chambers	20. external	32. lobes	44. pain
9. choroid	21. eyes	33. macula lutea	45. photo
10. ciliary body	22. focus	34. malleus	46. pupils
11. cochlea	23. fovea centralis	35. membranous	47. refraction
12. concave	24. hammer	36. middle	48. retina

49. rods
50. round
51. salt
52. sclera
53. semicircular canals
54. sensation
55. sight
56. smell
57. sound waves
58. sour
59. stapes
60. stirrups
61. sweet
62. taste
63. tears
64. touch
65. tunics
66. tympanic membrane
67. vision
68. vitreous
69. windows

CHAPTER

19

Endocrine System

LESSON ONE: MATERIALS TO BE LEARNED

Classification and Function of the Endocrine System
Disorders of the Endocrine System
Miscellaneous Terms

LESSON TWO: PROGRESS CHECK

Multiple Choice
Matching: Disorders of the Endocrine System
Fill-in
Definitions
Compare and Contrast
Word Puzzle on the Endocrine System

OBJECTIVES

After completing this chapter and the exercises, the student should be able to:

1. Locate and name the endocrine glands and list the hormones produced by each gland.
2. Describe the major function(s) of each of the endocrine glands.
3. Build and define medical words related to the endocrine system.
4. Define and explain various pathologic conditions of the endocrine system.
5. Differentiate between diabetes mellitus, diabetes insipidus, and gestational diabetes.
6. Identify laboratory tests and clinical procedures related to endocrinology.
7. Identify and define abbreviations related to endocrinology.

ALLIED HEALTH PROFESSIONS

Emergency Medical Technicians and Paramedics

People's lives often depend on the quick reaction and competent care of emergency medical technicians (EMTs) and paramedics. Incidents as varied as automobile accidents, heart attacks, slips and falls, childbirth, and gunshot wounds all require immediate medical attention. EMTs and paramedics provide this vital service as they care for and transport the sick or injured to a medical facility.

In an emergency, EMTs and paramedics are typically dispatched by a 911 operator to the scene, where they often work with police and firefighters. Once they arrive, EMTs and paramedics assess the nature of the patient's condition while trying to determine whether the patient has any preexisting medical conditions. Following medical protocols and guidelines, they provide appropriate emergency care and, when necessary, transport the patient. Some paramedics are trained to treat patients with minor injuries on the scene of an accident, or they may treat them at their home, without transporting them to a medical facility. Emergency treatment is carried out under the medical direction of physicians. EMTs and paramedics may use special equipment, such as backboards, to immobilize patients before placing them on stretchers and securing them in the ambulance for transport to a medical facility.

These healthcare workers generally go out in teams. During the transport of a patient, one EMT or paramedic drives while the other monitors the patient's vital signs and gives additional care as needed. Some paramedics work as part of a helicopter's flight crew to transport critically ill or injured patients to hospital trauma centers.

At the medical facility, EMTs and paramedics help transfer patients to the emergency department, report their observations and actions to emergency department staff, and may provide additional emergency treatment. After each run, EMTs and paramedics replace used supplies and check equipment. If a transported patient had a contagious disease, EMTs and paramedics decontaminate the interior of the ambulance and report cases to the proper authorities.

INQUIRY

National Association of Emergency Medical Technicians: PO Box 1400, Clinton, MS 39060-1400. www.naemt.org
National Highway Traffic Safety Administration, Office of Emergency Medical Services: 1200 New Jersey Ave., SE, NTI-140, Washington, DC 20590. www.ems.gov
National Registry of Emergency Medical Technicians: Rocco V. Morando Bldg., 6610 Busch Blvd., PO Box 29233, Columbus, OH 43229. www.nremt.org

Data from Stanfield, Peggy S., Cross, Nanna, and Hui, Y.H. *Introduction to the Health Professions*, 6th ed. Burlington, MA: Jones & Bartlett Learning; 2012.

The endocrine system interacts with the nervous system to regulate and coordinate body activities (see **Figure 19–1**). *Endocrine glands* have no ducts. They secrete hormones directly into the tissue fluid that surrounds their cells. In contrast, *exocrine* glands, such as salivary glands, secrete their products into ducts. Endocrine control is regulated by chemical messengers (hormones). The word *hormone* comes from the Greek *hormon*, which means to excite or stimulate. A *hormone* is a chemical product produced and released by the endocrine glands and transported by the blood to cells and organs of the body on which it has a specific regulatory effect. Hormones produce their effects by binding to receptors that are recognition sites in the various target cells. The target cells are very selective and respond only to specific hormones. They usually secrete more than one hormone. The parathyroid gland is the exception, secreting only parathyroid hormone.

Glands of the endocrine system include the following:

1. Anterior and posterior pituitary gland
2. Thyroid gland
3. Four parathyroid glands
4. Two adrenal glands
5. Islets of Langerhans in the pancreas
6. Two ovaries

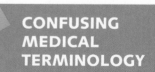

CONFUSING MEDICAL TERMINOLOGY

anter/o Versus antr/o

anter/o = front, e.g., anterior (an-<u>teer</u>-ee-er) refers to situated before or at the front of body (as opposed to posterior)

antr/o = a cavity, e.g., nasoantritis (nazo-an-<u>try</u>-tis) refers to inflammation of the nose antrum (cavity)

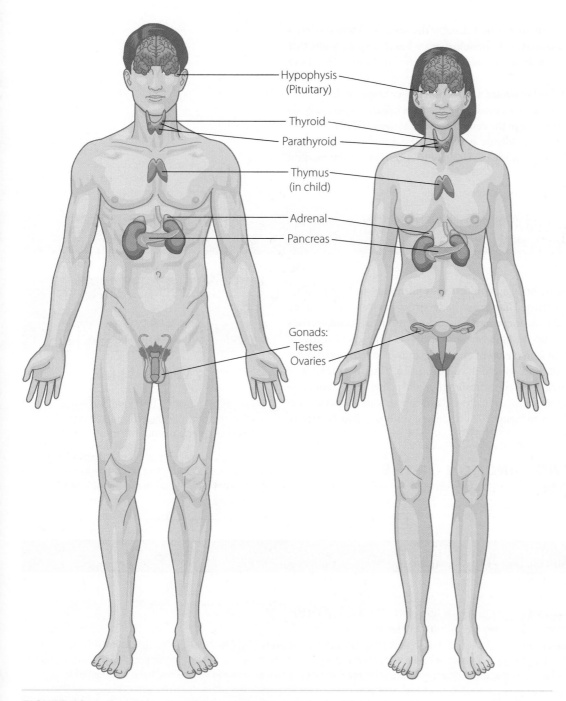

Hypophysis
(Pituitary)

Thyroid

Parathyroid

Thymus
(in child)

Adrenal

Pancreas

Gonads:
Testes
Ovaries

FIGURE 19–1 General location of the major endocrine glands of the body

7. Two testes
8. Pineal gland
9. Thymus gland

Many activities are regulated or influenced by the endocrine glands, including (1) reproduction and lactation; (2) immune system; (3) acid–base balance; (4) fluid intake and fluid balance; (5) carbohydrate, protein, lipid, and nucleic acid metabolism; (6) digestion, absorption, and nutrient distribution; (7) blood pressure; (8) stress resistance; and (9) adaptation to environmental change. The specific function of each of the glands can be found in anatomy and physiology texts because space limits that discussion in this chapter. The glands are defined and classified in Lesson One (also see Figure 19–1).

The endocrine system is cyclical in nature. Cycles occur over hours or days rather than seconds or minutes. Integration of nervous and endocrine influences on the body occurs in the *hypothalamus,* a structure of the central nervous system (CNS).

Endocrinology is the study of the endocrine system and the disorders and diseases that affect the system. An *endocrinologist* is a physician who specializes in the medical practice of endocrinology.

<table>
<tr><td>**LESSON ONE**</td><td>**Materials to Be Learned**</td></tr>
</table>

The endocrine system is a unique body system that uses hormones to help regulate practically all facets of body activity. Glands are body structures (organs) and are divided into two types. A gland may or may not have a duct. A ducted gland secretes its materials by way of the duct into the bloodstream. In this case, the gland is an *exocrine gland.* The exocrine system is made up of all such glands. A ductless gland has no duct and secretes its materials directly into the bloodstream. Thus, the gland is an *endocrine gland,* and the endocrine system is made up of all such glands. Endocrine glands secrete important hormones. Occasionally, a gland contains an endocrine section *and* an exocrine section. Refer to Figure 19–1 when you study the classification of the endocrine system.

CLASSIFICATION AND FUNCTION OF THE ENDOCRINE SYSTEM

<table>
<tr><td>**CONFUSING MEDICAL TERMINOLOGY**</td></tr>
<tr><td>

thym/o Versus thyr/o

thym/o = thymus, thymus gland, e.g., thymectomy (thi-<u>mek</u>-to-me) refers to excision of the thymus gland

thyr/o = thyroid, thyroid gland, shield, e.g., thyrotoxicosis (thi-ro-tok-sih-<u>ko</u>-sis) refers to a toxic condition of the thyroid gland or thyroid crisis
</td></tr>
</table>

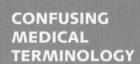

TABLE 19-1

Gland	Pronunciation	Definition
pituitary gland	pe-<u>tu</u>-i-tar-ee	also known as the hypophysis, the pituitary gland is about the size of a pea and is located on the underside of the brain in a depression at the base of the skull called the *sella turcica* and protected by the brain above it and the nasal cavities below it; it is connected by a thin stalklike projection to the hypothalamus. The pituitary is a very complex gland that secretes many hormones that affect body functions; it is often referred to as the master gland as it contains two major parts, the anterior pituitary and the posterior pituitary lobes
thyroid	<u>thi</u>-royd	consisting of a right and left lobe, the thyroid gland is a U- or H-shaped gland located in front of the neck just below the larynx; the lobes are connected by a narrow piece of thyroid cartilage that produces the prominence on the neck known as the Adam's apple. The thyroid gland produces three hormones: 1. Thyroxin (T4) helps maintain normal body metabolism. 2. Triiodthyronine (T3), a chemically similar compound, helps regulate growth and development and control metabolism and body temperature. 3. Calcitonin regulates the level of calcium in the blood. It lowers the blood calcium level by inhibiting the release of calcium from the bones by a negative feedback loop when blood calcium levels are high.

TABLE 19-1 *(continued)*

Gland	Pronunciation	Definition
parathyroid	par'-ah-<u>thi</u>-royd	the parathyroid glands are four small nodules of tissue embedded in the back side of the thyroid glands; they secrete a hormone known as parathyroid hormone or parathormone (PTH), which increases blood calcium levels
adrenal	ah'-<u>dre</u>-nal	also called suprarenal glands, the two adrenal glands sit one atop each kidney; each consists of two portions, the central region, or adrenal medulla, and the outer region, or adrenal cortex. The adrenal cortex is the largest portion of the gland, and it secretes three types of steroid hormones called corticosteroids. Each has different functions. 1. Glucocorticoids affect glucose metabolism and maintain blood glucose levels. 2. Mineralocorticoids are involved in electrolyte balance. The most important is aldosterone, whose main function is to control sodium and potassium ion concentration in the kidney. 3. Gonadocorticoids are sex hormones released from the adrenal cortex instead of the gonads, but the small amounts secreted by the adrenal cortex contribute to the secondary sex characteristics, such as breast and beard development, and are necessary for reproduction. The adrenal medulla, the inner portion of the adrenal gland, secretes two nonsteroid hormones called catecholamines. The two hormones, adrenaline (epinephrine) and noradrenaline (norepinephrine), are the stress hormones that exert physiologic changes during times of stress (the fight-or-flight response)
pancreas	<u>pan</u>-kree-as	an elongated structure located behind the stomach in the left upper quadrant. The specialized cells that produce hormones are called the islets of Langerhans; these cells produce two hormones, insulin and glucagon, and both play a role in glucose levels in the body. The islets of Langerhans carry on the endocrine functions of the pancreas; other cells within the organ carry on its exocrine functions. • Insulin, produced in the beta cells of the pancreas, is necessary for glucose to pass from the blood into the cells and be used for energy. Skeletal muscles are virtually impermeable to glucose in the absence of insulin. Insulin also promotes the conversion of glucose into glycogen for storage (glycogenesis) in the liver. When blood sugar is high (hyperglycemia), the pancreas is stimulated to release insulin and convert the excess glucose into glycogen. • Glucagon, produced in the alpha cells, increases blood levels of glucose by stimulating the breakdown of glycogen stored in the liver cells; glycogen is the major carbohydrate in the body. This process, called glycogenolysis, helps maintain blood glucose levels between meals, and it also helps synthesize glucose from amino acids and glycerol derived from triglycerides (gluconeogenesis) and elevates blood glucose levels
ovaries	<u>oh</u>-vah-reez	two small glands located in the upper pelvic cavity, on either side of the uterine wall, near the fallopian tubes of the female; each of the pair is almond-shaped and held in place by ligaments. Ovaries are the female sex glands, also known as female gonads; they produce mature ova as well as two hormones responsible for female sex characteristics and regulation of the menstrual cycle. The hormones are estrogen and progesterone. • Estrogen promotes maturation of the ova in the ovary and prepares the uterine lining for implantation of a fertilized egg, should fertilization occur. It is also responsible for the development and maintenance of secondary female characteristics that occur in puberty, such as breast development, growth of pubic and axillary hair, widened pelvis, general growth spurt, and onset of menstruation • Progesterone is responsible for preparation and maintenance of the uterus in pregnancy, and for the development of the placenta after implantation of a fertilized ovum

(continues)

| TABLE 19-1 | | (continued) |

Gland	Pronunciation	Definition
testes	<u>tes</u>-teez	male gonads, also known as testicles, are two small ovoid glands suspended from the inguinal region of the male by the spermatic cord and surrounded by the scrotal sac. After descending from high in the abdominal cavity during fetal growth, they descend shortly before birth into the scrotum and remain there. Testes are the primary organs of the male reproductive system. The testes produce male sperm cells and secrete *androgens*, the male steroid hormone; they also produce *testosterone*, the male hormone necessary for secondary sex characteristics that appear in the male during puberty, such as growth of the beard and pubic hair, growth of skeletal muscles, deepening of the voice, and enlargement of the testicles, penis, and scrotum. Testosterone is also responsible for sperm maturation
pineal	<u>pin</u>-e-al	the pineal gland is a cone-shaped structure attached by a stalk to the posterior wall of the cerebrum. Its exact function is unclear, but it is thought to function as a light receptor and to play a part in regulation of the "biological clock" (patterns of sleeping, eating, and reproduction). It secretes melatonin, the hormone believed to induce sleep
thymus	<u>thi</u>-mus	a single gland located behind the sternum in the mediastinum; it resembles a lymph gland in structure because it is part of the lymphatic system, but it also is a hormone-secreting endocrine gland. The thymus is large in children but shrinks with age until there is only a trace of active tissue in older adults; the gland secretes thymosin and thymopoietin which stimulate the production of T cells, the specialized lymphocytes involved in the immune response

DISORDERS OF THE ENDOCRINE SYSTEM

| TABLE 19-2 | | |

Clinical Condition	Pronunciation	Definition
acromegaly	ak'-ro-<u>meg</u>-ah-le	abnormal enlargement of the extremities of the skeleton, nose, jaws, fingers, and toes; caused by hypersecretion of the pituitary growth hormone after maturity (see **Figure 19–2**)
Addison's disease	<u>ad</u>-i-sonz di-<u>zez</u>	bronzelike pigmentation of the skin, severe prostration, progressive anemia, low blood pressure, diarrhea, and digestive disturbance, caused by adrenal hypofunction _extreme exhaustion, lack energy_
adrenalectomy	ah-dre-nal-<u>ect</u>-omy	surgical excision of the adrenal gland

TABLE 19-2 *(continued)*

Clinical Condition	Pronunciation	Definition
adrenogenital syndrome	ah-<u>dre</u>-no-jen'-i-tal <u>sin</u>-drom	group of symptoms associated with alterations in sex characteristics caused by abnormally increased production of androgens
adrenomegaly	ah-dre-no-<u>meg</u>-ah-le	enlargement of the adrenal gland
cretinism	<u>kre</u>-ti-nizm	arrested physical and mental development owing to congenital lack of thyroid secretion
Cushing's disease	<u>koosh</u>-ingz di-<u>zez</u>	obesity, weakness, moon face, edema, and high blood pressure; caused by hyperfunction of the adrenals
diabetes insipidus	dye-ah-<u>bee</u>-tez in-<u>sip</u>-ih-dus	a condition caused by insufficient excretion of antidiuretic hormone (ADH) (vasopressin) by the posterior pituitary gland. Deficient ADH causes the kidney tubules to fail to reabsorb needed water and salts. Clinical symptoms include polyuria (increased urination) and polydipsia (increased thirst); the person complains of excessive thirst and drinks large volumes of water, and the urine is very dilute with a low specific gravity. Synthetic preparations of ADH are administered as treatment for diabetes insipidus
diabetes mellitus	dye-ah-<u>bee</u>-tez mel-<u>li</u>-tus	inability to metabolize sugar because of abnormal insulin function; high blood sugar, excessive urination, thirst, hunger, emaciation, and weakness are cardinal symptoms of the most severe type (type 1)
exophthalmic goiter	ek'-sof-<u>thal</u>-mic <u>goi</u>-ter	toxic goiter; Graves' disease; protrusion of the eyeballs, swollen neck, weight loss, shaking, and mental deterioration are symptoms
gestational diabetes	jes-<u>tay</u>-shun-al dye-ah-<u>bee</u>-tez	a condition in which pregnant women sometimes show abnormal glucose levels during the course of pregnancy (hyperglycemia)
goiter (simple)	<u>goi</u>-ter	enlargement of the thyroid gland; swelling in the front part of the neck, mostly caused by dietary deficiency of iodine (see **Figure 19–3** and **Figure 19–4**)
Hashimoto's disease	hash'-i-<u>mo</u>-toz di-<u>zez</u>	a progressive disease of the thyroid gland with degeneration of its epithelium and replacement by lymphoid and fibrous tissue
hyperglycemia	hi-per-gli-<u>se</u>-me-ah	blood sugar (glucose) level above normal
hyperthyroidism	hi-per-<u>thi</u>-roi-dizm	excessive activity of the thyroid gland
hypothyroidism	<u>high</u>-poh-thigh-royd-ism	underactivity of the thyroid gland; shortage of thyroid hormones causes a low body metabolism because of the body's reduced use of oxygen. Any one of several conditions can produce hypothyroidism, such as endemic goiter, thyroidectomy, faulty hormone synthesis, and congenital thyroid defects, a condition that is called cretinism, and which results in a child lacking normal mental and physical growth (see **Figure 19–5**)
myxedema	mik'-se-<u>de</u>-mah	a dry, waxy type of swelling with deposits of mucin in the skin, swollen lips, and thickened nose; myxedema is the advanced form of hypothyroidism in adults (see **Figure 19–6**)

(continues)

TABLE 19-2	*(continued)*	
Clinical Condition	**Pronunciation**	**Definition**
ovariorrhexis	o-va'-re-o-<u>rek</u>-sis	rupture of an ovary
pancreaticogastrostomy	pan-kre-at'-i-ko-gas-<u>tros</u>-to-me	anastomosis of the pancreatic duct to the stomach
pancreatitis	pan'-kre-ah-<u>ti</u>-tus	inflammation of the pancreas caused by autodigestion of pancreatic tissue by its own enzymes
pheochromocytoma	fe'-o-kro'-mo-si-<u>to</u>-mah	"pheochromo" means dusky color; tumor of the medulla characterized by hypertension, weight loss, and personality changes
Simmonds' disease (panhypopituitarism)	<u>sim</u>-ondz di-<u>zez</u> (pan-hi'-po-pi-<u>tu</u>-i-tar-izm)	generalized hypopituitarism owing to absence of or damage to the pituitary gland; exhaustion, emaciation, and cachexia are symptoms
tetany	<u>tet</u>-ah-ne	sharp flexion of the wrist and ankle joints, muscle twitching, cramps, and convulsion; caused by abnormal calcium metabolism
thyroidectomy	thi-roi-<u>dek</u>-to-me	surgical excision of the thyroid gland
thyrotherapy	thi-ro-<u>ther</u>-ah-pe	treatment with thyroid preparations
thyrotomy	thi-<u>rot</u>-o-me	surgical division of thyroid cartilage

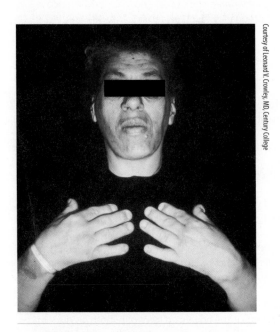

Courtesy of Leonard V. Crowley, MD, Century College

FIGURE 19–2 The appearance of a subject with advanced acromegaly

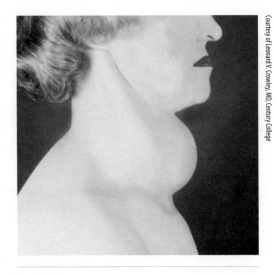

Courtesy of Leonard V. Crowley, MD, Century College

FIGURE 19–3 Large nodular goiter

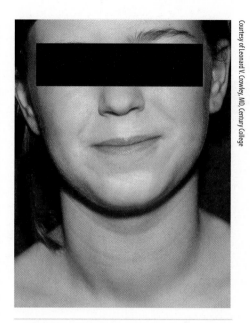

Courtesy of Leonard V. Crowley, MD, Century College

FIGURE 19–4 Small diffuse toxic goiter in a young woman

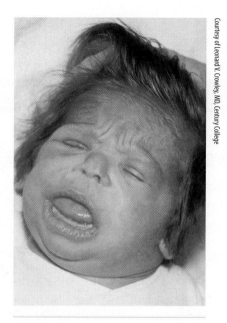

Courtesy of Leonard V. Crowley, MD, Century College

FIGURE 19–5 The characteristic appearance of neonatal hypothyroidism (cretinism) as a result of a congenital absence of thyroid gland; treatment with thyroid hormone reversed manifestations of hypothyroidism

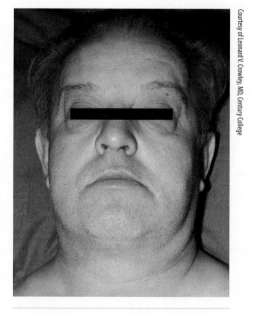

Courtesy of Leonard V. Crowley, MD, Century College

FIGURE 19–6 The appearance of a patient with myxedema

CONFUSING MEDICAL TERMINOLOGY

aden/o Versus adren/o

aden/o = gland, e.g., adenohypophysis (ad-en-o-<u>hi</u>-pof-ih-sis) refers to lack of growth in the glands

adren/o = adrenal gland, e.g., adrenocortical hyperplasia (ad-re-no-<u>cor</u>-tih-ko hi-per-<u>pla</u>-se-ah) refers to excessive development of the adrenal cortex

MISCELLANEOUS TERMS

TABLE 19-3

Term	Pronunciation	Definition
acidosis	as'-i-<u>do</u>-sis	a pathologic condition caused by accumulation of acid in, or loss of base from, the body
anorexia	an'-o-<u>rek</u>-se-ah	lack or loss of appetite for food
cachexia	kah-<u>kek</u>-se-ah	malnutrition, wasting, and emaciation
cataract	<u>kat</u>-ah-rakt	clouding of the eye lens
convulsions	kon-<u>vul</u>-shunz	involuntary muscular contractions
diaphoresis	di'-ah-fo-<u>re</u>-sis	profuse perspiration
emaciation	e-ma'-se-<u>a</u>-shun	excessive leanness; a wasted condition
endocrine	<u>en</u>-do-krin	ductless gland that secretes directly into the bloodstream
exocrine	<u>eks</u>-oh-krin	a ducted gland that secretes into various organs
gangrene	<u>gang</u>-grēn	death of tissue from lack of circulation and consequent loss of nutrients
gland	gland	an organ that secretes a metabolic substance; may be endocrine or exocrine
hypoglycemia	hi'-po-gli-<u>se</u>-me-ah	blood sugar (glucose) level is below normal
hypoglycemic agent	hi'-po-gli-<u>se</u>-mik	drug for the diabetic to decrease the amount of glucose in the blood
hypophysectomy	hi-pof'-i-<u>sek</u>-to-me	excision of the pituitary gland (hypophysis)
insulin	<u>in</u>-su-lin	a protein hormone produced by the pancreatic islets of Langerhans that is secreted into the blood in response to a rise in concentration of blood glucose; insulin promotes the entrance of glucose from the blood into cells. A diabetic patient is deficient in insulin or insulin receptors, leading to a rise in blood glucose
ketoacidosis	ke-to-as-i-<u>do</u>-sis	accumulation of ketone bodies in the blood that results in metabolic acidosis (*ketosis* and *ketoacidosis* are often used interchangeably)
ketosis	ke-<u>to</u>-sis	accumulation of excessive amounts of ketone bodies in body tissues and fluids; a complication in some diabetic patients
neuropathy	nu-<u>rop</u>-ah-the	any functional disturbances and/or pathologic changes in the peripheral nervous system; a complication in some diabetic patients

PHARMACOLOGY AND MEDICAL TERMINOLOGY

Drug Classification	antidiabetic (an-tih-dye-ah-<u>bet</u>-ik)	hormone (<u>hor</u>-mohn)
Function	helps control the blood sugar level	treats deficiency states where a specific hormone level is abnormally low
Word Parts	**anti-** = against, **diabetic** = pertaining to diabetes	pertaining to a natural chemical substance in the body
Active Ingredients (examples)	chlorpropamide (Diabenese); tolazamide (Tolinase) insulin	estrogen, conjugated (Premarin); glucagon (Glucagon)

LESSON TWO   Progress Check

MULTIPLE CHOICE

Circle the letter of the correct answer:

1. Which of the following statements *best* describes the endocrine glands?
   a. They are small bodies in the region of the neck.
   b. They secrete hormones that regulate the body's activity.
   c. They secrete materials into the gastrointestinal tract to help digest food.
   d. They prevent chronic degenerative diseases.

2. Glands are body structures that
   a. are classified as endocrine or exocrine
   b. are not organs, but are attached to them
   c. are classified as exogenous or endogenous
   d. exert little influence over other body systems

3. A gland that secretes its fluids into a duct and then into the bloodstream is a(n) _____ gland.
   a. endogenous
   b. exogenous
   c. endocrine
   d. exocrine

4. The endocrine system is composed of
   a. the adrenal and thyroid glands
   b. ducted and ductless glands
   c. glands that secrete to the outside of the body
   d. ductless glands

5. The endocrine gland at the base of the brain is the
    a. pituitary
    b. parathyroid
    c. pineal
    d. pancreas

6. The endocrine gland with a lobe on each side of the trachea is the
    a. pituitary
    b. pancreas
    c. thyroid
    d. adrenal

7. The two small glands atop the kidneys are the
    a. pituitary
    b. adrenal
    c. thyroid
    d. thymus

8. The large organ situated transversely behind the stomach is the
    a. adrenal
    b. thymus
    c. sex
    d. pancreas

9. The organ situated in the pleural cavity that is believed to be part of the body's immune system is the
    a. pancreas
    b. pituitary
    c. thymus
    d. thyroid

10. The *islets (islands) of Langerhans* refers to
    a. small bodies in the pituitary gland
    b. the endocrine part of the pancreas
    c. the testes and ovaries
    d. the exocrine part of the adrenals

◆ MATCHING: DISORDERS OF THE ENDOCRINE SYSTEM

Match the disease with the malfunctioning gland that causes it (answers may be used more than once):

1. acromegaly	**a.** parathyroid
2. Addison's disease	**b.** pituitary
3. cretinism	**c.** adrenal
4. Cushing's disease	**d.** thyroid
5. goiter (simple)	**e.** pancreas
6. Graves' disease	
7. diabetes mellitus	
8. Simmonds' disease	
9. tetany	

FILL-IN

From the word pool following the descriptions, fill in the correct phrase(s) to make a true sentence:

1. Inability to metabolize sugar because of a lack of insulin leads to _____.

2. Arrested mental and physical growth is a sign of _____ caused by congenital lack of thyroxine.

3. Swollen neck, weight loss, shaking, and mental deterioration are symptoms of _____.

4. _____ is characterized by hypertension, weight loss, and personality changes.

5. _____ is characterized by muscle twitching, cramps, and convulsions.

6. A dry, waxy swelling with swollen lips and thickened nose is diagnosed as _____.

7. Obesity, weakness, moon face, edema, and high blood pressure characterize _____.

Word Pool: cretinism, Cushing's disease, diabetes mellitus, Graves' disease, myxedema, pheochromocytoma, tetany

DEFINITIONS

Define the following terms:

1. convulsion _____

2. diaphoresis _____

3. emaciation _____

4. insulin _____

5. ketosis _____

6. neuropathy _____

7. hypoglycemic agent _____

8. goiter _____

9. hyperthyroidism _____

10. Cushing's disease _____

COMPARE AND CONTRAST

Explain the *differences* in the following terms:

1. acidosis/anorexia _____

2. cachexia/cataract _____

3. gangrene/gland _____

4. hypoglycemia/hypophysectomy _____

◆ WORD PUZZLE ON THE ENDOCRINE SYSTEM

Find the 50 words related to the endocrine system by reading forward, backward, up, down, and diagonally. When you have circled the 50 listed words, the remaining letters will spell TO ALWAYS MAINTAIN HOMEOSTASIS.

```
A  L  L  U  D  E  M  T  P  I  T  C  O  R  T  I  S  O  N  E
C  D  T  E  S  T  E  S  N  I  T  C  A  L  O  R  P  O  N  N
T  L  R  A  L  P  H  A  C  E  L  L  S  P  T  H  R  D  A  O
H  A  L  E  N  O  M  R  O  H  H  T  W  O  R  G  O  W  C  R
K  E  P  I  N  E  P  H  R  I  N  E  A  T  E  C  G  B  I  E
C  S  A  N  I  O  V  A  R  Y  A  D  H  N  R  A  E  E  T  T
A  Y  D  S  O  Y  C  S  R  N  I  Y  O  I  M  L  S  T  E  S
B  H  R  U  D  A  I  O  D  O  R  R  N  N  G  C  T  A  R  O
D  P  E  L  I  T  I  R  R  O  E  E  R  N  M  I  E  C  U  D
E  O  N  I  N  R  O  Y  I  T  S  O  I  U  M  T  R  E  I  L
E  P  A  N  E  G  H  D  S  Y  I  Z  I  C  A  O  O  L  D  A
F  Y  L  T  E  T  A  O  S  R  I  C  I  H  S  N  N  L  I  F
E  H  N  N  A  S  T  T  E  N  L  N  O  O  T  I  E  S  T  O
V  A  S  R  D  S  E  T  I  A  H  L  H  T  E  N  O  M  N  L
I  E  A  A  E  M  S  E  C  G  L  A  N  D  R  A  D  H  A  L
T  P  N  T  O  O  T  S  U  M  A  L  A  H  T  O  P  Y  H  I
A  O  H  S  P  U  G  H  S  A  E  R  C  N  A  P  P  T  A  C
G  F  S  H  L  D  U  C  T  L  S  F  E  M  A  L  E  I  I  L
E  S  T  R  O  G  E  N  S  E  S  O  X  Y  T  O  C  I  N  E
N  S  E  B  O  L  D  N  A  L  G  Y  R  A  T  I  U  T  I  P
```

Words to Look for in the Word Puzzle

1.	ACTH	**14.**	cortisone	**27.**	hypothalamus	**40.**	parathyroid
2.	ADH	**15.**	duct	**28.**	insulin	**41.**	pit
3.	adrenal	**16.**	endocrine system	**29.**	iodine	**42.**	pituitary gland
4.	adrenocorticotropin	**17.**	epinephrine	**30.**	LH	**43.**	posterior
5.	aldosterone	**18.**	estrogens	**31.**	lobes	**44.**	progesterone
6.	alpha cells	**19.**	female	**32.**	luteinizing	**45.**	prolactin
7.	androgens	**20.**	follicle	**33.**	male	**46.**	PTH
8.	anterior	**21.**	FSH	**34.**	master	**47.**	testes
9.	antidiuretic	**22.**	GH	**35.**	medulla	**48.**	testosterone
10.	beta cells	**23.**	gland	**36.**	negative feedback	**49.**	thyroid
11.	calcitonin	**24.**	gonads	**37.**	ovary	**50.**	TSH
12.	calcium	**25.**	growth hormone	**38.**	oxytocin		
13.	CHO	**26.**	hypophyseal	**39.**	pancreas		

CHAPTER

20

Cancer Medicine

LESSON ONE: MATERIALS TO BE LEARNED

Medical Terms in Cancer Medicine
Cancer: Classification, Terminology, and Types
Basic Classification
Cancer with Specific Names
Screening and Early Detection
Medical Terms Related to the Diagnosis of Cancer
Special Cancer Diagnostic Tests
Methods of Cancer Treatment
Cancer Treatment
Medical Terms Related to the Treatment of Cancer
Different Surgical Procedures Used to Treat Cancer
Breast Cancer and Medical Illustrations
Medical Terms Related to Types of Cancer

LESSON TWO: PROGRESS CHECK

Write In
Matching: Diagnosis
Multiple Choice
Definitions

OBJECTIVES

After completing this chapter and the exercises, the student should be able to:

1. Define cancer.
2. Classify cancer.
3. Identify rules and exceptions in naming cancer.
4. Describe the types of cancer normally affecting men and women.
5. Explain the two major clinical phases in cancer medicine: diagnosis and treatment.
6. Describe the details of screening, detection, and diagnosis of cancer.
7. Present the methods of treating cancer.

ALLIED HEALTH PROFESSIONS

Veterinary Technologists and Technicians and Animal Care and Service Workers

Veterinary technologists and technicians typically conduct clinical work in a private practice under the supervision of a licensed veterinarian. They often perform various medical tests, as well as treat and diagnose medical conditions and diseases in animals. Besides working in private clinics and animal hospitals, veterinary technologists and technicians may work in research facilities.

Many people like animals, but as pet owners can attest, taking care of them is hard work. Animal care and service workers—who include animal caretakers and animal trainers—train, feed, water, groom, bathe, and exercise animals. They also clean, disinfect, and repair their cages. They play with the animals, provide companionship, and observe behavioral changes that could indicate illness or injury. Boarding kennels, pet stores, animal shelters, veterinary hospitals and clinics, stables, laboratories, aquariums, natural aquatic habitats, and zoological parks all house animals and employ animal care and service workers. Job titles and duties vary by employment setting.

INQUIRY

American Association for Laboratory Animal Science: www.aalas.org

Data from Stanfield, Peggy S., Cross, Nanna, and Hui, Y.H. *Introduction to the Health Professions*, 6th ed. Burlington, MA: Jones & Bartlett Learning; 2012.

Cancer is the second leading cause of death from disease in the United States. Skin cancer is the most common type of cancer; however, lung cancer is the leading cause of death from cancer, followed by colon cancer in men and breast cancer in women. Brain cancer and leukemia are the most common cancers in children and young adults.

Normally, cells divide to produce more cells only when the body needs them. Normal life processes are characterized by continuous growth and maturation of cells that are subject to control mechanisms that regulate growth. This ongoing growth process serves the purpose of replacing cells that have been injured or have undergone degenerative changes. If cells keep dividing when new cells are not needed, a tumor or neoplasm is formed. A neoplasm (neo- = new + plasm = growth) is an overgrowth of cells that serves no useful purpose. Neoplasms appear not to be subject to the control mechanisms that normally regulate cell growth and differentiation. The terms *neoplasm* and *tumor* have essentially the same meaning and may be used interchangeably.

A malignant neoplasm is composed of less well differentiated cells that grow rapidly and infiltrate surrounding tissues. The process by which a tumor spreads (meta = change) and the secondary deposits (+ stasis = standing) are called metastatic tumors. See **Figures 20–1, 20–2,** and **20–3.**

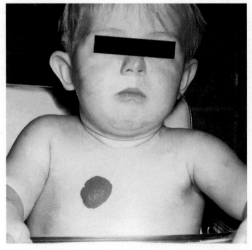

Courtesy of Leonard V. Crowley, MD, Century College

FIGURE 20–1 Clinical appearance of benign blood vessel tumor (angioma) of skin

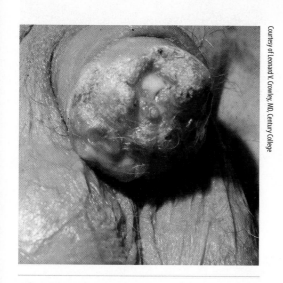

Courtesy of Leonard V. Crowley, MD, Century College

FIGURE 20–2 Large carcinoma of penis involving foreskin

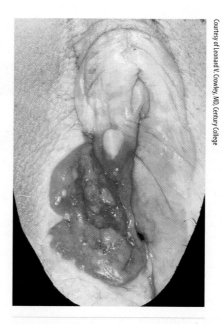

Courtesy of Leonard V. Crowley, MD, Century College

FIGURE 20–3 Large carcinoma of the vulva; the white appearance of the skin adjacent to the carcinoma is caused by preexisting vulva dystrophy

---

LESSON ONE | **Materials to Be Learned**

MEDICAL TERMS IN CANCER MEDICINE

The medical terms associated with cancer medicine are grouped as follows:

1. Those associated with the word *cancer*
2. Those associated with the cancer site (organ or tissue)
3. Those associated with the diagnosis
4. Those associated with the treatment

CANCER: CLASSIFICATION, TERMINOLOGY, AND TYPES

Basic Classification

There are two large classes of neoplasms, benign and malignant, with characteristics of each described in Table 20-1.

CONFUSING MEDICAL TERMINOLOGY

hematoma Versus hematoma

hematoma (hee-ma-<u>toh</u>-muh) = blood tumor if interpreted according to word parts or word origin; this meaning is incorrect under standard clinical circumstances

hematoma (hee-ma-<u>toh</u>-muh) = a mass of blood that has leaked out of a vessel and pooled; this is the accepted meaning in clinical medicine

Comparison of Benign and Malignant Tumors

TABLE 20-1

Characteristic	Benign Tumor	Malignant
growth rate	slow	rapid
character of growth	expansion	infiltration
tumor spread	remains localized	metastasis by bloodstream and lymphatics
cell differentiation	well differentiated	poorly differentiated

General Principles of Naming Tumors

TABLE 20-2

General Term	Meaning
polyp, papilloma	any benign tumor projecting from surface epithelium
root word + -oma (suffix)	a benign tumor; root word designates primary tissue of origin
carcinoma	malignant tumor arising from surface, glandular, or parenchymal epithelium (but not endothelium or mesothelium)
sarcoma	malignant tumor of any primary tissue other than surface, glandular, and parenchymal epithelium
leukemia	neoplasm of blood cells
scirrhous	pertaining to a carcinoma with a hard structure

Most benign tumors are named by adding the suffix "-oma" to the prefix that designates the cell of origin, as shown in Table 20-3. For example, a benign tumor arising from glandular epithelium is called an adenoma. A benign tumor of blood vessels is an angioma, and one arising from cartilage is designated a chondroma.

Using Root Words to Name Tumors

TABLE 20-3

Combining Form	Meaning
aden/o	gland
angi/o	vessels (type not specified)
chondr/o	cartilage
fibr/o	fibrous tissue
hemangi/o	blood vessels
lip/o	fat
lymphangi/o	lymph vessels
my/o	muscle
neur/o	nerve
oste/o	bone

There are many types of malignant tumors, but all can be classified into three groups according to the cancer site and tissue type: (1) carcinomas, (2) sarcomas, and (3) leukemias. The term *cancer* is a word used to indicate any type of malignant tumor.

A *carcinoma* is any malignant tumor arising from surface, glandular, or parenchymal epithelium and is classified further by designating the type of epithelium from which it arose. For example, a carcinoma arising from the glandular epithelium of the pancreas is termed an adenocarcinoma of the pancreas (aden = gland).

Sarcoma is a general term referring to a malignant tumor arising from primary tissues other than surface, glandular, or parenchymal epithelium. The exact type of sarcoma is specified by using the prefix that designates the cell of origin. For example, a malignant tumor of bone is designated as an osteosarcoma.

The term *leukemia* is applied to any neoplasm of blood-forming tissues. Neoplasms arising from the precursors of white blood cells usually do not form solid tumors but, instead, the abnormal cells proliferate within the bone marrow where they overgrow and crowd out the normal blood-forming cells. The abnormal cells also "spill over" into the bloodstream, and large numbers of abnormal cells circulate in the blood.

Tumors are named and classified according to the cells and tissues from which they originate. However, when cancer spreads, the new tumor has the same kind of abnormal cells and the same name as the primary tumor. For example, if lung cancer spreads to the liver, the cancer cells in the liver are lung cancer cells. The disease is called metastatic lung cancer (not liver cancer).

Cancer with Specific Names

This section explores some tumors with specific names. They do not follow the "rules" discussed earlier.

TABLE 20-4

Tumor	Explanation for Nomenclature
lymphoid tumors	all neoplasms of lymphoid tissue are called lymphomas and are malignant: Hodgkin's disease and non-Hodgkin's lymphomas
skin tumors	<ul><li>*pigment-producing cells of the epidermis*</li><li>*benign:* nervus, a Latin word that means "birthmark"</li><li>*malignant:* melanoma or malignant melanoma</li><li>*keratinocytes*</li><li>*benign:* basal cell carcinoma</li><li>*malignant:* squamous cell carcinoma (sometimes metastasizes)</li></ul>
teratoma tumors (of mixed components)	derived from cells that have the potential to differentiate into different types of tissue (bone, muscle, glands, epithelium, brain tissue, hair) and may be either benign or malignant; a common type of cystic benign teratoma arising in the ovary is usually called a dream cyst
embryonic tumors	derived from persisting groups of embryonic cells of the brain, retina, adrenal gland, kidney, liver, or genital tract. Named from the site of origin, with the suffix "-blastoma" added (blast = a primitive cell + oma = tumor); medulloblastoma: medulla of the brain; retinoblastoma: retina of the eye; hepatoblastoma: liver; Wilm's tumor: kidney, exception in naming (nephroblastoma not used)
noninfiltrating (in situ) carcinoma	noninfiltrating tumors are common in many locations, including the breast, cervix, colon, skin, and urinary tract; in situ carcinoma can be completely cured by surgical excision
precancerous conditions	refers to conditions that have a high likelihood of developing into cancer:<ul><li>*skin cancer:* actinic keratoses ("actinic" refers to sun rays) or lentigo maligna (a latin term meaning "malignant freckle")</li><li>*oral cancer:* leukoplakis (leuko- = white + plakia = patch) may develop in the mucous membranes of the mouth as a result of exposure to tobacco tars from smoking or use of smokeless tobacco</li><li>*colon polyps*</li></ul>

SCREENING AND EARLY DETECTION

The early detection of cancers relies on two conditions: the existence of a premalignant, or detectable, preclinical phase, and the availability of appropriate tests that can detect the tumor during the preclinical phase. On an individual basis, the standard history and physical examination provide a comprehensive format for early detection of cancer. Emphasis is placed on the following areas:

1. History and physical examination, including family history of cancer, personal habits—smoking, alcohol use, and sexual history—and occupational exposure to chemicals or radiation.

2. Signs and symptoms related to specific organ systems:

   a. *Bladder:* hematuria, dysuria
   b. *Breast:* nipple discharge, mass
   c. *Gastrointestinal:* change in bowel habits, bleeding
   d. *Gynecological:* abnormal vaginal bleeding or discharge, dyspareunia
   e. *Lymphadenopathy:* abnormal size or number of lymph nodes
   f. *Oropharynx:* hoarseness for more than 1 week, abnormal bleeding, pain
   g. *Prostrate cancer:* hematuria, dysuria
   h. *Pulmonary:* cough, pain, dyspnea, hemoptysis
   i. *Skin:* slow-healing sore, changing mole

The most common detection and diagnostic tools or tests are described in Table 20-5.

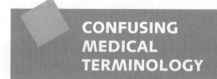

CONFUSING MEDICAL TERMINOLOGY

mallei Versus malleoli

mallei (mal-<u>ee</u>-ahy) = the outermost of a chain of three small bones in the middle ear of mammals; also called hammer

malleoli (mah-le´-o-<u>lahy</u>) = two rounded processes on the distal tibia and fibula

MEDICAL TERMS RELATED TO THE DIAGNOSIS OF CANCER

TABLE 20-5

Term	Pronunciation	Definition
aspirate	<u>as</u>-pi-rit	withdrawal of fluid from a lump, often a cyst
biopsy	<u>by</u>-ahp-see	removal of cells or tissues for examination under a microscope
Scope		a procedure in which a thin, lighted tube is inserted into the body part being examined and a tissue sample (biopsy) is taken to examine under a microscope to determine whether cancer cells are present
bronchoscopy	bron-<u>kos</u>-ko-pee	scope inserted through the nose or mouth to examine the inside of the trachea, bronchi, and lung
colonoscopy	ko-lun-<u>ahs</u>-ko-pee	scope inserted into the rectum to examine the colon
cystoscopy	sist-<u>ahs</u>-ko-pee	scope inserted into the urethra to examine the bladder
laryngoscopy	lair-in-<u>gos</u>-ko-pee	examination of the larynx (voice box) with a mirror (indirect laryngoscopy) or with a laryngoscope (direct laryngoscopy)
sigmoidoscopy	sig-moid-<u>oss</u>-ko-pee	scope inserted into the sigmoid part of the colon; also called proctosigmoidoscopy

SPECIAL CANCER DIAGNOSTIC TESTS

TABLE 20-6

Test	Purpose	Comments
Tumor Markers		obtained from blood sample
acid phosphatase	cancer of the prostate	may be used to monitor response to treatment or recurrence
AFP	hepatocellular carcinoma germ cell tumors	used to monitor treatment response
CA 19-9	cancers of the pancreas, colon, cervix, and ovary	a relatively specific tumor-associated antigen
CA 125	epithelial ovarian cancer	a tumor-associated antigen that might be used in conjunction with vaginal ultrasound for screening
CEA	cancers of the pancreas, colon, breast, lung, stomach, ovary	high levels correlate with high tumor burden
HCG/AFP	malignant germ cell tumors originating from ovaries or sperm; ovarian or uterine cancer in women and testicular cancer in men	return to normal indicates cure
monoclonal immunoglobulins	multiple myeloma	malignant clone can be IgG, IgM, or IgA
PSA	cancer of the prostate	used particularly to monitor response to treatment
Imaging		x-ray or computerized view with or without a contrast dye or radioactive substance
barium enema	cancer of the colon	series of x-rays of the colon taken after the person is given an enema that contains barium. Barium outlines the intestines on the x-rays
computed axial tomography (CAT, CT, ACTA)	cross-section images of internal structures	x-ray ± contrast dye with the creation of pictures by a computer linked to an x-ray machine; high specificity, especially for brain tumors
intravenous pyelogram or intravenous pyelography (IVP)	cancer of the kidneys, ureters, and bladder	dye is injected into a blood vessel and concentrated in the urine to visualize the kidneys, ureters, and bladder
lymphangiography	lymph node involvement, especially Hodgkin's disease, lymphoma, cancer of testes	blue dye, injected into lymphatic channel, visualizes abdominal lymph nodes
radionuclide scan	shows function and size of specific organ (brain, bone, liver, spleen, kidney)	used for staging because of specificity; radioactive material is injected or swallowed and radioactivity measured with a scanner
ultrasound	visualizes structural changes, mass (stomach, pancreas, kidney, uterus, ovary)	uses high-frequency sound waves

TABLE 20-6 *(continued)*

Test	Purpose	Comments
Microscopic Examination		obtained from a tissue sample
bone-marrow aspirate	tumor involvement, especially by leukemia or lymphoma	needle aspirate of marrow from iliac crest or sternum
estrogen/progesterone receptors	cancer of the breast	cells taken from breast tissue; defines certain tumors that may be more responsive to hormonal therapy
Pap smear	cancer of the cervix or uterus	cells obtained by swab of vagina, endocervical canal, and exocervix
sentinel lymph node biopsy	tumor metastasis, for example, breast cancer	dye or radioactive substance injected near a tumor flows into the sentinel lymph node(s)—the first lymph node(s) to which that cancer is likely to spread from the primary tumor
sputum cytology	bronchogenic cancer	examination of mucus coughed up from the lungs; used to detect abnormal lung cells
Other		
stool guaiac	cancer of the colon/rectum	a test to check for blood in stool (*fecal* refers to stool, *occult* means hidden)

Note: AFP, alpha-fetoprotein; CEA, carcinoembryonic antigen; HCG, human chorionic gonadotropin; PSA, prostate-specific antigen; CA 125 and CA 19-9, special antigens.

METHODS OF CANCER TREATMENT

Cancer Treatment

Cancer is treated with surgery, radiation therapy, chemotherapy, hormone therapy, or biological therapy, or a combination of these treatments. Treatment may be prophylactic for precancerous lesions, palliative to reduce the size of a tumor when the tumor has metastasized, or reconstructive after a mastectomy for breast cancer. Patients with cancer are often treated by a team of specialists, which may include a medical oncologist (specialist in cancer treatment), a surgeon, a radiation oncologist (specialist in radiation therapy), and others. The choice of treatment depends on the type and location of the cancer, the stage of the disease, the patient's age and general health, and other factors.

CONFUSING MEDICAL TERMINOLOGY

calic/o Versus calc/o

calic/o (cali/o) = calyx, cup, e.g., calices or calyces (kal-uh-seez) refers to areas inside the kidney

calc/o = calcium, e.g., calciuria (kal-sey-u-rea) refers to calcium in the urine

MEDICAL TERMS RELATED TO THE TREATMENT OF CANCER

TABLE 20-7

Term	Pronunciation	Definition
Biological		treatment to stimulate or restore the ability of the immune system to fight infection and disease (also, immunotherapy or biological response modifier [BRM] therapy)
autologous bone marrow transplantation	aw-<u>tahl</u>-o-gus	a procedure in which bone marrow is removed from a person, stored, and then given back to the person following intensive treatment
BCG vaccine		an anticancer drug, bacille Calmette-Guérin (BCG), that activates the immune system
colony-stimulating factors		substances that stimulate the production of blood cells; granulocyte colony-stimulating factors (G-CSF); granulocyte-macrophage colony-stimulating factors (GM-CSF)
peripheral stem cell transplantation	per-<u>if</u>-er-al	replacing blood-forming cells destroyed by cancer treatment; immature blood cells (stem cells) are given after treatment to help the bone marrow recover and produce healthy blood cells. Sources of stem cells are bone marrow and are allogeneic, autologous, or syngeneic
allogeneic	al-o-jen-<u>ay</u>-ik	stem cells donated by someone else
autologous	aw-<u>tahl</u>-o-gus	stem cells removed from a person, stored, and then given back to the person following intensive treatment
syngeneic	sin-juh-<u>nay</u>-ik	stem cells donated by an identical twin
Chemotherapy	kee-mo-<u>ther</u>-a-pee	treatment with anticancer drugs to destroy cancer cells by stopping them from growing or multiplying
Radiation Therapy	ray-dee-<u>ay</u>-shun	radiotherapy uses high-energy radiation from x-rays, neutrons, and other sources to kill cancer cells and shrink tumors
external		uses a machine to aim high-energy rays at the cancer
internal		given internally by placing radioactive material that is sealed in needles, seeds, wires, or catheters directly into or near the tumor
systemic radiation therapy		giving a radioactive substance, such as a radiolabeled monoclonal antibody, that circulates throughout the body
Surgery		a procedure to remove a part of the body because of the presence of cancer
cystectomy	sis-<u>tek</u>-toe-mee	surgical removal of the bladder

TABLE 20-7	(continued)	

Term	Pronunciation	Definition
cryosurgery	kyre-o-sir-jer-ee	treatment performed with an instrument that freezes and destroys abnormal tissues
fulguration	ful-gyoor-ay-shun	destroying tissue using an electric current
hysterectomy	hiss-ter-ek-toe-mee	surgical removal of the uterus
laryngectomy	lair-in-jek-toe-mee	an operation to remove all or part of the larynx (voice box)
laser	lay-zer	a device that concentrates light into an intense, narrow beam used to cut or destroy tissue. It is used in microsurgery, photodynamic therapy, and for a variety of diagnostic purposes
lumpectomy	lump-ek-toe-mee	surgery to remove the tumor and a small amount of normal tissue around it
mastectomy	mas-tek-toe-mee	surgery to remove the breast (or as much of the breast tissue as possible)
modified radical mastectomy		surgical procedure in which the breast, some of the lymph nodes in the armpit, and the lining over the chest muscles are removed
orchiectomy	or-kee-ek-toe-mee	surgical removal of one or both testicles
pneumonectomy	noo-mo-nek-toe-mee	surgical removal of an entire lung
prostatectomy	pros-ta-tek-toe-mee	surgical removal of part or all of the prostate
salpingo-oophorectomy	sal-pin-go-o-o-for-ek-toe-mee	surgical removal of the fallopian tubes and ovaries
Hormone Therapy		treatment of cancer by removing, blocking, or adding hormones. Also called endocrine therapy
antiandrogens	an-tee-an-dro-jens	drugs used to block the production or interfere with the action of male sex hormones
luteinizing hormone-releasing hormone agonist	loo-tin-eye-zing ag-o-nist	a substance that closely resembles luteinizing hormone-releasing hormone (LH-RH), which controls the secretion of sex hormones; given to decrease secretion of sex hormones

DIFFERENT SURGICAL PROCEDURES USED TO TREAT CANCER

TABLE 20-8

Approach	Example
palliative	cytoreduction; oncologic emergencies; neurosurgical procedures/pain control; nutritional support
prophylactic	excision of premalignant lesions
primary/definitive	local excision; en bloc dissection
rehabilitative	cosmetic and functional restoration
resection of metastases	lung; liver
supportive	insertion of access devices such as a porta catheter for infusion of drugs for chemotherapy; radiation implants

BREAST CANCER AND MEDICAL ILLUSTRATIONS

This chapter is unable to discuss medical terms associated with each type of cancer. **Figures 20–4** to **20–8** serve as illustrations for breast cancer.

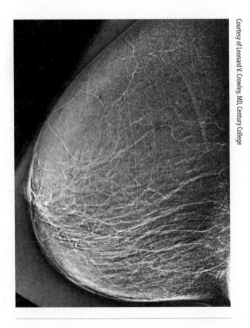

Courtesy of Leonard V. Crowley, MD, Century College

FIGURE 20–4 A normal mammogram

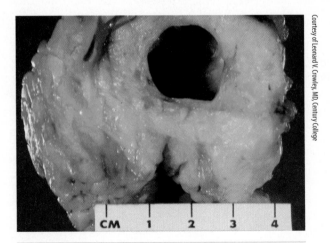

Courtesy of Leonard V. Crowley, MD, Century College

FIGURE 20–5 A benign cyst in the breast viewed in cross-section; a cyst is filled with fluid that escapes when the cyst is excised

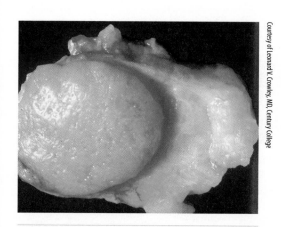

Courtesy of Leonard V. Crowley, MD, Century College

FIGURE 20–6 Benign fibroadenoma of the breast; the tumor is well circumscribed and readily separates from adjacent tissue

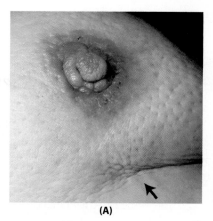
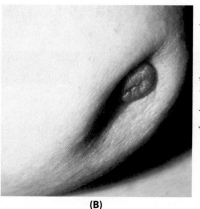

(A)   **(B)**

Courtesy of Leonard V. Crowley, MD, Century College

FIGURE 20–7 Changes in the breast caused by advanced carcinoma. (A) Skin retraction (arrow) and orange-peel appearance of the skin. (B) Nipple retraction.

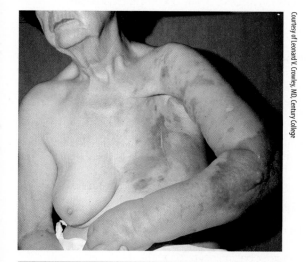

Courtesy of Leonard V. Crowley, MD, Century College

FIGURE 20–8 Severe edema of arm resulting from long-standing lymphatic obstruction. The patient had a radical operation for breast carcinoma many years previously. Scarring in the axilla blocked lymphatic drainage from the arm, leading to chronic edema. The dark discolored areas in the skin of the chest wall and upper limb are caused by a malignant tumor of lymphatic vessels (lymphosarcoma), which sometimes complicates chronic lymphedema.

CONFUSING MEDICAL TERMINOLOGY

-ectomy Versus -stomy Versus -tomy

-ectomy = removal, cutting out, excision, e.g., blepharectomy (blef-ah-<u>rek</u>-to-me) refers to excision of a lesion of the eyelid

-stomy = furnish with a mouth or outlet, new opening, e.g., salpingostomy (sal-pin-<u>jos</u>-to-me) refers to creation of an artificial opening in the fallopian tube

-tomy = cutting, incision, e.g., prostatolithotomy (pros-tat-o-<u>lith</u>-o-to-me) refers to incision in the prostate gland to remove a stone

MEDICAL TERMS RELATED TO TYPES OF CANCER

TABLE 20-9

Term	Pronunciation	Definition
adenocarcinoma	ad-in-o-kar-sin-o-ma	cancer that begins in cells that line certain internal organs
atypical hyperplasia	hy-per-play-zha	benign (noncancerous) condition in which cells have abnormal features and are increased in number
benign	beh-nine	not cancerous; does not invade nearby tissue or spread to other parts of the body
cancer		a term for diseases in which abnormal cells divide without control; cancer cells can invade nearby tissues and spread through the bloodstream and lymphatic system to other parts of the body
carcinogen	kar-sin-o-jin	any substance that causes cancer
carcinoma	kahr-suh-noh-muh	cancer that begins in the skin or in tissues that line or cover internal organs
cyst	sist	a sac or capsule filled with fluid
ductal carcinoma in situ	duk-tal kahr-suh-noh-muh in sye-too	abnormal cells that involve only the lining of a duct; the cells have not spread outside the duct to other tissues in the breast
epidermoid carcinoma	ep-i-der-moyd kahr-suh-noh-muh	a type of cancer in which the cells are flat and look like fish scales; also called squamous cell carcinoma
familial polyposis	pah-li-po-sis	an inherited condition in which numerous polyps (tissue masses) develop on the inside walls of the colon and rectum; it increases the risk for colon cancer
fibroid	fye-broyd	a benign smooth muscle tumor, usually in the uterus or gastrointestinal tract; also called leiomyoma
hyperplasia	hye-per-play-zha	an abnormal increase in the number of cells in an organ or tissue
Kaposi's sarcoma	kap-oh-seez sar-koh-mah	an uncommon malignant disorder, beginning as soft purple-brown nodules or plaques on the feet that gradually spread throughout the skin
large cell carcinomas	kahr-suh-noh-muhs	a group of lung cancers in which cells are large and look abnormal when viewed under a microscope
lobular carcinoma in situ	lob-yoo-lar kahr-suh-noh-muh in sye-too	abnormal cells found in the lobules of the breast. This condition seldom becomes invasive cancer; however, having lobular carcinoma in situ increases one's risk of developing breast cancer in either breast
malignant	ma-lig-nant	cancerous; a growth with a tendency to invade and destroy nearby tissue and spread to other parts of the body
non-small cell lung cancer		a group of lung cancers that includes squamous cell carcinoma, adenocarcinoma, and large cell carcinoma

TABLE	20-9	*(continued)*

Term	Pronunciation	Definition
oat cell cancer		a type of lung cancer in which the cells look like oats when viewed under a microscope; also called small cell lung cancer
polyp	<u>pol</u>-ip	a growth that protrudes from a mucous membrane
sarcoma		a cancer of the bone, cartilage, fat, muscle, blood vessels, or other connective or supportive tissue
small cell lung cancer		a type of lung cancer in which the cells appear small and round when viewed under the microscope; also called oat cell lung cancer
squamous cell carcinoma	<u>skway</u>-mus sell kahr-suh-<u>noh</u>-muh	cancer that begins in squamous cells, which are thin, flat cells resembling fish scales. Squamous cells are found in the tissue that forms the surface of the skin, the lining of the hollow organs of the body, and the passages of the respiratory and digestive tracts; also called epidermoid carcinoma
tumor	<u>too</u>-mer	an abnormal mass of tissue that results from excessive cell division; tumors may be either benign (not cancerous) or malignant (cancerous)
Wilm's tumor	wilmz <u>too</u>-mer	a malignant tumor of the kidney occurring predominately in childhood

PHARMACOLOGY AND MEDICAL TERMINOLOGY

Drug Classification	antibiotic (anti-infective) (an-tih-<u>bye</u>-ot-ik)	antineoplastic (an-tih-nee-oh-<u>plass</u>-tik)	immunosuppressant (im-voo-noh-suh-<u>press</u>-ant)
Function	stops or controls the growth of infection-causing microorganisms	prevents the development, growth, or reproduction of cancerous cells	suppresses the body's natural immune response to an antigen, as in treatment for transplant patients
Word Parts	**anti-** = against; **bi/o** = life; **-tic** = pertaining to	**anti-** = against; **ne/o** = new; **plas/o** = formation; **-tic** = pertaining to	**immun/o** = immunity, **suppressant** = pertaining to lower, to control
Active Ingredients (examples)	phenoxymethyl-penicillin sodium (Pen-Vee-K, Penicillin VK, Veetids, V-Cillin K)	fluorouracil (Adrucil); methotrexate (Rheumatrex Dose Pack)	cyclosporine (Sandimmune); azathioprine (Imuran)

| LESSON TWO | Progress Check |

◆ WRITE IN

For the type of cancer described, write in the correct term:

1. _____ benign cancer of the colon

2. _____ benign skin cancer

3. _____ cancer of the blood cells

4. _____ embryonic tumor of the brain

5. _____ malignant cancer of the lymph system

6. _____ malignant tumor of cartilage

7. _____ malignant tumor of the skin

8. _____ malignant cancer of the bone

9. _____ benign tumor of the uterus

10. _____ cancer cells appear the size and shape of oats

◆ MATCHING: DIAGNOSIS

Match the following diagnostic procedure to its function:

1. biopsy	**a.**	used to detect abnormal lung cells
2. barium enema	**b.**	using a dye to visualize kidneys, ureters, and bladder
3. PSA	**c.**	visualization of abdominal lymph nodes
4. Pap smear	**d.**	tissue sample taken for microscopic examination
5. sputum cytology	**e.**	tissue sample taken near a breast tumor
6. bone marrow aspiration	**f.**	screen for gastrointestinal bleeding
7. estrogen/progesterone receptors	**g.**	tissue sample taken for diagnosis of uterine cancer
8. lymphangiography	**h.**	used to detect and monitor treatment of prostate cancer
9. stool guaiac	**i.**	diagnostic tool for detecting cancer of the blood cells
10. IVP	**j.**	outline of the colon on x-ray

◆ MULTIPLE CHOICE

Circle the letter of the correct answer:

1. A biopsy is not used in the diagnosis of this cancer.
   a. leukemia
   b. breast
   c. lung
   d. bladder

2. Radiation therapy with a radioactive substance given intravenously is
   a. external
   b. internal
   c. prophylactic
   d. systemic

3. Surgical removal for treatment of bladder cancer is called
   a. orchiectomy
   b. cystectomy
   c. intravenous pyelogram
   d. cystoscopy

4. A procedure that would not be used to diagnose or treat lung cancer is
   a. hormone therapy
   b. bronchoscopy
   c. sputum cytology
   d. pneumonectomy

5. Cancer cells in the liver in someone with metastatic cancer of the colon are described as
   a. liver cancer
   b. colon cancer
   c. colon and liver cancer
   d. lymph cancer

6. Cryosurgery is a method of surgery using
   a. electricity
   b. light
   c. freezing
   d. radioisotopes

7. Carcinoma of the breast would be treated by any of the following except which method?
   a. computed axial tomography
   b. hormone therapy
   c. radiation therapy
   d. modified radical mastectomy

8. Surgical excision of basal cell carcinoma of the skin is a type of treatment described as
   a. definitive
   b. palliative
   c. prophylactic
   d. resection

9. This diagnostic test is used to monitor treatment of cancer of the prostate.
   a. AFP
   b. CEA
   c. HCG
   d. PSA

10. Stem cell transplantation when the source of the cells is oneself is called
   a. allogeneic
   b. autologous
   c. syngeneic
   d. internal

11. Bone marrow aspiration is a diagnostic tool for
   a. leukemia
   b. lymphoma
   c. leukemia and lymphoma
   d. neither leukemia nor lymphoma

12. A common symptom of cancer of the bladder or prostrate is
   a. hemoptysis
   b. dyspnea
   c. lymphadenopathy
   d. hematuria

◆ DEFINITIONS

Define the following symptoms of cancer.

1. malignant _____

2. metastasis _____

3. fungating _____

4. proliferation _____

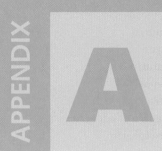
Answer Keys

Unit I: Word Parts and Medical Terminology

Answer Key to Chapter 2: Word Parts

◆ MATCHING

1. f
2. d
3. a
4. g
5. b
6. h
7. c
8. e

◆ SPELLING AND DEFINITION

1. (a) ovary
2. (b) rectum or anus
3. (c) kidney
4. (b) nose
5. (a) testicle
6. (c) sacrum
7. (b) fallopian tube
8. (a) eardrum
9. (b) pharynx
10. (c) vertebra
11. (c) ureter
12. (a) cartilage
13. (b) rib
14. (b) vessel
15. (a) vein
16. (a) red

DEFINING MEDICAL WORD ELEMENTS

1. andr/o
2. gyne
3. cardi/o
4. cephal/o
5. steth/o
6. dent/o or odont/o
7. encephal/o
8. gastr/o
9. hepat/o or hep/a
10. cholecyst/o
11. stomat/o
12. lingua
13. mast/o or mamm/o
14. my/o or myos
15. neur/o

BUILDING MEDICAL WORDS

1. tendinitis, tendonitis
2. thyroidectomy
3. tracheotomy
4. enteropathy
5. neuralgia
6. cystitis
7. arthritis
8. splenectomy
9. ophthalmologist
10. angiogram
11. cholelithiasis
12. arteriosclerosis
13. pneumonectomy
14. myelogram
15. otoscope
16. phlebotomy
17. prostatectomy
18. cerebrovascular accident
19. esophagitis
20. thoracotomy
21. hyperglycemia

MATCHING

1. i
2. j
3. g
4. h
5. f
6. e
7. c
8. d
9. a
10. b

◆ SPELLING AND DEFINITION

1. (a) centesis: surgical puncture
2. (b) clasis: to break down; refracture
3. (c) ectasis: to expand, dilate
4. (d) malacia: softening
5. (a) plegia: paralysis (stroke)
6. (b) ptosis: prolapse, falling, drooping
7. (c) sclerosis: hardening
8. (d) megaly: enlargement
9. (a) cele: hernia, swelling
10. (b) iasis: abnormal condition: presence of, formation of

◆ BUILDING MEDICAL WORDS

1. cephalgia or cephalodynia
2. roentgenography
3. gastritis
4. cholelithiasis
5. polycythemia
6. osteomalacia
7. arthrocentesis
8. phlebotomy
9. rhinoplasty
10. biology
11. hepatomegaly
12. dermatosis
13. appendectomy
14. psychiatry
15. encephalotomy
16. chemotherapy
17. hemostasis
18. carcinogen
19. nephropathy
20. aphasia

◆ DEFINING MEDICAL TERMS

1. surgical fracture or refracture of a bone
2. surgical separation of intestinal adhesions
3. crushing of a stone in the bladder and washing out the fragments
4. death of cells or tissue
5. removal of the foreskin from the penis
6. a gland tumor
7. difficulty in swallowing
8. reduced number of white blood cells
9. paralyzed on one side of the body
10. morbid fear of heights

Unit II: Root Words, Medical Terminology, and Patient Care

Answer Key to Chapter 3: Bacteria, Color, and Some Medical Terms

MULTIPLE CHOICE

1. c
2. c
3. b
4. d
5. b
6. a

MATCHING

1. h
2. e
3. j
4. i
5. f
6. g
7. a
8. h
9. c
10. d
11. h
12. b
13. a

WRITE IN THE PREFIX

1. acro-
2. aniso-
3. hetero-
4. dys-
5. homo-
6. iso-
7. mal-
8. megaly-
9. pan-
10. post-
11. hemo-

DEFINE THE PREFIX

1. bad, poor
2. bad, painful, difficult
3. enlarged, large
4. excessive, beyond, above normal
5. fast
6. under, below normal
7. slow
8. take away, remove
9. put back
10. water
11. beside
12. around

13. many
14. before
15. before, preceding
16. through
17. together, united
18. night
19. night
20. through
21. around
22. producing pus

Answer Key to Chapter 4: Body Openings and Plural Endings

SPELLING AND DEFINITION

1. (c) aperture: opening (orifice)
2. (a) constriction: closed, narrowed
3. (b) foramen: a natural opening or passage
4. (d) hiatus: a gap, cleft, or opening
5. (a) orifice: any opening (aperture)
6. (b) introitus: vaginal cavity (opening)
7. (c) ventricle: a small cavity or chamber (especially in the brain or heart)
8. (b) lumen: opening within a hollow tube or organ

WORD CONSTRUCTION

1. ae
2. aces
3. ina
4. es (or) a
5. ices
6. inges
7. ges
8. a
9. a
10. i
11. ora
12. ies
13. vertebra
14. thorax
15. lumen
16. crisis
17. ovary
18. artery
19. diverticulum
20. nucleus
21. meninx
22. diagnosis
23. spermatozoon
24. femur
25. appendix
26. ovum
27. thrombus

BUILDING MEDICAL TERMS

1. cavity
2. dilated
3. foramen
4. lumen
5. stoma
6. ventricle
7. patent
8. vaginal canal
9. alimentary canal
10. hiatus (hernia)
11. quadriplegia

DEFINITIONS

1. thigh bone
2. a membrane covering the brain
3. chest
4. small cavity that prevents friction between tissues
5. any bone of the finger or toe
6. blood vessel
7. cavity (orifice) in the body
8. female gonad
9. slender outgrowth from the small intestine
10. male seed (germ) (semen)
11. red blood cell
12. outgrowth (pouch) on large intestine (colon)
13. mouth (oral cavity)
14. general term for the entrance to a cavity or space, e.g., vaginal cavity
15. a small cavity in a chamber

Answer Key to Chapter 5: Numbers, Positions, and Directions

COMPARE AND CONTRAST

1. circum—around/contra —against
2. ecto—outside/endo—inside
3. infra—below/ipsi—same
4. para—near/peri—about (around)
5. uni—one/bi—two/tri—three
6. prima—first/multi—many
7. semi—half/hemi—one-sided (half)
8. ambi—both (sides)/quadri—four
9. meso—middle/meta—after (beyond)
10. retro—behind (backward)/trans—across (through)

IDENTIFY THE LOCATION

1. anterior
2. posterior
3. cephalic
4. caudal
5. supine or prone
6. eversion
7. extension
8. oblique
9. medial
10. adjacent

◆ MATCHING: POSITIONS

1. m
2. o
3. n
4. j
5. a
6. l
7. b
8. c
9. k
10. d
11. i
12. e
13. f
14. h
15. g

◆ DEFINE THE TERM

1. the system for weighing and measuring drugs and solutions, precious metals, and precious stones
2. the English system of weights and measures for all commodities except drugs, stones, and metals
3. system of measures and weights based on the meter and based on multiples of 10
4. monster
5. small
6. degree of heat or cold based on a specific scale
7. a temperature scale where H_2O boils at 100° and freezes at 0°
8. a temperature scale where H_2O boils at 212° and freezes at 32°
9. change from one scale or system to another
10. conversions that are equal to each other

◆ MATCHING: METRIC UNITS

1. d
2. c
3. g
4. e
5. f
6. a
7. b

◆ SHORT ANSWER

1. 1,000
2. 1,000
3. 100
4. 10
5. 100
6. 1,000
7. 1,000
8. 1
9. 2.2
10. 2.5
11. 1,000; 1,000
12. 9, 5, 32
13. 32, 5, 9

◆ **SHORT ANSWER** (*continued*)

14. 4.18
15. 3
16. 30
17. 240
18. 4.2
19. 1

◆ **FILL-IN**

1. milligram
2. microgram
3. kilogram
4. drops
5. dram
6. fluid dram
7. giga
8. liter
9. joule
10. tera
11. degrees Celsius
12. gram
13. elevated, high
14. take; prescription
15. without
16. with
17. infinity
18. before
19. after
20. female

Answer Key to Chapter 6: Medical and Health Professions

◆ **MULTIPLE CHOICE: SCIENTIFIC STUDIES**

1. d
2. b
3. c
4. a
5. c
6. d
7. c

◆ **MATCHING**

1. h
2. d
3. e
4. i
5. f
6. g
7. j
8. c
9. b
10. a

SHORT ANSWER

1. care and treatment of the teeth and related structures. Dentist (DMD) (DDS)
2. use of diet in promotion of health, and disease prevention and its treatment. Registered Dietitian (RD)
3. care and treatment of the foot. Podiatrist (DMP)
4. care of women throughout pregnancy, delivery, and postpartum. Registered Nurse, Midwife (RN)
5. routine care for persons in acute and chronic institutional facilities or community settings. Licensed Practical Nurse or Licensed Vocational Nurse (LPN or LVN)
6. use of a variety of techniques with persons who have disturbed mental faculties and/or behavior problems. Psychologist (title depends on degree; usually MS or PhD)
7. interpretation and dispensing of drugs. Pharmacist (RPh)
8. direct care of ill persons in a variety of settings under the supervision of a physician. May also function independently. Registered Nurse (RN) or Public Health Nurse (PHN)
9. the practice of medicine and/or surgery as well as research on animals. Veterinarian (DVM)

COMPLETION

1. oral surgeon
2. periodontist
3. dental hygienist
4. dietetic technician
5. podiatrist
6. medical technician
7. physical therapist
8. psychologist
9. pharmacist
10. optometrist

MULTIPLE CHOICE: PROFESSIONS

1. a, b, c, d
2. a, b, c, d
3. a, b, c, d
4. a, b, c, d

ABBREVIATIONS

1. OTR
2. RPT
3. PHN
4. RD
5. LPN/LVN
6. RN or PHN
7. RMT
8. RT
9. DDS/DMD
10. DVM
11. OD
12. MD
13. MS/PhD
14. MD
15. RPh
16. ARRT
17. DO
18. MD

◆ **DESCRIBE THE SPECIALTY**

1. administration of medications to kill pain sensation
2. study of the endocrine gland functions and illness
3. study of the blood and blood-forming tissue
4. the use of x-ray and radioactive substances to diagnose disease
5. study of body tissues for diagnosis of all diseases, and the nature of disease
6. study of bacteria, especially disease-producing bacteria (pathogens)
7. study of living organisms
8. study of the care of the aging and elderly adults
9. study of the care of children
10. care of the foot
11. promotion of health, and disease prevention and treatment as related to nutrition
12. care of the pregnant woman through delivery
13. practicing medicine and performing surgery on animals
14. assisting families with personal problems resulting from illness

Unit III: Abbreviations

Answer Key to Chapter 7: Medical Abbreviations

◆ **IDENTIFY THE DEPARTMENT**

1. admitting and discharge
2. central service
3. operating room
4. physical medicine and rehabilitation
5. radiology
6. laboratory
7. obstetrics
8. pediatrics
9. outpatient department
10. emergency room
11. social service
12. intensive care unit
13. food service

◆ **IDENTIFY THE PRESCRIPTION**

1. 2 grams by mouth three times a day
2. 60 milliequivalents by rectal suppository at bedtime
3. 6 drops under the tongue every 4 hours
4. 2 liters intravenously every day
5. 30 units intramuscularly before meals
6. 10 milliliters under the skin as needed
7. 2 grains in 10 cubic centimeters of normal saline by needle under the skin once a day
8. one-half of a 5-milligram tablet by mouth after meals

◆ **IDENTIFY THE DIET ORDER**

1. nothing by mouth
2. diet as tolerated
3. carbohydrate or consistent carbohydrate diet
4. 2 g sodium medical soft
5. mechanical soft
6. clear liquid
7. regular high fiber, force fluids
8. full liquid with interval nourishment at 10 AM to 2 PM and at bedtime; intake and output recorded
9. after meals
10. as required

◆ MATCHING

1. f
2. d
3. g
4. h
5. c
6. e
7. b
8. a
9. i
10. j

◆ SPELL OUT THE ABBREVIATION

1. prepare preoperatively
2. dead on arrival
3. with; without; temperature, pulse, respiration
4. cardiopulmonary resuscitation
5. blood pressure; millimeters; mercury
6. tender loving care
7. discontinue; intravenous (line); as soon as possible
8. carbon dioxide and water
9. treatment; symptoms
10. sodium; potassium
11. diagnosis; iron

Answer Key to Chapter 8: Diagnostic and Laboratory Abbreviations

◆ IDENTIFY THE DISEASE

1. arteriosclerotic heart disease
2. coronary heart disease
3. congestive heart failure
4. cardiovascular disease
5. cerebrovascular accident
6. chronic brain syndrome
7. chronic obstructive pulmonary disease
8. myocardial infarction
9. rheumatoid arthritis
10. transient ischemic attack
11. sexually transmitted diseases

◆ SHORT ANSWER

1. auscultation and percussion
2. pupils equal, round, react to light, and accommodation
3. percussion and auscultation
4. rule out
5. systems review
6. tonsillectomy and adenoidectomy
7. physical examination
8. prescription
9. head, eyes, ears, nose, throat
10. diagnosis
11. red blood cell (count)

◆ **MATCHING**

1. c
2. h
3. f
4. b
5. a
6. e
7. g
8. d
9. m
10. p
11. q
12. o
13. n
14. j
15. r
16. l
17. i
18. k

◆ **DEFINE THE ABBREVIATION**

1. chief complaint
2. complains of
3. family history
4. fever of undetermined origin
5. history
6. short of breath
7. upper respiratory infection
8. urinary tract infection
9. murmur
10. present illness
11. symptoms
12. past history

Unit IV: Review

Answer Key to Chapter 9: Review of Word Parts from Units I, II, and III

◆ **COMPARE AND CONTRAST**

1. lipo: a term for fat; litho: stone
2. para: to bear; pathy: any disease
3. phagia: swallowing; phasia: speech; phonia: voice
4. schizo: split; sclero: hardening
5. thrombo: clot; thermo: heat; trauma: injury
6. abscess: pus; adnexa: accessory structure
7. axilla: armpit; anomaly: defect
8. cervical: neck; coccyx: tailbone
9. edema: excess fluid; embolus: clot in a vessel
10. emesis: vomiting; enema: fluid injected into rectum
11. icterus: jaundice; ischemia: lack of blood to a part
12. palpable: felt by touch; parietal: walls of a cavity
13. prolapse: falling downward; prophylaxis: preventive treatment
14. suture: stitch; sputum: expectorate
15. viscera: interior organ; virus: infectious agent

◆ **BUILDING MEDICAL TERMS**

1. chondritis
2. colpitis or vaginitis
3. laryngitis
4. paronychia
5. pancreatitis
6. phlebitis
7. salpingitis
8. otitis
9. pleurisy (pleuritis)
10. spondylitis
11. stomatitis
12. ureteritis
13. urethritis
14. esophagitis
15. neuritis
16. aphasia
17. dysphagia
18. carcinoma
19. necrosis
20. lipid
21. scleroderma
22. hemostasis
23. trauma
24. acute
25. anomaly
26. chronic
27. embolus
28. emesis
29. voiding
30. edema
31. coccyx
32. cervical vertebrae
33. excreting
34. exacerbation
35. incontinence
36. inflammation
37. ischemia
38. hemorrhage
39. metastasis
40. obesity
41. palpable
42. prophylaxis
43. sputum
44. virus
45. suture

◆ **FILL-IN**

1. metacarpals
2. laparotomy (celiotomy)
3. oophorectomy (or) ovariectomy
4. podiatry
5. rhinoplasty
6. metatarsals
7. thoracentesis
8. cryptorchidism
9. primigravida
10. multipara
11. salpingitis

◆ **DEFINE THE TERM**

1. expulsion of the fetus from the uterus before it is viable
2. listening for sounds within the body
3. strand of collagen from a mammal, used to suture
4. a flexible tube to be passed into body channels
5. stretching; expanding
6. a clot or other plug taken by the blood to a smaller vessel
7. increase in severity of a disease or symptoms
8. deep band of fibrous tissue
9. transfer of disease from one organ or body to another area not connected directly
10. striking a part with short, sharp blows
11. existing at the time of birth

◆ **MATCHING**

1. e
2. d
3. a
4. h
5. j
6. i
7. b
8. c
9. f
10. g

◆ **SHORT ANSWER: ROOT WORDS**

1. carp/o
2. cervic/o
3. dent/o, odont
4. esophag/o
5. lapar/o, celi/o
6. onych/o
7. ophthalm/o
8. pancreat/o
9. soma
10. pod/o
11. pubis
12. rhin/o
13. stomat/o
14. tarslo
15. thorac/o

SHORT ANSWER: BODY PARTS

1. vagina
2. vein
3. pleura
4. vertebra
5. mouth

Unit V: Medical Terminology and Body Systems

Answer Key to Chapter 10: Body Organs and Parts

SPELLING AND DEFINITION

1. integumentary; skin, nails, hair, oil and sweat glands
2. cardiovascular; heart and blood vessels
3. musculoskeletal; bones, joints, ligaments, cartilage, and muscles
4. gastrointestinal; mouth, esophagus, stomach, intestines, and accessory organs
5. respiratory; nose, pharynx, larynx, trachea, bronchi, and lungs
6. genitourinary; kidneys, bladder, ureters, urethra, gonads, genitalia, and internal organs
7. endocrine; ductless glands and supporting structures
8. nervous; brain, spinal cord, cranial and spinal nerves

FILL-IN

1. cell
2. genetic
3. mitosis
4. multiplying
5. membrane
6. tissues
7. epithelial tissue
8. connective tissue
9. muscle tissue
10. nerve tissue
11. organ
12. systems
13. cavity
14. planes
15. diaphragm
16. chromosomes
17. pancreas, liver, gallbladder, and salivary glands

DEFINITIONS

1. sum of physical and chemical processes that convert food into elements for growth, repair, and energy as well as recycling and excretion
2. when the body systems maintain a balance optimal for survival: a steady state

SHORT ANSWER

1.
   a. epithelial: protects, absorbs, secretes
   b. connective: binds all tissue together
   c. muscle: contracts and relaxes
   d. nerve: controls and coordinates body activity
2. serves as the wall or outer covering; allows some substances to go into the cell but keeps others out
3. contains genes and chromosomes for reproduction

Answer Key to Chapter 11: Integumentary System

◆ SPELLING AND DEFINITION

1. (a) epidermis: the outermost nonvascular layer of skin
2. (d) subcutaneous: beneath the skin
3. (b) biopsy: removal of tissue from the body for examination
4. (c) debridement: removal of devitalized tissue
5. (a) escharotomy: removal of burn scar tissue
6. (b) keratosis: any horny growth
7. (c) steatoma: a fatty mass within an oil gland
8. (d) verruca: a wart
9. (b) impetigo: a staphylococcal or streptococcal skin infection marked by vesicles that become pustular
10. (a) pediculosis: infestation with lice
11. (c) eczema: redness in the skin
12. (b) psoriasis: chronic, hereditary, recurrent dermatosis
13. (d) erysipelas: a contagious skin disease
14. (a) varicella: chickenpox
15. (b) actinic: referring to ultraviolet rays reacting on the skin

◆ WRITE IN

1. albinism
2. alopecia
3. dermatology
4. erythema
5. eschar
6. nummular
7. papule
8. urticaria
9. pustule
10. cicatrix
11. keratosis
12. herpes genitalis

◆ MATCHING: SKIN TERMS

1. h
2. g
3. f
4. e
5. d
6. c
7. b
8. a

◆ DEFINITIONS

1. a test for tuberculosis (TB)
2. a test for scarlet fever
3. a test for diphtheria
4. a test for the presence of cystic fibrosis
5. a test for valley fever
6. a test for systemic fungal disease

◆ MATCHING: SKIN DISEASES

1. d
2. g
3. e

4. c
5. f
6. b
7. a
8. i
9. h

◆ **LIST THE FUNCTIONS**

1. a protective barrier from many things
2. enables the body to sense heat, cold, or pain
3. assists in regulating body temperature by insulating
4. eliminates body wastes through perspiration
5. synthesizes vitamin D

◆ **ANSWER TO THE WORD PUZZLE ON THE INTEGUMENTARY SYSTEM**

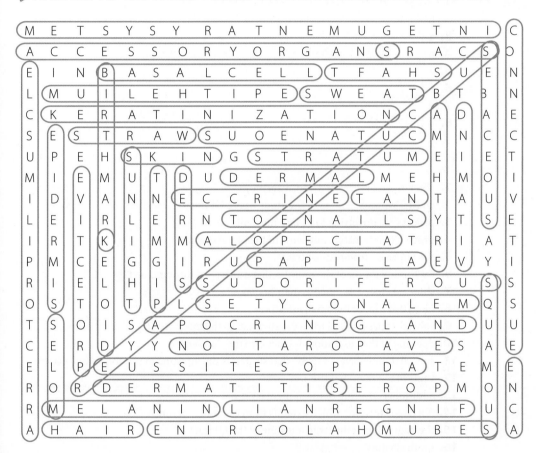

Answer Key to Chapter 12: Digestive System

◆ **WRITE IN**

1. adhesions
2. botulism
3. carcinoma
4. cholelithiasis
5. colitis
6. diverticula
7. gastric ulcer

◆ **WRITE IN** (*continued*)

8. gastritis/gastroenteritis
9. glossitis
10. hernia
11. intussusception
12. strangulated
13. hepatitis
14. nausea and vomiting
15. obesity
16. pancreatitis
17. peritonitis
18. pyloric stenosis
19. steatorrhea
20. cirrhosis

◆ **MATCHING: DIGESTIVE TRACT**

1. c
2. h
3. a
4. g
5. e
6. f
7. d
8. i
9. j
10. b

◆ **DEFINITIONS**

1. chief organ of digestion and absorption
2. an MD who specializes in the study of the GI tract
3. process of converting food into nutrients
4. process that transfers nutrients to the bloodstream
5. the entire gastrointestinal tract
6. rhythmic motion of the muscles that move food through the GI tract
7. slime produced in mucous membranes
8. first 10–12 in. of the small intestine
9. valve that passes food from the stomach to the intestine in one direction only
10. opening of the common bile duct into the duodenum
11. special double-layered tissue that suspends the intestine in the abdominal cavity
12. veins in the region of the anus
13. additional covering of the alimentary canal
14. the large intestine, which extends from cecum to rectum
15. the beginning of the large intestine of the GI tract
16. tooth cavities
17. having or ending in two points, e.g., bicuspid teeth
18. a malignant tumor
19. forced feeding, especially through a tube into the stomach
20. loop of bowel twisting on itself resulting in a bowel obstruction

WORD POOL: STRUCTURE OF THE DIGESTIVE TRACT

1. mouth or oral cavity
2. small intestine
3. duodenum
4. cecum
5. liver, gallbladder, pancreas
6. deciduous
7. rectum
8. anus
9. greater omentum
10. duodenum, jejunum, ileum
11. palate
12. periodontal disease

MATCHING: SURGICAL PROCEDURES

1. g
2. f
3. h
4. j
5. e
6. a
7. b
8. d
9. c
10. i

ANSWER TO THE WORD PUZZLE ON THE DIGESTIVE SYSTEM

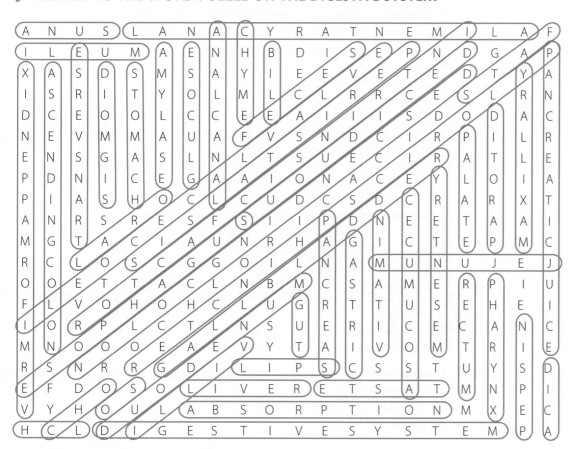

Answer Key to Chapter 13: Respiratory System

◆ MATCHING

1. j
2. i
3. e
4. g
5. a
6. b
7. h
8. d
9. c
10. f

◆ MULTIPLE CHOICE

1. c
2. a
3. b
4. d
5. b
6. b
7. c
8. a
9. c
10. d

◆ DEFINITIONS

1. the throat; the cavity between nasal passages and mouth; passageway for food and liquid (also airway)
2. voice box; contains the vocal cords
3. the windpipe; a long tube extending from the trachea to the chest
4. a cluster of air sacs whose walls exchange oxygen and carbon dioxide
5. the main branches conveying air from the trachea to the lungs
6. between the ribs
7. pockets (cavities) in the face and skull bones
8. organs of respiration where blood and air meet and mix
9. chief muscle of respiration; separates the lungs from the abdomen
10. sudden infant death syndrome; the dying during sleep of healthy infants, cause unknown; also called crib death
11. chronic obstructive pulmonary disease (also COLD: chronic obstructive lung disease); a group of chronic, progressively debilitating lung diseases including emphysema, bronchitis, and asthma
12. inflammation of the pleura, the lining that encases the lungs
13. hereditary disorder present from birth associated with malfunction of the pancreas and frequent respiratory infections
14. contagious inflammation of the upper respiratory tract
15. pathological accumulation of air in tissues or organs
16. acute (adult) respiratory distress syndrome; faulty gaseous exchange leading to shock lung
17. very rapid breathing
18. surgical repair of the nose

◆ ABBREVIATIONS

1. upper respiratory infection
2. shortness of breath
3. intermittent positive pressure breathing
4. submucous resection

5. complete blood count
6. temperature, pulse, and respiration
7. purified protein derivative (TB test)
8. cardiopulmonary resuscitation
9. endotracheal tube
10. auscultation and percussion

◆ NAMING

1. hypercapnia
2. orthopnea
3. dyspnea
4. cyanosis
5. hemoptysis
6. hypoxia
7. pyothorax; empyema
8. stridor
9. dysphonia
10. hemothorax

◆ MATCHING: BREATH SOUNDS

1. f
2. a
3. b
4. e
5. d
6. c

◆ ANSWER TO THE WORD PUZZLE ON THE RESPIRATORY SYSTEM

Answer Key to Chapter 14: Cardiovascular System

◆ DEFINITIONS

1. x-ray examination of vessels
2. a balloon-type catheter is used to exert pressure on the plaque in a vessel, opening up a blocked area
3. medication to delay blood clotting
4. catheter passed into the heart through a vein in the arm and used to detect abnormal blood flow in arteries
5. cutting of a heart valve that is defective
6. medication that reduces intravascular blood volume, thus lowering blood pressure
7. ultrasonic probe that checks blood flow
8. picture of electrical impulses of the heart
9. boring out the inner lining of an artery to increase the size of the lumen
10. having a body temperature below normal; may be induced as a therapeutic measure
11. a battery-powered device implanted to regulate heartbeat
12. normal heart rhythm originating in the SA node
13. adjunct treatment used to help reduce edema and blood pressure
14. a drug that causes a vessel to dilate
15. a drug that causes a vessel to constrict
16. puncture of a vein

◆ NAMING

1. right lymphatic duct
2. adenoids
3. thymus gland
4. lymph capillaries
5. lymph nodes
6. thoracic duct
7. interstitial fluid
8. spleen

◆ MATCHING: DIAGNOSTIC PROCEDURES

1. c
2. g
3. j
4. e
5. b
6. a
7. i
8. h
9. f
10. d

◆ MULTIPLE CHOICE

1. a
2. d
3. a
4. c
5. b
6. b
7. a
8. b
9. d
10. c

ABBREVIATIONS

1. atrial septal defect
2. blood pressure
3. complete blood count
4. coronary care unit
5. congestive heart failure
6. carbon dioxide
7. cardiopulmonary resuscitation
8. cerebrovascular accident (stroke)
9. electrocardiogram
10. myocardial infarction (heart attack)
11. oxygen
12. premature ventricular contraction
13. red blood cell/red blood cell count
14. transient ischemic attack
15. white blood cell/white blood cell count

ANSWERS TO THE WORD PUZZLE ON THE HEART

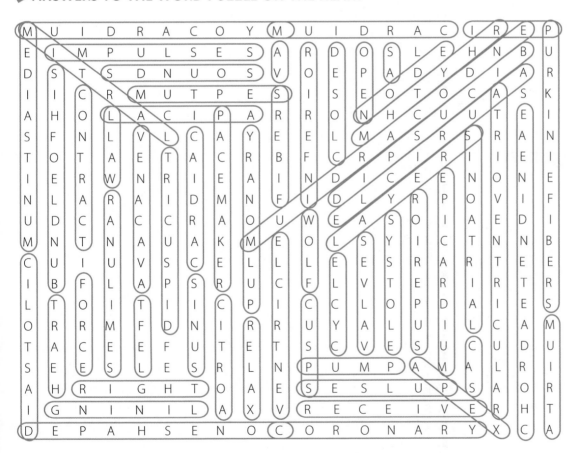

Answer Key to Chapter 15: Nervous System

◆ FILL-IN

1. central
2. central
3. autonomic
4. ventricles
5. plexus
6. sulcus
7. limbic
8. ganglion
9. hemisphere
10. encephalon
11. opening in the occipital bone through which the spinal cord passes
12. cauda equina
13. cerebellum
14. dura mater
15. sympathetic

◆ MATCHING: NERVES

1. g
2. e
3. a
4. b
5. c
6. f
7. d

◆ MATCHING: DISEASE STATES

1. a
2. f
3. e
4. g
5. h
6. d
7. c
8. b

◆ TRUE OR FALSE

1. T
2. F
3. T
4. F
5. T
6. F
7. F
8. T
9. T
10. F

◆ DEFINITIONS

1. conflicting emotional attitude
2. complete withdrawal
3. a false personal belief
4. illusions, excitement, hallucinations (short duration)
5. automatic repetition of what is said

6. imaginary illness
7. belief in one's greatness, power
8. a person abnormally suspicious of others
9. abnormal dread or fear
10. a group of severe emotional disorders characterized by delirium, delusion, hallucinations, and other bizarre behaviors
11. pretending to be ill
12. a person who is very suspicious of people and things

◆ SPELLING AND DEFINITION

1. (a) cerebrum. The largest portion of the brain; divided into left and right hemispheres; located in the upper part of the cranial cavity
2. (c) meninges. The three membranes covering the brain and spinal cord
3. (b) arachnoid. The delicate membrane between the pia mater and dura mater
4. (d) trochlear. Muscle of the eyes
5. (a) olfactory. Sense of smell
6. (b) hypoglossal. Beneath the tongue
7. (c) anencephaly. Congenital absence of a brain
8. (a) hydrocephalus. Accumulation of cerebrospinal fluid within the skull
9. (d) meningocele. Hernial protrusion of the meninges through a defect in the skull or vertebrae
10. (a) poliomyelitis. An acute viral disease

◆ ANSWERS TO THE WORD PUZZLE ON THE NERVOUS SYSTEM

Answer Key to Chapter 16: Genitourinary System

◆ **LISTS**

1.
- **a.** (two) kidneys
- **b.** (two) ureters
- **c.** (one) bladder
- **d.** (one) urethra

2.
- **a.** remove water and wastes, convert to urine, transport, excrete
- **b.** reabsorb substances the body wants to keep
- **c.** maintain body system equilibrium by regulation of pH, RBC production, blood pressure, blood glucose

3. perpetuating the species

4.
- **a.** (two) testes
- **b.** (three) glands
- **c.** (four) ducts
- **d.** (one) penis
- **e.** (one) scrotum
- **f.** (one) urethra

5.
- **a.** (two) ovaries
- **b.** (two) fallopian tubes
- **c.** (two) breasts
- **d.** (one) uterus
- **e.** (one) vagina
- **f.** (one) vulva

◆ **MULTIPLE CHOICE**

1. b
2. a
3. c
4. d

◆ **COMPARE AND CONTRAST**

1. albuminuria is the presence of protein (albumin) in the urine; anuria is no (without) urine

2. enuresis is bed-wetting while asleep; diuresis is increased excretion of urine

3. incontinence is inability to control bowel or bladder excretion; urinary retention is inability to excrete urine

4. hydronephrosis is distention of the renal pelvis because of the inability to urinate; nephrolithiasis is kidney (renal) stones

5. nycturia is excessive night urination; oliguria is diminished urine secretion; and dysuria is painful or difficult urination

6. pyelitis is inflammation of the renal pelvis; glomerulonephritis is inflammation of the capillary loops in the glomeruli

MATCHING: CLINICAL PROCEDURES

1. e
2. d
3. f
4. h
5. g
6. c
7. a
8. b

COMPLETION

1. testis
2. external genitalia
3. vas deferens
4. prostate
5. epididymis
6. seminal duct
7. ovaries
8. fallopian tube
9. uterus
10. vagina
11. dystocia
12. hydrosalpinx

MATCHING: MALE CLINICAL CONDITIONS

1. c
2. d
3. e
4. b
5. a

MATCHING: FEMALE CLINICAL CONDITIONS

1. c
2. e
3. d
4. a
5. b

DEFINITIONS

1. amniocentesis
2. Apgar test
3. cephalopelvic disproportion (CPD)
4. dystocia
5. ectopic or extrauterine
6. gestation
7. gravida
8. neonatal period
9. postpartum
10. placenta

ANSWERS TO THE WORD PUZZLE ON THE GENITOURINARY SYSTEM

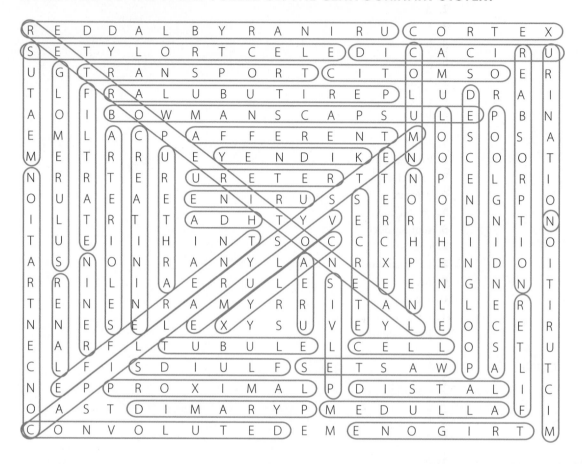

Answer Key to Chapter 17: Musculoskeletal System

LIST THE FUNCTION

1. Support and protection—vital organs protected
2. Movement—all body movements
3. Red blood cell turnover—bone marrow is the site
4. Storage—minerals and nutrients

MATCHING: LOCATIONS

1. f
2. g
3. i
4. h
5. j
6. a
7. b
8. c
9. d
10. e

MULTIPLE CHOICE

1. b
2. b
3. a
4. c
5. d
6. c

7. b
8. c
9. d

NAME THE STRUCTURE

1. bursa
2. fascia
3. lamina
4. ligament
5. aponeurosis
6. hinges
7. sutures
8. ball and socket
9. tendon
10. meniscus

MATCHING: MUSCLES

1. c
2. d
3. e
4. b
5. a
6. d
7. a
8. b
9. e
10. c
11. g
12. f
13. d
14. e
15. b
16. c
17. a

COMPARE AND CONTRAST

1. kyphosis is humpback (or hunchback); lordosis is curvature of the lumbar spine (swayback)
2. gout is a form of arthritis; rickets is a deficiency of vitamin D
3. carpal tunnel syndrome is a painful disorder of the wrist and hand; collagen disease is a disease of connective tissue
4. muscular dystrophy is progressive atrophy of the skeleton; myasthenia gravis is lack of muscle strength
5. osteomalacia is softening of the bones; osteoporosis is brittle porous bones
6. sarcoma is a malignant bone tumor; scoliosis is lateral curvature of the spine
7. spina bifida is a congenital defect in the spine; spondylitis is inflammation of the vertebra
8. in a closed fracture, the bone is broken with no open wound; an open fracture involves a broken bone and an external wound, with bone fragments sometimes protruding through the skin
9. a complicated fracture occurs when a broken bone has injured some internal organ; a comminuted fracture occurs when a bone breaks and splinters into pieces
10. an impacted fracture occurs when a bone is broken and one edge is wedged into another bone; an incomplete fracture occurs when the fracture does not include the whole bone

◆ ANSWERS TO THE WORD PUZZLE ON THE MUSCULOSKELETAL SYSTEM

Answer Key to Chapter 18: Eyes and Ears

◆ MATCHING: EYE STRUCTURES

1. e
2. f
3. g
4. h
5. i
6. d
7. a
8. b
9. c

◆ MULTIPLE CHOICE: EYE

1. c
2. b
3. d
4. c
5. b
6. c
7. a
8. c
9. a

IDENTIFICATION: STRUCTURES OF THE EAR

1. ear canal
2. separated from the external ear by the tympanic membrane
3. membrane labyrinth
4. partition between external and middle ear
5. between the nasopharynx and tympanic cavity
6. earwax in the ear

MULTIPLE CHOICE: EAR

1. a
2. b
3. c
4. d
5. a

ABBREVIATIONS

1. peripheral nervous system
2. with correction
3. oculus sinister left eye
4. oculus dexter right eye
5. oculus uterque both eyes or each eye
6. pupils equal, round, react to light, accommodation
7. visual acuity
8. auris dextra
9. auris sinistra
10. auris unitas

ANSWERS TO THE WORD PUZZLE ON THE SENSORY SYSTEM

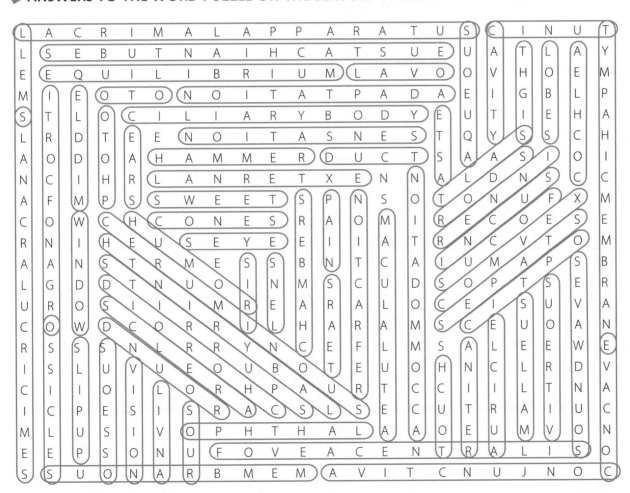

Answer Key to Chapter 19: Endocrine System

◆ MULTIPLE CHOICE

1. b
2. a
3. d
4. d
5. a
6. c
7. b
8. d
9. c
10. b

◆ MATCHING: DISORDERS OF THE ENDOCRINE SYSTEM

1. b
2. c
3. d
4. c
5. d
6. d
7. e
8. b
9. a

◆ FILL-IN

1. diabetes mellitus
2. cretinism
3. Graves' disease
4. pheochromocytoma
5. tetany
6. myxedema
7. Cushing's disease

◆ DEFINITIONS

1. involuntary muscle contraction
2. profuse perspiration
3. wasted condition; excessive leanness
4. protein hormone produced by the islets of Langerhans
5. accumulation of excess ketone bodies in tissues and fluids
6. any functional disturbance or pathologic condition in the nervous system
7. a group of drugs prescribed for the diabetic to reduce circulating glucose
8. enlargement of the thyroid gland
9. excessive activity of the thyroid gland
10. obesity, moon face, edema, and high blood pressure caused by hyperfunction of adrenal gland

◆ COMPARE AND CONTRAST

1. acidosis is a pathologic condition resulting from accumulation of acid or loss of base; anorexia is loss of appetite
2. cachexia is extreme wasting of body tissue; cataracts are clouding of the lenses of the eye
3. gangrene is death of a tissue from lack of circulation of nutrients; a gland is an organ that secretes
4. hypoglycemia is blood sugar that falls below the normal range; hypophysectomy is excision of the pituitary gland

ANSWERS TO THE WORD PUZZLE ON THE ENDOCRINE SYSTEM

A L L U D E M T P I T C O R T I S O N E
C D T E S T E S N I T C A L O R P O N N
T L R A L P H A C E L L S P T H R D A O
H A L E N O M R O H H T W O R G O W C R
K E P I N E P H R I N E A T E C G B I E
C S A N I O V A R Y A D H N R A E E T T
A Y D S O Y C S R N I Y O I M L S T U S
B H R U D A I O D O R R N G C T A E R O
D P E L I T I R R O E E R N M I R C U D
E E N R O Y I T S O I U M I T E L I L A
E P A N E G H D S Y I Z I C A N E D I F
F Y L T E T A O S R I C I H S I N D I O
V A H N N A S T T E N L N O O T N O M N L
I E A A E M S E C G L A N D R A D H A L
P N T O O T S U M A L A H T O P Y H I
A O H S P U G H S A E R C N A P P T A C
G F S H L D U C T L S F E M A L E I L E
E S T R O G E N S E S O X Y T O C I N E
N S E B O L D N A L G Y R A T I U T I P

Answer Key to Chapter 20: Cancer Medicine

WRITE IN

1. polyp, papilloma
2. basal cell carcinoma
3. leukemia
4. medullablastoma
5. lymphoma
6. chrondosarcoma
7. melanoma
8. osteosarcoma
9. fibroid
10. oat cell carcinoma

MATCHING: DIAGNOSIS

1. d
2. j
3. h
4. g
5. a
6. i
7. e
8. c
9. f
10. b

◆ **MULTIPLE CHOICE**

1. a
2. d
3. b
4. a
5. b
6. c
7. a
8. c
9. d
10. b
11. c
12. d

◆ **DEFINITIONS**

1. neoplasm that is cancerous as opposed to benign
2. movement of cancer cells from one part of the body to another
3. growing rapidly
4. reproducing repeatedly by cell division

Bibliography

Barton-Burke, Margaret, and Gail M. Wilkes. *Cancer Therapies.* Sudbury, MA: Jones and Bartlett Publishers; 2006.

Bonow, Robert, Douglas Mann, Douglas Zipes, and Peter Libby. *Braunwald's Heart Disease: A Textbook of Cardiovascular Medicine, Single Volume,* 9th ed. Philadelphia: Elsevier; 2011.

Donnersberger, Anne B. *A Laboratory Textbook of Anatomy and Physiology: Cat Version,* 9th ed. Sudbury, MA: Jones and Bartlett Publishers; 2010.

Dorland, W. A. Newman. *Dorland's Illustrated Medical Dictionary.* Philadelphia: Elsevier; 2011.

Hall, John, John E. Hall, and Arthur C. Guyton. *Textbook of Medical Physiology,* 12th ed. Philadelphia: Elsevier; 2010.

Hawkes, Christopher, Jaime Bosch, Guadalupe Garcia-Tsao, and Francis Chan. *Clinical Gastroenterology and Hepatology,* 2nd ed. Malden, MA: Wiley-Blackwell; 2012.

Hay, David W. *Little Black Book of Gastroenterology,* 3rd ed. Burlington, MA: Jones & Bartlett Learning; 2011.

Mason, Robert J., V. Broaddus, Thomas Martin, Talmadge King, Dean Schraufnagel, John Murray, and Jay Nadel. *Murray and Nadel's Textbook of Respiratory Medicine,* 4th ed. Philadelphia: Elsevier; 2010.

Mosby's Dictionary of Medicine, Nursing & Health Professions, 9th ed. St. Louis, MO: Elsevier; 2013.

Pagana, Kathleen D., Timothy J. Pagana, and Sandra McDonald. *Mosby's Canadian Manual of Diagnostic and Laboratory Tests.* Philadelphia: Elsevier; 2012.

Patton, Kevin, Gary Thibodeau, and Matthew Douglas. *Anatomy & Physiology Outline for Essentials of Anatomy & Physiology (User Guide and Access Code).* Philadelphia: Elsevier; 2011.

Ropper, Allan H., and Martin Samuels. *Adams and Victor's Principles of Neurology,* 9th ed. Columbus, OH: McGraw-Hill; 2009.

Stanfield, Peggy S. *Nutrition and Diet Therapy: Self-Instruction Modules,* 5th ed. Sudbury, MA: Jones and Bartlett Publishers; 2010.

Wilkes, Gail M., and Margaret Barton-Burke. *2013 Oncology Nursing Drug Handbook.* Burlington, MA: Jones & Bartlett Learning; 2013.

Wu, Alan. *Tietz Clinical Guide to Laboratory Tests*, 4th ed. Philadelphia: Elsevier; 2006.

Yamada, Tadataka, William L. Hasler, John M. Inadomi, Michselle A. Anderson, and Robert S. Brown, Jr. *Handbook of Gastroenterology*, 2nd ed. Philadelphia: Lippincott Williams & Wilkins; 2005.

Index

Note: Page numbers followed by *f* or *t* indicate material in figures and tables, respectively.

A

AB. *See* abortion
abbreviations
    activity and toiletry, 76*t*
    administering substances, 74*t*–75*t*
    cardiovascular, 195, 195*t*–196*t*
    diagnostic, 82*t*–87*t*
    diet orders, 75*t*–76*t*
    frequencies, 73*t*
    laboratory, 84*t*–87*t*
    laboratory tests, x-rays, and pulmonary function, 76*t*–77*t*
    miscellaneous, 77*t*–78*t*
    musculoskeletal system, 269*t*
    services or units in a healthcare facility, 72*t*
    weights and measurements, 47, 47*t*–49*t*, 73*t*–74*t*
abdomen, 100*t*
    flat plate of, 150*t*
    quadrants and division of, 151*f*, 151*t*
abdominal cavity, 100*t*, 115*t*, 141
abdominal reference terms, digestive system, 151*t*
abdominal regions, 115*f*
abducens, 211*t*
abduction, 264*t*
abortion (AB), 100*t*, 238*t*
abscess, 100*t*, 238*t*
    brain, 212*t*
    lung, 165*t*
absorption, digestive system, 139, 151*t*
accessory glands, 236*t*
accommodation, 283*t*
accredited record technician (ART), 62*t*
acetabulum, 261*t*
achalasia, 153*t*

acid phosphatase, 314*t*
acidosis, 302*t*
acne vulgaris, 126*t*
acoustic meatus, 286*t*
acoustic neuroma, 285*t*
acquired immunodeficiency syndrome (AIDS), 240*t*
acromegaly, clinical condition, 298*t*, 300*f*
actinic, 129*t*
activity, abbreviations for, 76*t*
acute, 101*t*
AD. *See* auris dextra
Addison's disease, 298*t*
adduction, 264*t*
adenocarcinoma, 320*t*
adenoids, 197*t*
adenoma, 310
adhesion, 101*t*, 146*t*
administering substances, abbreviations for, 74*t*–75*t*
adnexa, 101*t*, 237*t*
adrenal gland, 227, 297*t*
adrenalectomy, 298*t*
adrenogenital syndrome, 299*t*
adrenomegaly, 299*t*
adult/acute respiratory distress syndrome (ARDS), 165*t*
advanced practice nurse (APN), 62*t*
aerosol, 168*t*
affect, 217*t*
AFP. *See* alpha-fetoprotein
aggression, 217*t*
agranulocytes, 189*t*
AIDS. *See* acquired immunodeficiency syndrome
albinism, 129*t*
albuminuria, 233*t*
alcoholism, 146*t*

alimentary tract. *See* digestive system
allergy, skin, 128*t*
allogeneic, 316*t*
alopecia, 129*t*
alpha-fetoprotein (AFP), 314*t*
ALS. *See* amyotrophic lateral sclerosis
alveoli, 161
alveolus, 165*t*
Alzheimer's disease, 212*t*
ambivalence, 217*t*
amblyopia, 280*t*
amenorrhea, 230
amnesia, 217*t*
amniocentesis, 241*t*
amniotic fluid, 241*t*
amniotic sac, 241*t*
amputation, 268*t*
amyotrophic lateral sclerosis (ALS), 212*t*
ANA. *See* antinuclear antibodies
anabolism, 151*t*
anasarca, 153*t*
anastomosis, 148*t*
anatomical position, 111
anemia, 191*t*
anencephaly, 212*t*
anesthesia (OB), 241*t*
aneurysm, 191*t*
angina pectoris, 191*t*
angiogram, 215*t*
angiography, 193*t*
angioplasty, 193*t*
anisocoria, 283*t*
ankylosing disorder, 266*t*
anogenital area, 121
anomaly, 101*t*
anorexia nervosa, 146*t*, 302*t*
anoxia, 168*t*
ANS. *See* autonomic nervous system
antepartum, 241*t*
anthracosis, 165*t*
antiandrogens, 317*t*
antibodies, 197*t*
anticoagulant, 193*t*
antihypertensive drug, 193*t*
antinuclear antibodies (ANA), 269*t*
antistreptolysin O (ASO), 269*t*
anuria, 233*t*
anus, 145*t*
aorta, 189*t*
aortic, 188*t*
apex, 187*t*
Apgar, 241*t*
aphasia, 218*t*
APN. *See* advanced practice nurse
apnea, 168*t*
aponeurosis, 260*t*
apothecaries weight, 47*t*
appendectomy, 148*t*
appendicitis, 146*t*

appendicular skeleton, 251, 257*t*
aqueous humor, 279*t*
arachnoid, 207–208, 211*t*
arbor vitae, 210
ARDS. *See* adult/acute respiratory distress syndrome
areola, 237*t*
arrhythmia, 191*t*
ART. *See* accredited record technician
arteries, 179*f*, 180*f*, 182, 186*f*
arteriogram, 215*t*
arterioles, 182
arteriosclerosis, 191*t*
arthritis, 265*t*
arthrocentesis, 268*t*
arthroscopy, 268*t*
arthrotomy, 268*t*
AS. *See* auris sinistra
asbestosis, 165*t*
ascending colon, 145*t*
ascites, 153*t*
ASO. *See* antistreptolysin O
asphyxiation, 165*t*
aspirate, 313*t*
asthma, 165*t*
astigmatism, 280*t*
asystole, 191*t*
ataxia, 218*t*
atelectasis, 165*t*
atherosclerosis, 191*t*
atrioventricular node, 188*t*
atrium, 187*t*
atypical hyperplasia, 320*t*
AU. *See* aures unitas
audiometer, 286*t*
audiometrist, 286*t*
auditory, 212*t*, 286*t*
auditory tube. *See* Eustachian tube
aures unitas (AU), 286*t*
auris dextra (AD), 286*t*
auris sinistra (AS), 286*t*
auscultation, 101*t*, 193*t*
autism, 217*t*
autoclave, 101*t*
autologous, 316*t*
autologous bone marrow transplantation, 316*t*
autonomic nervous system (ANS), 210, 211*t*–212*t*
avoirdupois weight, 47*t*
axial skeleton, 251
axilla, 101*t*, 121
axis, 257*t*
azoturia, 232*t*

B

Babinski's sign, 215*t*
bacteria
    root words for, 24
        skin infection, 126*t*–127*t*
bacteriuria, 233*t*

balanoplasty, 238t
ball and socket, 259t
balloon angioplasty, 193t
barium enema, 314t
barium swallow, 149t
Bartholin's cyst, 238t
Bartholin's glands, 237t
basophils, 189t
BCG vaccine, 316t
Bell's palsy, 212t
benign, 320t
benign prostatic hypertrophy (BPH), 238t
biceps brachii, 263t
bifurcation, 169t
biofeedback, 218t
biologic agents, 126t–127t
    and skin infection, 126t–127t
biopsy, 101t, 125t, 148t, 149t, 313t
bipolar disorder, 217t
bladder distention, 233t
blepharitis, 280t
blepharoptosis, 280t
blood chemistries, 233t
blood components, 189t–190t
blood gases, 169t
blood pressure, 190t
blood tests, 149t
blood urea nitrogen (BUN), 233t
blood vessels, 178, 181f, 182, 185f
    tumor, 308f
    types of, 189t
bloody show, 241t
body cavities, 115t
body openings, 34t
body parts
    abdominal regions, 115f
    cavities, 114, 115t–116t
    diagrams, 115f
    digestive system, 139–144
    planes, 114, 114f, 116t
    root words for, 97, 97t–99t
    sagittal section of, 115f
    structural units of, 112t–113t
body planes, 116t
bolus, 140
bone-marrow aspirate, 315t
bones
    body, 258t
    disorders, 265t–266t
    functions of, 250–251
    head, 259t
    injuries, 265t
    joints and accessory parts, 259t–260t
    medical management, 268t–269t
    overview of, 250–253
    processes, depressions, and holes, 260, 261t
borborygmus, 146t
botulism, 146t
Bowman's capsule, 231t

BPH. See benign prostatic hypertrophy
bradycardia, 193t
bradypnea, 165t
braille, 283t
brain, 206–208, 210, 211t
brain stem, 211t
brain tumor, 215t
breasts, 124t
bronchi, 161
    anterior aspect of, 163f
bronchiectasis, 165t
bronchioles, 161, 165t
bronchitis, 165t
bronchodilator, 169t
bronchoscope, 169t
bronchoscopy, 169t, 313t
bronchospasm, 169t
bronchus, 165t
buccal cavity, 139, 140f, 153t
buccinator, 263t
bulla, 129t
BUN. See blood urea nitrogen
bundle of His, 188t
burn, 129t
burr holes, 215t
bursa, 260t
bursitis, 265t
bypass, 149t, 193t
byssinosis, 165t

C

CA 19-9, 314t
CA 125, 314t
cachexia, 153t, 302t
caesarean, 241t
calculus, renal, 232t
callus, 129t
calyx, 231t
canal of schlemm, 283t
cancer, 320t
    benign vs. malignant, 310t
    biological terms, 316t
    diagnostic and test terms, 314t–315t
    gender differences and death rates, 308
    medical illustrations of breast, 318f–319f
    medical terms, 309
    naming principles, 310t
    overview of, 308–309
    root words of name, 311t
    screening and early detection, 312–313
    sites and tissue type, 311
    skin, 126f
    specific names, 312t
    surgical terms, 318t
    terms, 320t–321t
    treatment, 315, 316t–317t
canthus, 283t
capillaries, 182, 197t

carbon dioxide (CO$_2$), 169*t*
carbuncle, furuncle, 126*t*
carcinoembryonic antigen (CEA), 314*t*
carcinogen, 320*t*
carcinoma, 125*t*, 146*t*, 165*t*, 310*t*, 311, 320*t*
    of penis, 309*f*
    of vulva, 309*f*
cardiac arrest, 191*t*
cardiac catheterization, 193*t*
cardiac enzyme test, 193*t*
cardiac muscle, 263*t*
cardiopulmonary resuscitation (CPR), 169*t*
cardiovascular system, 113*t*, 187*t*
    abbreviations, 195, 195*t*–196*t*
    arteries, 182, 183
    blood vessels, 178, 181*f*, 182, 185*f*, 189*t*
    diagrams, 179*f*–182*f*, 184*f*–187*f*
    disorders affecting, 191*t*–192*t*
    functions of, 183, 197*t*
    heart, 178, 181*f*, 182–183
        anterior structure of, 184*f*
        diagram of, 184*f*
        failure, 193*f*
        parts of, 183
        posterior structure of, 185*f*
    overview of, 178–183
    surgery, lab, and medical tests, 193*t*–195*t*
    veins, 182–183
cardiovascular technologists and technicians, 178
carinii pneumonia, 198*t*
carpal tunnel syndrome, 213*t*, 265*t*
cartilage, 265*t*
CAT. *See* computed axial tomography
catabolism, 159*t*
cataract disorder, 280*t*, 302*t*
cataract extraction, 282*t*
catatonia, 217*t*
catgut, 101*t*
catheter, 101*t*, 231*t*
catheterization, 233*t*
cauda equina, 218*t*
cautery, 125*t*
CC, 283*t*
CEA. *See* carcinoembryonic antigen
cecum, 145*t*
celiac disease, 146*t*
cell, 112*t*
cell membrane, 112*t*
cellulitis, 127*t*
central nervous system (CNS), 206, 210, 296
cephalopelvic disproportion (CPD), 241*t*
cerebellum, 210, 211*t*
cerebral cortex, 208
cerebral palsy, 213*t*
cerebrospinal fluid, 208, 211*t*
cerebrovascular accident (CVA), 192*t*, 213*t*
cerebrum, 208, 211*t*
cerumen, 121, 284*t*

cervical, 101*t*
cervix, 237*t*
chalazion, 280*t*
cheiloplasty, 149*t*
chemotherapy, 316*t*
Cheyne-Stokes, 169*t*
CHF. *See* congestive heart failure
chiropractor (DC), 61*t*
chlamydia, 240*t*
cholangiography, 150*t*
cholecystectomy, 149*t*
choledochoduodenostomy, 149*t*
cholelithiasis, 146*t*
cholesteatoma, 285*t*
choroid, 277, 279*t*
chromosomes, 112*t*
chronic, 101*t*
chronic brain syndrome, 214*t*
chronic obstructive pulmonary disease (COPD), 166*t*
cicatrix, 129*t*
ciliary body, 277
ciliary muscle, 279*t*
circulation, 188*t*
circulatory system, 183, 186, 187*t*–188*t*
    blood components, 189*t*–190*t*
    blood pressure, 190*t*
    blood vessels, 178, 182, 185*f*
circumcision, 238*t*
cirrhosis, 146*t*
clavicle, 258*t*
cleft lip/palate, 146*t*
climacteric, 230
clinical disorders
    affecting cardiovascular system, 191*t*–192*t*
        digestive system, 146*t*–148*t*
        muscular system, 265*t*–266*t*
clinical laboratory scientist, 62*t*
clinitest, 234*t*
clitoris, 237*t*
CNA. *See* nursing assistant
CNS. *See* central nervous system
coarctation, 191*t*
coccidioidin, 129*t*
coccidioidomycosis, 166*t*
coccyx, 101*t*
cochlea, 278
colitis, 146*t*
collagen disease, 265*t*
collateral circulation, 193*t*
colonoscopy, 150*t*, 313*t*
colony-stimulating factors, 316*t*
color
    blindness, 280*t*
    prefixes for, 24, 25*t*
colostomy, 149*t*
colporrhaphy, 239*t*
colposcopy, 239*t*
comatose, 218*t*

combining forms, roots and, 9–12
commissurotomy, 193*t*
compound words, 6
computed axial tomography (CAT), 194*t*, 314*t*
computerized tomography (CT), 215*t*
concussion, 213*t*
conduction deafness, 285*t*
congenital defects, 101*t*, 191*t*
congestive heart failure (CHF), 191*t*
conjunctiva, 278, 279*t*
conjunctivitis, 280*t*
connective tissue, 113*t*
consolidation, 169*t*
continent, 234*t*
contracture, 264*t*
contrecoup, 218*t*
convulsion, 213*t*, 302*t*
Coombs' test, 242*t*
COPD. *See* chronic obstructive pulmonary disease
copulation, 227
cor pulmonale condition, 166*t*
cord tumor, 215*t*
cordotomy, 215*t*
cornea, 276, 279*t*
corneal ulcer, 280*t*
coronal, 116*t*
coronary arteries, 189*t*
coronary artery bypass graft, 194*t*
coronary thrombosis, 192*t*
cortex, 231*t*
coryza, 166*t*
cough, 166*t*
Cowper's glands, 235*t*
CPD. *See* cephalopelvic disproportion
CPR. *See* cardiopulmonary resuscitation
cranial cavity, 116*t*
cranial nerves, 211*t*
craniotomy, 215*t*
C-reactive protein (CRP), 269*t*
cretinism, 299*t*
croup condition, 166*t*
CRP. *See* C-reactive protein
cryoextraction, 282*t*
cryoprobe, 283*t*
cryoretinopexy, 282*t*
cryosurgery, 317*t*
cryptitis, 146*t*
cryptorchidism, 238*t*
CT. *See* computerized tomography
culdocentesis, 242*t*
Cushing's disease, 299*t*
cuticle, 121, 123*t*
CVA. *See* cerebrovascular accident
cyanosis, 169*t*, 191*t*
cyst, 129*t*, 320*t*
cystectomy, 316*t*
cystic fibrosis, 166*t*
cystitis, 232*t*

cystitome, 283*t*
cystocele, 239*t*
cystoscopy, 234*t*, 313*t*
cytoplasm, 112*t*

D

dacryoadenitis, 280*t*
dacryocystitis, 280*t*
dacryocystotomy, 282*t*
dacryolith, 280*t*
DC. *See* chiropractor
deafness, 285*t*
debridement, 125*t*
decibel, 286*t*
deciduous, 152*t*
deep tendon reflex (DTR), 218*t*
defecation, digestive system, 139
defibrillator, 101*t*
degenerative joint disease (DJD), 269*t*
deglutition, 152*t*
delirium, 217*t*
deltoid, 263*t*
delusion, 217*t*
dental assistant, 61*t*, 120
dental caries, 153*t*
dental hygienist, 61*t*, 120
dental technician, 61*t*
dentist, 61*t*
depression, 217*t*
dermabrasion, 125*t*
dermatologist, 123
dermatology, 123, 129*t*
dermatome, 125*t*
dermis, 120
    components of, 121*f*
    corium, 123*t*
descending colon, 145*t*
descriptive word elements, 99*t*–100*t*
detached retina, 280*t*
deviated septum, 166*t*
diabetes insipidus, 299*t*
diabetes mellitus, 128*t*, 299*t*
diagnoses and symptoms, suffixes for, 13–15
diagnostic
    abbreviations, 82*t*–87*t*
    cancer terms, 313*t*
    eye terms, 282*t*
    genitourinary system terms, 233*t*–235*t*
    nervous system, 215*t*–216*t*
dialysate, 232*t*
dialysis, 232*t*
diaphoresis, 302*t*
diaphragm, 116*t*, 165*t*, 178
diarthrodial joints, 257*f*
diastolic pressure, 190*t*
dick test, 129*t*

diet orders, abbreviations for, 75*t*–76*t*
dietetic technician, registered (DTR), 62*t*, 112
dietitians, 112
digestion, 139, 152*t*
digestive system, 113*t*, 138
    abdominal cavity, 141
    abdominal reference terms, 151*t*
    clinical disorders, 146*t*–148*t*
    diagrams, 139, 140, 142–144
    function of, 138–139
    miscellaneous terms, 153*t*–154*t*
    organs of, major and accessory, 145*t*
    pathologies of, 144*f*
    processes, 138–139, 151*t*–152*t*
    tests, 149*t*–150*t*
digital examination, 150*t*
digitalize, 194*t*
dilatation, 101*t*
dilatation and curettage (D&C), 239*t*
dilation, 101*t*
diopter, 283*t*
diphtheria, 166*t*
distal, 264*t*
diuresis, 234*t*
diuretic, 194*t*
diverticulitis, 146*t*
division of abdomen, 151*f*, 151*t*
DJD. *See* degenerative joint disease
Doppler, 194*t*
DTR. *See* deep tendon reflex; dietetic technician, registered
ductal carcinoma in situ, 320*t*
ducts, 197*t*
duodenum, 145*t*
dura mater, 208, 211*t*
dyscrasia, 194*t*
dysentery, 146*t*
dysphonia, 169*t*
dyspnea, 169*t*
dystocia, 242*t*
dysuria, 234*t*

E

eardrum, 278
ears
    diagram of, 277*f*, 278
    disorders, 285*t*
    medical terms, 286*t*–287*t*
    overview of, 278
    structure of, 284*t*
    surgical terms, 286*t*
ecchymosis, 129*t*
echocardiography, 194*t*
echoencephalogram (EEG), 215*t*
echolalia, 217*t*
ECT. *See* electroconvulsive therapy
ectopic pregnancy, 242*t*
eczema, 128*t*
EDC. *See* expected date of confinement

edema, 101*t*
EEG. *See* echoencephalogram
effacement, 242*t*
effusion, 166*t*
egestion, digestive system, 139
ejaculatory duct vesicle, 236*t*
EKG. *See* electroencephalogram
electrical stimulation, 268*t*
electrocardiogram, 194*t*
electroconvulsive therapy (ECT), 217*t*
electrodesiccation, 125*t*
electroencephalogram (EKG), 216*t*
electromyogram, 268*t*
electromyography, 268*t*
electronystagmography, 283*t*
elimination substance, 152*t*
emaciation, 146*t*, 302*t*
embolism, 191*t*
embolus, 101*t*, 191*t*
embryonic tumors, 312*t*
emergency medical technicians, 178
emesis, 101*t*, 146*t*
emmetropia, 283*t*
emphysema, 166*t*
encephalitis, 213*t*
encephalon, 211*t*, 218*t*
endarterectomy, 194*t*
endocarditis, 191*t*
endocardium, 188*t*
endocrine cells, 141
endocrine glands, 294, 295*f*, 296, 302*t*
endocrine system, 113*t*
    classification and functions of, 296*t*–298*t*
    disorders, 298*t*–300*t*
    glands of, 294, 296
    overview of, 294–296
    terms, miscellaneous, 302*t*
endocrinology, 296
endodontist, 61*t*
endometriosis, 239*t*
endotracheal (ET) tube, 169*t*
enema, 101*t*, 153*t*
enteropath, 153*t*
enucleation, 282*t*
enuresis, 234*t*
enzyme, 153*t*
eosinophils, 189*t*
epicardium, 188*t*
epidermis, 120, 123*t*
    components of, 121*f*
epidermoid carcinoma, 320*t*
epididymis, 236*t*
epididymitis, 238*t*
epiglottis, 152*t*, 161
epilepsy, 213*t*
episiotomy, 242*t*
epistaxis, 166*t*
epithelial tissue, 113*t*
erosion, 129*t*

eructation, 152t
eruption, 130t
erysipelas, 128t
erythema, 130t
erythrocyte sedimentation rate (ESR), 269t
eschar, 130t
escharotomy, 125t
esophageal atresia, 146t
esophageal varices, 147t
esophagitis, 147t
esophagogastroduodenoscopy (EGD), 150t
esophagus, 141, 145t
ESR. *See* erythrocyte sedimentation rate
estrogen/progesterone receptors, 230, 315t
ET tube. *See* endotracheal tube
ethmoid, 257t
Eustachian salpingitis, 285t
Eustachian tube, 278, 284t
exacerbation, 102t
exanthem, 130t
excoriation, 130t
excretion, 102t, 152t
excretory system, organs of, 228f
exercise stress test, 194t
exfoliation, 130t
exocrine glands, 141, 294, 296, 302t
exophthalmic goiter, 299t
expected date of confinement (EDC), 242t
expectorant, 169t
expectoration, 166t
extension, 264t
external ear, 284t
external fixation, 268t
external genitalia, 236t
external term, cancer treatment, 316t
extracorporeal shock wave lithotripsy (ESWL), 150t
eye bank, 283t
eyes
    diagnostic and surgery terms, 282t
    disorders, 280t–281t
    medical terms, 283t–284t
    structure of, 276–278, 277f, 279t

F

facial, 212t
fallopian tubes (oviducts), 237t
familial polyposis, 320t
fascia, 102t, 260t
febrile, 102t
fecal impaction, 147t
female(s)
    anatomy, 230
    clinical conditions, 238t–239t
    conditions, 240–241, 240t
    organs, 237t
    pregnancy and birth, 241t–243t
    reproductive system, 230
    sexually transmitted diseases, 240–241

femoral, 147t
femur, 258t
fenestration, 286t
fertilization, 227
fetal heart tones (FHT), 242t
fibrillation, 102t, 191t
fibrinogen, 190t
fibroid, 239t, 320t
fibrosis, 166t
fibula, 258t
fingernails, 121
fissure, 130t, 218t
fistula, 153t, 239t
flaccid, 219t
flail chest, 166t
flat plate of abdomen, 150t
flexion, 264t
flexure, 147t
floaters (in vitreous), 280t
floating kidney, 232t
flu, 166t
fluid, 197t
fluid-filled canals, 278
fluoroscopy, 150t
foramen magnum, 219t
foramen structure, 261t
forceps delivery, 242t
foreign body in the eye, 280t
fossa, 260t
fracture, 265t
    reduction, 268t
    skull, 213t
    types of, 262f
frequency
    abbreviations for, 73t
    urgency, 234t
frontal, 258t, 259t
fulguration, 125t, 317t
functions of skin, 124t
fundoscope, 283t
fundoscopy, 282t
fundus, 283t
fungal infection, skin, 127t
furunculosis, 285t

G

gallbladder, 141, 145t
gamma globulins, 153t
ganglion, 219t
gangrene, 130t, 302t
    of foot, 131f
gastrectomy, 149t
gastric bypass, 149t
gastric ulcers, 147t
gastritis, 147t
gastrocnemius, 263t
gastroenteritis, 147t
gastroenterologist, 138

gastroesophageal reflux disease (GERD), 147*t*

gastrointestinal series (GIs), 150*t*

gastrointestinal (GI) system. *See* digestive system

gastroscopy, 150*t*

gavage, 153*t*

genital herpes, 240*t*

genital warts, 240*t*

genitourinary system, 113*t*
    clinical conditions, 232*t*–233*t*
    female, 238*t*–239*t*
    male, 238*t*
    diagnostic terms, 233*t*–235*t*
    organs
        female, 237*t*
        male, 235*t*–236*t*
    overview of, 226–230
    pregnancy and birth, 241*t*–243*t*
    reproductive system
        female, 229*f*, 230
        male, 227–229, 229*f*
    sexually transmitted diseases, 240–241
    urinary system, 226–227, 227*f*

gestation, 242*t*

gestational diabetes, 299*t*

glands, 302*t*
    endocrine, 294, 295*f*, 296
    exocrine, 294, 296
    salivary, 140, 145*t*
    skin, 121

glans penis, 235*t*

glaucoma, 280*t*

glomerulonephritis, 232*t*

glomerulus, 231*t*

glossal, 153*t*

glossitis, 147*t*

glossopharyngeal, 212*t*

gluteus maximus, 263*t*

glycosuria, 234*t*

goiter (simple), 299*t*

gonads, 228, 235*t*

gonioscopy, 282*t*

gonorrhea, 240*t*

Goodell's sign, 242*t*

gout, 265*t*

graft, 125*t*

grand mal seizure, 213*t*

granulocytes, 189*t*

gravida, 242*t*

groove, 261*t*

guide dogs, 283*t*

gynecology, 230

gyrus, 219*t*

H

hair, 120, 121
    nails, 124*t*

hallucination, 217*t*

hamstring, 263*t*

Hashimoto's disease, 299*t*

hay fever, 166*t*

HCG. *See* human chorionic gonadotropin

health professions, 112
    additional, 64, 64*t*–65*t*
    list of terms, titles, and pronunciations for, 61*t*–63*t*

healthcare social worker, 63*t*

hearing aid, 286*t*

hearing-ear dogs, 286*t*

heart. *See* cardiovascular system

heart block, 192*t*

heart murmur, 192*t*

hematoma, 213*t*

hematuria, 234*t*

hemisphere, 219*t*

hemoglobin, 162, 194*t*

hemophilia, 192*t*

hemoptysis, 169*t*

hemorrhage, 102*t*
    subconjunctival, 280*t*

hemothorax, 166*t*

heparin, 194*t*

hepatitis, 147*t*

hernia, 147*t*

herniated nucleus pulposus, 265*t*

herniorrhaphy, 149*t*

herpes genitalis, 127*t*

herpes ophthalmicus, 127*t*

herpes simplex, 127*t*

herpes zoster, 127*t*, 213*t*
    ophthalmic, 280*t*
    hiatal hernia, 147*t*, 166*t*
    hiatus, 169*t*
    hiccup condition, 166*t*
    hilus, 169*t*
    hinge, 259*t*
    Hirschsprung's disease, 147*t*
    hirsutism, 130*t*
    histoplasmosis, 128*t*, 166*t*
    Hodgkin's disease, 192*t*
    Holter monitor, 194*t*
    homeostasis, 116, 116*t*, 227
    hormone therapy, 317*t*
    hormones, 294, 296
    human chorionic gonadotropin (HCG), 314*t*

humerus, 258*t*

Huntington's chorea, 213*t*

hyaline, 167*t*

hyaline membrane disease, 167*t*

hydrocele, 238*t*

hydrocephalus, 213*t*

hydronephrosis, 232*t*

hydrosalpinx, 239*t*

hyfracator, 125*t*

hymen, 237*t*

hyoid, 259*t*

hyperalimentation, 153*t*

hypercapnia, 169*t*

hyperglycemia, 299*t*

hyperopia, 280t
hyperplasia, 320t
hypersplenism, 198t
hypertension, 190t, 192t
hyperthyroidism, 299t
hyperventilation, 169t
hypochondria, 217t
hypoglossal, 212t
hypoglycemia, 302t
hypoglycemic agent, 302t
hypophysectomy, 302t
hyposensitization, 169t
hypothalamus, 210, 296
hypothyroidism, 299t
hypoxia, 169t
hysterectomy, 239t, 317t
hysteria, 217t
hysterosalpingogram, 239t

I

ICN. *See* intensive care nursery
icterus, 102t
ileostomy, 149t
ileum, 145t
imaging, cancer diagnostic tests, 314t
immunization, 102t
impacted cerumen, 285t
impaction, fecal, 147t
impetigo, 127t
incisors, 152t
incontinence, 102t
incontinent, 234t
induction, 242t
infarction, 192t
infections and biologic agents, skin, 126t–127t
inflammation, 102t
influenza, 167t
ingestion, digestive system, 138, 152t
inguinal, clinical disorder, 147t
injury, eye, 280t
inner ear, 284t
insemination, 242t
insulin, 302t
intake and output (I&O), 234t
integumentary system, 113t
    hair, 120, 121
    nails, 121
    overview of, 120–123
    skin
        allergy, 128t
        diagrams of, 122f, 123f
        disorders from systemic diseases, 128t
        functions of, 121–122, 124t
        glands, 121
        growths, 125t
        infections and biologic agents, 126t–127t
        parts of, 123t–124t
        surgical processes, 125t

tests, 129t
    vocabulary terms, 129t–131t
intensive care nursery (ICN), 242t
intermittent positive pressure breathing (IPPB), 170t
internal term, cancer treatment, 316t
interphalangeal, 260t
intervertebral, 260t
intrapartum, 242t
intravenous pyelogram/pyelography (IVP), 234t, 314t
intussusception, 147t
IPPB. *See* intermittent positive pressure breathing
ipsilateral, 219t
iridectomy, 282t
iridencleisis, 282t
iris, 277, 279t
iritis, 281t
irritable bowel syndrome (IBS), 147t
ischemia, 102t, 192t
islets of Langerhans, 141
IVP. *See* intravenous pyelogram/pyelography

J

jaundice, 102t
jejunum, 145t
joints and accessory parts, 259t–260t

K

Kaposi's sarcoma, 198t, 320t
keloid, 130t
keratoconus, 281t
keratoplasty, 282t
keratosis, 125t
ketoacidosis, 302t
ketonuria, 234t
ketosis, 302t
kidney, ureter, and bladder (KUB), 234t
kidneys, 226, 231t
Korsakoff's syndrome, 213t
KUB. *See* kidney, ureter, and bladder
Kussmaul breathing, 170t
kyphosis, 265t

L

labia majora, 237t
labia minora, 237t
laboratory abbreviations, 84t–87t
    tests, screenings, and procedures, 76t–77t
laboratory procedures, 216t
laboratory tests, 149t
labyrinthitis, 285t
laceration, 130t
lachrymal, 259t
lacrimal glands, 278
lacrimation, 283t
lamina, 260t
laminectomy, 216t
    with diskectomy, 268t

Landsteiner types, 190*t*

laparoscopy, 239*t*

laparotomy, 149*t*

large cell carcinomas, 320*t*

large intestine, 143*f*
    functions, 141

laryngectomy, 170*t*, 317*t*

laryngitis, 167*t*

laryngopharynx, 160–161

laryngoscopy, 170*t*, 313*t*

laryngotracheobronchitis, 167*t*

larynx, 161, 163*f*, 164*t*
    anterior aspect of, 163*f*

laser, 283*t*, 317*t*

laser photocoagulation, 282*t*

last menstrual period (LMP), 242*t*

latissimus dorsi, 263*t*

lavage, 153*t*
    of sinuses, 170*t*

LE. *See* lupus erythematosus

Legg-Calvé-Perthes disease, 265*t*

lens, 279*t*

lensometer, 283*t*

lesion, 130*t*

leukemia, 192*t*, 310*t*, 311

leukorrhea, 239*t*

licensed practical nurse (LPN), 63*t*

licensed vocational nurse (LVN), 63*t*

ligament, 260*t*

limbic system, 219*t*

linea nigra, 242*t*

lingual, 153*t*

liver, 144*f*, 145*t*
    body functions, 141

LMP. *See* last menstrual period

lobectomy, 170*t*

lobular carcinoma in situ, 320*t*

lochia, 242*t*

lordosis, 265*t*

low-salt diet, 194*t*

LP. *See* lumbar puncture

LPN. *See* licensed practical nurse

lumbar puncture (LP), 216*t*

lumbar sympathectomy, 216*t*

lumen, 194*t*

lumpectomy, 317*t*

lung, 161–162, 164*t*
    internal structure of, 164*f*

lung abscess, 167*t*

lung pleura, 178

lunula, 121

lupus erythematosus (LE), 128*t*, 265*t*

luteinizing hormone-releasing hormone agonist, 317*t*

LVN. *See* licensed vocational nurse

lymph system, pathologic conditions of, 198*t*

lymphadenopathy, 198*t*

lymphangiography, 314*t*

lymphatic system, 182*f*, 196–197
    components of, 197
    parts and functions of, 197*t*
    pathologic conditions, 198*t*

lymphocytes, 189*t*, 197*t*

lymphoid tumors, 312*t*

lymphoma, 198*t*

M

macrophage, 197*t*

macular degeneration, 281*t*

macule, 130*t*

magnetic resonance imaging (MRI), 150*t*, 194*t*, 216*t*

major depression, 217*t*

male(s)
    clinical conditions, 238*t*, 240–241, 240*t*
    organs, 235*t*–236*t*
    reproductive system, 227–229, 229*f*
    sexually transmitted diseases, 240–241

malignant, 320*t*

malingering, 217*t*

malleolus, 261*t*

malleus (hammer), 278

mammary glands, 121, 237*t*

mandible, 152*t*, 258*t*, 259*t*

manometer, 219*t*

mantoux, 129*t*, 170*t*

masseter, 263*t*

mastectomy, 317*t*

mastication, 152*t*

mastoidectomy, 286*t*

mastoiditis, 285*t*

maxilla, 152*t*, 258*t*, 259*t*

meatus, 231*t*

meconium, 242*t*

mediastinum, 115*t*

medical assistant, 62*t*

medical librarian (MLA), 62*t*

medical record administrator, 62*t*

medical technologist, 62*t*

medical terms, review of, 100, 100*t*–103*t*

medulla structure, 231*t*

megalomania, 217*t*

meibomian cyst, 281*t*

melanocytes, 121

melena, 148*t*

Meniere's disease, 285*t*

meninges, 207, 211*t*

meningitis, 213*t*

meningocele, 214*t*

meniscectomy, 268*t*

meniscus, 260*t*

menopause, 230

metabolism, 116, 116*t*, 124*t*

metastasis, 102*t*

metastatic lung cancer, 311

metastatic tumors, 308

metric system, 47*t*

MG. *See* myasthenia gravis
microscopic examination, special cancer diagnostic tests, 315*t*
micturate, 234*t*
middle ear, 284*t*
midsagittal, 116*t*
midsternum, 178
miotic/myotic, 283*t*
miscarriage, 239*t*
miscellaneous terms, endocrine system, 302*t*
mitral, 188*t*
MLA. *See* medical librarian
molars substance, 152*t*
monilia, 239*t*
moniliasis, 239*t*
monoclonal immunoglobulins, 314*t*
monocytes, 189*t*
mononucleosis, 198*t*
mons pubis, 237*t*
motion, 264*t*
mouth, 140, 145*t*
MRI. *See* magnetic resonance imaging
MS. *See* multiple sclerosis
mucus, 102*t*
multigravida, 242*t*
multipara, 242*t*
multiple sclerosis (MS), 214*t*
muscle atrophy, 264*t*
muscle hypertrophy, 264*t*
muscle system, clinical disorders, 265*t*–266*t*
muscle tissue, 113*t*
muscle tone, 264*t*
muscles, 254*f*–256*f*
    categories of, 261
    disorders, 265*t*–266*t*
    injuries, 265*t*
    medical management, 268*t*–269*t*
    motion, 264*t*
    physiological status of, 264*t*
    properties of, 253
    role of, 253
muscular dystrophy, 266*t*
musculoskeletal system, 113*t*. *See also* bones; muscles; skeleton
    abbreviations, 269*t*
    overview of, 250–255
myasthenia gravis (MG), 214*t*, 266*t*
mydriatic, 283*t*
myelin, 219*t*
myelogram, 216*t*, 269*t*
myelography, 216*t*
myelomeningocele, 214*t*
myocardial infarction, 192*t*
myocarditis, 192*t*
myocardium, 188*t*
myogram, 269*t*
myositis, 266*t*
myringitis, 285*t*
myringotomy, 286*t*
myxedema, 299*t*, 301*f*

N

Nagele's rule, 243*t*
nails, 121
nasal, 259*t*
nasal cavity, 164*t*
nasogastric (ng), 153*t*
nasopharynx, 160
nausea and vomiting (N&V), 148*t*
neonatal hypothyroidism, 301*f*
neonatal period, 243*t*
neoplasm, 308
nephrolithiasis, 232*t*
nephron, 231*t*
nephroptosis, 232*t*
nephrorrhaphy, 232*t*
nerve block, 216*t*
nerve cells (neurons), 216*t*
nerve tissue, 113*t*
nervous system (NS), 113*t*
    anatomy and physiology, 206
    brain, 206–208, 210, 211*t*
    central, 206, 210
    clinical disorders, 212*t*–215*t*
    diagnostic and surgical terms, 215*t*–216*t*
    diagrams, 207*f*–209*f*
    disorders, 212*t*–215*t*
    overview of, 206–210
    peripheral, 206–207, 210, 211*t*–212*t*
    special terms, 218*t*–219*t*
    spinal cord, 206, 207, 209*f*, 210, 211*t*
neurasthenia, 217*t*
neurilemma (sheath of Schwann), 219*t*
neurodermatitis, 128*t*
neurologist, 206
neurology, 206
neuropathy, 214*t*, 302*t*
neurosis, 217*t*
neurosurgeon, 206
neutrophils, 189*t*
nevus, 125*t*
nocturia, 234*t*
nodes, 197*t*
nodular goiter, 300*f*
nodule, 130*t*
noninfiltrating (in situ) carcinoma, 312*t*
non-small cell lung cancer, 320*t*
normal BP, 190*t*
nose, 160
nostrils, 160
nothing per os (NPO), 153*t*
NS. *See* nervous system
nuclear medicine technologists, 178
nucleus, 112*t*
numbers, prefixes for, 41, 42*t*
nummular, 130*t*
nurse practitioner, 62*t*
nursing assistant (CNA), 63*t*

nycturia, 234*t*
nystagmus, 281*t*

O

oat cell cancer, 321*t*
OB index. *See* obstetrical index
obese, 102*t*
obesity, 102*t*, 148*t*
obstetrical index (OB index), 243*t*
occipital, 258*t*, 269*t*
occupational therapist (OTR), 63*t*
oculomotor, 211*t*
oculus dexter, 283*t*
oculus sinister (OS), 284*t*
oculus uterque (OU), 284*t*
OD. *See* oculus dexter
olecranon, 261*t*
olfactory, 211*t*
oliguria, 234*t*
oophorectomy, 239*t*
open reduction internal fixation (ORIF), 269*t*
ophthalmic disorder, 280*t*
ophthalmoscope, 283*t*, 284*t*
opportunistic infections, 238*t*
optic nerve, 211*t*, 278
optometrist, 63*t*
oral cavity, 139, 140*f*
oral leukoplakia, 148*t*
oral surgeon, 61*t*
orbicularis occuli, 263*t*
orbicularis oris, 263*t*
orchiectomy, 238*t*, 317*t*
orchiopexy, 238*t*
orchitis, 238*t*
organ, 113*t*
organ of Corti, 278
organic brain syndrome, 214*t*
ORIF. *See* open reduction internal fixation
oropharynx, 160
orthodontist, 61*t*
orthopedist, 253
orthopnea, 167*t*, 170*t*
OS. *See* oculus sinister
Osgood-Schlatter disease, 266*t*
osteochondritis, 266*t*
osteochondrosis, 266*t*
osteogenic disorder, 266*t*
osteomalacia, 266*t*
osteomyelitis, 266*t*
osteoporosis, 266*t*
otitis externa, 285*t*
otitis media, 285*t*
otoplasty, 286*t*
otosclerosis, 285*t*
otoscope, 287*t*
otoscopy, 287*t*
OTR. *See* occupational therapist
OU. *See* oculus uterque

ovaries, 237*t*, 297*t*
ovariorrhexis, 300*t*
oximetry, 170*t*
oxygen (O$_2$), 170*t*

P

PA. *See* physician assistant
pacemaker, 194*t*
palate, 152*t*
palatine, 259*t*
palliative approach, 318*t*
palpable, 102*t*
palpation, 170*t*
pancreas, 141, 145*t*, 297*t*
pancreaticogastrostomy, 300*t*
pancreatitis, 148*t*, 300*t*
panhypopituitarism, 300*t*
Pap smear, 315*t*
papillae, 140, 152*t*
papilledema, 281*t*
papulae, 130*t*
paralysis, 102*t*, 219*t*, 264*t*
paralyzed, 102*t*
paramedics, 178
paranoid, 218*t*
parasitic infection, skin, 127*t*
parasympathetic component, 212*t*
parathyroid gland, 294, 297*t*
parenchyma (lung), 170*t*
paresis condition, 219*t*, 264*t*
paresthesia, 219*t*
parietal, 102*t*, 258*t*, 259*t*
parietal peritoneum, 141
parietal pleura, 162, 164*t*
Parkinson's disease, 214*t*
paronychia, 130*t*
parotid, 153*t*
parts of skin, 123*t*–124*t*
patent ductus arteriosus, 191*t*
pathologic conditions of lymph system, 198*t*
peak expiratory flow rate, 170*t*
pectoralis major, 263*t*
pedodontist, 61*t*
PEG. *See* pneumoencephalogram
pelvic cavity, 115*t*
pelvic examination, 239*t*
pelvic inflammatory disease (PID), 239*t*
pelvimeter (pelvimetry), 243*t*
penis, 235*t*
percussion, 102*t*
percussion and auscultation (P&A), 170*t*
percutaneous transhepatic cholangiography (PTC), 150*t*
percutaneous transluminal coronary angioplasty (PTCA), 195*t*
perfusion, 170*t*
pericarditis, 192*t*
pericardium, 178, 188*t*
perineum, 102*t*, 235*t*, 237*t*
periodontal disease, 152*t*

periodontist, 61*t*
peripheral nervous system (PNS), 206–207, 210, 211*t*–212*t*, 276
peripheral stem cell transplantation, 316*t*
peripheral vision, 284*t*
perirenal fat, 227
peristalsis, digestive system, 138, 152*t*
peritoneal cavity, 115*t*
peritoneum, 102*t*, 153*t*
peritonitis, 148*t*, 232*t*
PERRLA/PERLA, 284*t*
pertussis, 167*t*
PET. *See* positron emission tomography
petechia, 130*t*
petit mal seizures, 214*t*
phagocytes, 197*t*
pharmacist, 63*t*
pharmacology medical terminology, 132
pharyngitis, 167*t*
pharynx, 140, 145*t*, 160–161, 164*t*
phenylketonuria (PKU), 148*t*
pheochromocytoma, 300*t*
phlebotomy, 194*t*
PHN. *See* public health nurse
phobia, 218*t*
physical therapists, 63*t*, 206
physician assistant (PA), 63*t*
pia mater, 207, 211*t*
PID. *See* pelvic inflammatory disease
pineal, 298*t*
pinna, 278
pituitary gland, 296*t*
placenta, 243*t*
plaque, 130*t*, 192*t*
plasma, 190*t*
platelet, 190*t*
pleural cavity, 103*t*, 115*t*
pleural effusion, 167*t*
pleurisy, 167*t*
plexus, 219*t*
plural endings, 35, 35*t*–36*t*
pneumoconiosis, 167*t*
pneumoencephalogram (PEG), 216*t*
pneumogastric vagus, 212*t*
pneumonectomy, 317*t*
pneumonocystic pneumonia, 198*t*
pneumothorax, 167*t*, 170*t*
PNS. *See* peripheral nervous system
podiatrist, 62*t*
poliomyelitis, 214*t*
polydipsia, 234*t*
polyp, 321*t*
    papilloma, 310*t*
polyposis, 148*t*
pons, 210
portacaval shunt, 149*t*
portal circulation, 188*t*
positions and directions
    prefixes for, 43, 43*t*–44*t*
    terms for, 45, 45*t*–46*t*

positron emission tomography (PET), 195*t*, 216*t*
postpartum, 243*t*
postural drainage, 170*t*
PPD. *See* purified protein derivative
precancerous conditions, 312*t*
prefixes
    for color, 24, 25*t*
    commonly used, 8–9, 25, 26*t*–28*t*
    defined, 5–6
    for numbers, 41, 42*t*
    for positions and directions, 43, 43*t*–44*t*
    review of, 95–97
    with roots and suffixes, 6
pregnancy and birth terms, 241*t*–243*t*
prenatal, 243*t*
prepuce, organ, 235*t*
presbycusis, 285*t*
presbyopia, 281*t*
presenile dementia, 212*t*
presentation, 243*t*
primary/definitive approach, 318*t*
primipara, 243*t*
proctoscopy, 150*t*
productive cough, 170*t*
progesterone, 230
prolapse, 103*t*
    of uterus, 239*t*
prominence, 261*t*
pronation, 264*t*
pronunciations, 3
prophylactic approach, 318*t*
prophylaxis, 103*t*
prostate gland, 235*t*
prostatectomy, 238*t*, 317*t*
prostate-specific antige, 314*t*
prosthodontist, 61*t*
protection process, 124*t*
proximal movement, 264*t*
pruritus, 130*t*
PSA. *See* prostate-specific antige
psoriasis, 128*t*
psychiatric social worker, 63*t*
psychiatric terms, 217*t*–218*t*
psychologist, 63*t*
psychosis, 218*t*
PTCA. *See* percutaneous transluminal coronary angioplasty
pterygium surgery, 282*t*
ptosis, 281*t*
public health nurse (PHN), 62*t*
pulmonary circulation, 183, 188*t*
pulmonary functions, 170*t*
    abbreviations for, 76*t*–77*t*
pulmonary parenchyma, 170*t*
pulmonary semilunar, 188*t*
pupil structure, 277, 279*t*
purified protein derivative (PPD), 170*t*
purulent, 103*t*
pustule, 130*t*

pyelitis, 233*t*
pyloric stenosis, 148*t*
pyuria, 234*t*

Q

quadrants of abdomen, 151*f*, 151*t*
quadriceps femoris, 263*t*
quickening, 243*t*

R

radiation therapy, cancer, 316*t*
radical mastectomy, modified, 317*t*
radiology technologist, 63*t*
radionuclide scan, 314*t*
radius, 258*t*
rales, 171*t*
rapid eye movements (REM), 218*t*
rarefaction, 171*t*
RBCs. *See* red blood cells
RD. *See* registered dietitian
receptor process, 124*t*
rectocele, 148*t*
rectum, 145*t*
red blood cells (RBCs), 189*t*
reflex, 219*t*
refractive error, 284*t*
registered dietitian (RD), 62*t*
registered nurse (RN), 62*t*
rehabilitative approach, 318*t*
REM. *See* rapid eye movements
remission, 103*t*
renal artery, 231*t*
renal capsule, 231*t*
renal failure, 233*t*
renal fascia, 227
renal pelvis, 231*t*
renal transplant, 233*t*
renal tubule, 231*t*
renal vein, 231*t*
replantation procedure, 269*t*
reproductive system
    female, 230
        clinical conditions, 238*t*–239*t*
        conditions, 240–241, 240*t*
        organs, 237*t*
        pregnancy and birth, 241*t*–243*t*
    male, 227–229, 229*f*
        clinical conditions, 238*t*–239*t*
        conditions, 240–241, 240*t*
        organs, 235*t*–236*t*
resection of metastases approach, 318*t*
residual air, 171*t*
respirator, 171*t*
respiratory system, 113*t*
    body parts, 164*t*–165*t*
    diagnostic, surgical, medical procedures and general terms, 168, 168*t*–171*t*
    diagrams, 162*f*–164*f*

disorders, 165*t*–168*t*
    overview of, 160–162
respiratory therapist (RRT), 63*t*, 160
respiratory therapy technicians, 160
reticulocytes, 190*t*
retina, 278, 279*t*
retinitis, 281*t*
retinoblastoma, 281*t*
retinopathy, 281*t*
retrograde pyelogram, 234*t*
retroperitoneal, 227
Rh factors, 190*t*
rheumatic heart disease, 103*t*, 192*t*
rheumatism disorder, 266*t*
rheumatoid arthritis (RA), 267*f*, 269*t*
    factor, 269
rhinitis rhinorrhea, 167*t*
rhinoplasty, 171*t*
rhizotomy, 216*t*
rhonchi, 171*t*
rib cage, 250
rickets, 266*t*
RN. *See* registered nurse
Romberg test, 216*t*
roots, 310*t*
    for bacteria, 24
    for body parts, review, 97, 97*t*–99*t*
    for cancer, 311*t*
    and combining forms, 9–12
    defined, 6
    for scientific studies, 58*t*–59*t*
    for specialties and specialists, 59*t*–61*t*
RRT. *See* respiratory therapist
rubella disease, 128*t*
rubeola disease, 128*t*
rugae, 154*t*

S

SA node. *See* sinoatrial node
sacculi, 278
sagittal body planes, 116*t*
salivary glands, 140, 145*t*
salpingectomy, 239*t*
salpingitis, 239*t*
salpingo-oophorectomy, 317*t*
sarcoidosis, 198*t*
sarcoma, 198*t*, 266*t*, 310*t*, 311, 321*t*
SC, 284*t*
scales, crusts, 130*t*
scan, 150*t*, 171*t*, 234*t*
scapula, 258*t*
scar, cicatrix, 130*t*
Schick test, 129*t*
schizophrenia, 218*t*
sciatica, 214*t*
scientific studies, roots and suffixes for, 58*t*–59*t*
scirrhous, 310*t*, 310*t*
sclera, 276, 279*t*

scoliosis, 266t
scrotum, 235t
sedimentation rate (SR), 269t
seizure, 213t
seminal duct, 236t
seminal vesicles, 235t
seminal vessels, 228
sensorineural deafness, 285t
sensory organ, 124t
sentinel lymph node biopsy, 315t
septum, 188t
serous layer, 103t, 178
serum, 190t
serum glutamic oxalacetic transaminase (SGOT), 150t
serum lipid test, 195t
sexually transmitted diseases (STDs), 240–241
shortness of breath (SOB), 171t
shunt, 214t
sialolith, 148t
SIDS. See sudden infant death syndrome
sigmoid colon, 145t
sigmoidoscopy, 313t
sign language, 287t
silicosis, 167t
Simmonds' disease, 300t
sinoatrial node (SA node), 188t
sinus, 260, 261t
sinus rhythm, 195t
sinusitis, 167t
skeletal muscle, 263t
skeleton, 251f, 252f
    body bones, 258t
    bone processes, depressions, and holes, 260, 261t
    disorders, 265t–266t
    division, 257t–258t
    functions of, 253
    head bones, 259t
    injuries, 265t
    joints and accessory parts, 259t–260t
    medical management, 168t–169t
    overview of, 250–255
skin. See also integumentary system
    allergy, 128t
    cancers, 126f
    diagrams of, 122f, 123f
    disorders from systemic diseases, 128t
    functions of, 124t
    glands, 121
    ___ns, 125t
    ___rection and biologic agents, 126t–127t
    parts of, 123t–124t
    surgical processes and, 125t
    tests, 129t
    tumors. 312t
    vocabulary terms and, 129t–131t
skull, 251, 255f
    fracture, 213t, 265t
SLE. See systemic lupus erythematosus
slit lamp, 282t

small cell lung cancer, 321t
small intestine, 141
smooth muscle, 263t
SMR. See submucous resection
sneeze, 167t
Snellen eye chart, 284t
SNS. See somatic nervous system
SOB. See shortness of breath
somatic nervous system (SNS), 210
spastic, 219t
spastic colon, 147t
specialties and specialists
    roots and suffixes for, 59t–61t
    terms for health professions, 61t–63t
spermatozoon, 227
sphenoid, 258t, 259t
sphygmomanometer, 190t
spina bifida, 266t
spinal accessory nerves, 212t
spinal cavity, 116t
spinal cord, 206, 207, 209f, 210, 211t
    injuries, 214t
    spinal cranial nerves, 212t
    spirometer, 171t
    spirometry, 171t
    spleen, 197t
    spondylitis disorder, 266t
    spondylolisthesis, 265t
    spondylosyndesis, 269t
    sputum, 103t, 171t
    sputum cytology, 315t
    squamous cell carcinoma, 321t
    squamous epithelium, 124t
    SR. See sedimentation rate
    stapedectomy, 286t
    STDs. See sexually transmitted diseases
steatoma, 125t
sternomastoid, 263t
sternum, 178, 258t
stillborn (sb), 243t
stimulus, 219t
stoma, 154t
stomach, 141, 145t
    external and internal anatomy, 143f
stomach stapling, 149t
stool guaiac, 315t
stool sample/specimen, 150t
strabismus, 281t
stratum basale, 124t
stratum corneum, 124t
streptococcal throat, 167t
stroke, 192t
structural units of body, 112t–113t
stye/hordeolum, 281t
subarachnoid space, 208
subconjunctival hemorrhage, 280t
subcutaneous skin, 124t
subcutaneous tissue, 120
    components of, 121f

subdural hematoma, 214t
subluxation, 265t
submucous resection (SMR), 171t
sudden infant death syndrome (SIDS), 167t
suffixes
    defined, 6
    for diagnoses and symptoms, 13–15
    review of, 94–95
    for scientific studies, 58t–59t
    for specialties and specialists, 59t–61t
    used in surgery, 12–13
sulcus, 219t
superfluous hair, 130t
supination, 264t
supportive approach, 318t
surgery
    cancer, 316t
    suffixes used in, 12–13
surgical procedures/tests/terms, 148t–149t
    cancer, 318t
    cardiovascular, 193t–195t
    ear, 286t
    eye, 282t
    nervous system, 215t–216t
    skin, 125t
    to treat cancer, 318t
surgical technologists, 178
sutures, 103t, 259t
sweat test, 129t
symbols, list of frequently used, 52, 52t
sympathetic, 212t
syncope, 219t
syngeneic, 316t
synovial fluid, 260t
synovial joint, 253
syphilis, 128t, 240t
system, 113t
systemic circulation, 183, 188t
systemic lupus erythematosus (SLE), 266t, 269t
systemic radiation therapy, 316t
systolic pressure, 190t

T

T cells, 197t
tachycardia, 195t
tachypena, 171t
Tay-Sach's disease, 215t
TB. *See* tuberculosis
teeth, 140, 145t
temperature, 49t
temperature regulator, 124t
temporal, 258t, 259t, 263t
tendinitis, 266t
tendon, 260t, 265t
teratoma tumors (of mixed components), 312t
terms, basic
    for health professions, 61t–63t

for positions and directions, 45, 45t–46t
    for weights and measurements, 47, 47t–49t
Testape, 234t
testes, 228, 235t, 298t
tests
    cancer, 314t–315t
    cardiovascular, 193t–195t
    digestive system, 149t–150t
    laboratory and diagnostic, 76t–77t
    skin, 129t
test-tube baby, 243t
tetany, clinical condition, 300t
tetralogy of Fallot, 191t
thallium stress test, 195t
theca, 260t
thoracentesis, 171t
thoracic cage, 251
thoracic cavity, 155t, 162, 178
throat, 160–161
thrombocytes, 190t
thrombolysis, 195t
thrombophlebitis, 192t
thrush, 154t
thymus gland, 197t, 298t
thyroid, 296t
thyroidectomy, 300t
thyrotherapy, 300t
thyrotomy, 300t
TIA. *See* transient ischemic attack
tibia, 258t
tine test, 171t
tinea, 127t
tinea barbae, 127t
tinea capitis, 127t
tinea corporis, 127t
tinea cruris, 127t
tinea pedis, 127t
tinea unguium, 127t
tinnitus, 287t
tissue, 113t
toenails, 121
toiletry, abbreviations for, 76t
tongue, 140, 145t
tonometer, 282t
tonometry, 282t
tonsillitis, 167t
tonsils, 197t
torn ligament, 265t
total hip replacement, 269t
total parenteral nutrition, 154t
toxemia, 243t
toxic goite, 301f
trabeculectomy, 282t
trachea, 152t, 161, 164t
    anterior aspect of, 163f
tracheostomy, 171t
tracheotomy, 171t
trachoma, 281t

traction, 269t
transient ischemic attack (TIA), 192t
transverse body planes, 116t
transverse colon, 145t
trapezius, 263t
trephination, 216t
triceps brachii, 263t
trichomonas infection, 239t
tricuspid, 188t
trigeminal, 211t
trimester, 243t
trochanter, 260
trochlear, 211t
tubal ligation, 239t
tubercle, 260
tuberculosis (TB), 168t
tuberosity, 261t
tumors, 130t, 321t
    marker, 314t
    naming, principles of, 310t
tuning fork, 287t
turbinate, 258t, 259t
20/20 vision, 284t
tympanic membrane, 278, 284t
tympanoplasty, 286t
tympanotomy, 286t
tympanum, 284t
type and crossmatch, 190t

U

UA. *See* urinalysis
ulcers, 131t, 148t
ulna, 258t
ultrasonography, 150t, 234t, 243t
ultrasound, 314t
umbilical clinical disorder, 148t
universal donor, 190t
universal recipient, 190t
upper respiratory infection (URI), 168t
uremia, 233t
ureterostomy, 233t
ureters, 226, 232t
urethra, 226, 232t, 236t
urethral orifice, 226
urethritis, 233t
URI. *See* upper respiratory infection
urinalysis (UA), 235t
urinary bladder, 232t
urinary meatus, 232t
urinary retention, 235t
urinary system, 226–227, 227f
    organs and structures, 231t–232t
urinary tract infection (UTI), 233t
urticaria, 131t
uterus, 237t
UTI. *See* urinary tract infection
utricle, 278

uvea, 276
uveitis, 281t
uvula, 140, 152t

V

VA. *See* visual acuity
vagina, 237t
vaginal speculum, 239t
vagotomy, 149t, 216t
valley fever, 168t
varicella, 128t
varicocele, 238t
varicose veins, 192t
vas deferens, 236t
vasectomy, 238t
vasodilator, 195t
vasopressor, 195t
veins, 179f, 180f, 182–183, 187f
vena cava, 189t
venipuncture, 195t
ventilator, 171t
ventricle, 187t, 210, 219t
ventriculography, 216t
vernix caseosa, 243t
verruca, 125t, 127t
vertebral column, 251, 252f, 258t
vertigo, 287t
vesicle, 131t
vestibular apparatus, 278
viral infection, skin, 127t
virus, 103t
viscera, 154t
visceral peritoneum, 141
visceral pleura, 162, 164t
viscus, 103t
visual acuity (VA), 284t
vital capacity, 171t
vitiligo, 131t
vitrectomy, 282t
vitreous humor, 279t
voice box. *See* larynx
void, 103t, 235t
volvulus, 154t
vomer, 259t
vulva, 237t

W

waste elimination, 124t
WBCs. *See* white blood cells
weights and measurements
    common, 51t
    converting from U.S. system to metric and from metric to U.S.
        system, 50t
    words and abbreviations, 47, 47t–49t, 73t–74t
wheal, 131t
wheeze, 168t, 171t

whiplash, 215*t*
white blood cells (WBCs), 189*t*
whooping cough, 168*t*
Wilm's tumor, 233*t*, 321*t*
windpipe. *See* trachea
words parts, listing of, 7–15

X

xanthoderma, 131*t*
xeroderma, 131*t*

x-rays
    abbreviations for, 76*t*–77*t*
    examination, 171*t*

Z

zygomatic, 259*t*